CONSULTANT PATHOLOGY

BRAIN TUMORS

Consultant Pathology Series

David E. Elder, MB, ChB
Series Editor

TUMORIGENIC MELANOCYTIC PROLIFERATIONS
David E. Elder

BRAIN TUMORS
Richard Prayson, Bette Kleinschmidt-DeMasters, and Mark L. Cohen

Forthcoming Volumes in the Series

THYROID PAPILLARY LESIONS
Virginia A. LiVolsi and Jennifer L. Hunt

URINARY BLADDER DIAGNOSIS
Robert O. Petersen

HEAD AND NECK PATHOLOGY
Leon Barnes, Raja Seethala, and Simion Chiosea

LIVER PATHOLOGY
Linda Ferrell and Sanjay Kakar

CONSULTANT PATHOLOGY

BRAIN TUMORS

Richard Prayson, MD
Section Head of Neuropathology
Cleveland Clinic Main Campus
Professor of Pathology
Lerner College of Medicine
Cleveland, Ohio

Bette K. Kleinschmidt-DeMasters, MD
Head of Neuropathology
University of Colorado
Professor of Pathology
University of Colorado School of Medicine
Denver, Colorado

Mark L. Cohen, MD
Director, Division of Neuropathology
University Hospital of Cleveland
Professor of Pathology
Case Western Reserve University School of Medicine
Cleveland, Ohio

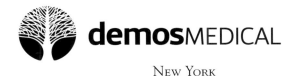

New York

Acquisitions Editor: Richard Winters

Cover Design: Joe Tenerelli

Compositor: Publication Services, Inc.

Printer: Sheridan Press

Visit our website at www.demosmedpub.com

Medicine is an ever-changing science. Research and clinical experience are continually expanding our knowledge, in particular our understanding of proper treatment and drug therapy. The authors, editors, and publisher have made every effort to ensure that all information in this book is in accordance with the state of knowledge at the time of production of the book. Nevertheless, the authors, editors, and publisher are not responsible for errors or omissions or for any consequences from application of the information in this book and make no warranty, express or implied, with respect to the contents of the publication. Every reader should examine carefully the package inserts accompanying each drug and should carefully check whether the dosage schedules mentioned therein or the contraindications stated by the manufacturer differ from the statements made in this book. Such examination is particularly important with drugs that are either rarely used or have been newly released on the market.

Library of Congress Cataloging-in-Publication Data

Prayson, Richard A.
  Brain tumors / Richard Prayson, Mark L. Cohen, Bette Kleinschmidt-DeMasters.
    p. ; cm. — (Consultant pathology)
  Includes bibliographical references and index.
  ISBN 978-1-933864-69-3 (hardcover)
  1. Brain — Tumors — Case studies. I. Cohen, Mark L., 1957- II. Kleinschmidt-DeMasters, Bette. III. Title. IV. Series: Consultant pathology.
  [DNLM: 1. Brain Neoplasms — diagnosis — Case Reports. 2. Brain Neoplasms — pathology — Case Reports. WL 358 P921b 2010]
  RC280.B7P725 2010
  616.99'481 — dc22   2009040379

Special discounts on bulk quantities of Demos Medical Publishing books are available to corporations, professional associations, pharmaceutical companies, health care organizations, and other qualifying groups. For details, please contact:

Special Sales Department

Demos Medical Publishing

11 W. 42nd Street, 15th Floor

New York, NY 10036

Phone: 800–532–8663 or 212–683–0072

Fax: 212–941–7842

E-mail: orderdept@demosmedpub.com

Made in the United States of America
09 10 11 12 13   5 4 3 2 1

To Beth, Brigid, and Nick for their unwavering support.

To my family—husband Bob, sons Tim and Tor, and daughter Julie—
without whom nothing in my career would have been possible.

To my parents, Beverly and Murray Cohen, without whom
my contribution would not have been possible.

To our patients, who have taught us so that
we may better help others.

CONTENTS

ix

CONTENTS

Series Foreword

Diagnostic surgical pathology remains the gold standard for diagnosis of most tumors and many inflammatory conditions in most, if not all, organ systems. The power of the morphologic method is such that, in many instances, a glance at a thin section of tissue stained with two vegetable dyes is sufficient to determine with absolute certainty whether a patient should undergo a major procedure or not, or whether a patient is likely to live a healthy life or die of an inoperable tumor. In such cases, the diagnostic process is one of "gestalt," a form of almost instantaneous pattern recognition that is similar to the recognition of faces, different brands of automobiles, or breeds of dogs. In other "difficult" cases, the diagnosis is not so obvious. In many of these cases, a diagnosis may be possible, but may be outside of the experience of the routine practitioner. In such a circumstance, it may be possible for a practitioner with more experience—a consultant—to make a diagnosis rather readily. In other cases, the problem may really not be suited to the histologic method. In these cases as well, a consultant may be invaluable in determining that it is simply not possible to make a reliable diagnosis with the materials available. In yet other cases, the diagnosis may be ambiguous, and again a consultant's opinion can be important in establishing a differential diagnosis that may guide clinical investigation.

There are many fine consultants available to the practicing surgical pathology community. Many of them have authored textbooks, and many of them give presentations at national meetings. However, these materials can offer only a superficial insight into the vast amount of knowledge that is embedded in these individuals' cerebral cortices—and in their filing cabinets. This series represents an effort to enable the dissemination of this hitherto-inaccessible knowledge to the wider community. Our authors are individuals who have accumulated large collections of difficult cases and are willing to share their material and their knowledge. The cases are based on actual consultations, and the indications for the consultation, when available, are presented, because these are the records of the manner in which these cases presented themselves as being problematic. We have asked the consultants, when possible, to present their consultation letters in much the same form (albeit edited to some degree) as that in which they were first presented, because these represent the true records of the clinical encounter. In addition, we asked the authors to amplify upon these descriptions, with brief reference to the literature, and to richly illustrate the case reports with high-quality digital images. The images from the book, as well as additional images to amplify the presentation of the case, are available on a website for downloading, study, and use in education. These images, in some cases, have been derived from virtual slides, which also may be made available in the future from a digital repository for their additional educational value.

David E. Elder, MB, ChB, FRCPA
Professor of Pathology and Laboratory Medicine
Hospital of the University of Pennsylvania
Philadelphia, Pennsylvania

PREFACE

The practice of surgical neuropathology is challenging. In part, this is related to the relative lack of experience most pathologists have in this arena as compared with other areas of surgical pathology. Thus, a selection of neuropathology cases fits well into the Consultant Pathology series—a series of texts that will cover the spectrum of surgical pathology and will examine topics in a case-based format, similar to the real practice of pathology.

The focus of this text is on brain tumors. Examples of over 100 brain tumors, running the gamut from the very common to the rare, are presented in a case-based format. The cases were taken from our surgical neuropathology practices. We attempt to share with the reader our approaches and thought processes in evaluating the spectrum of central nervous system neoplasms. The wide variety of cases presented covers the entire scope of brain tumors and offers both an opportunity to review the basics for the beginner or relatively inexperienced pathologist, and a chance to see some of the rare entities. When relevant, current practical applications of immunohistochemistry and molecular pathology are discussed.

Each case is formatted as if it were a consult case and includes a brief clinical history, a description of the pathologic findings with numerous illustrations, the line diagnosis, a discussion of the entity and the diagnostic thought process, and a few pertinent references for further reading.

Our hope is that by sharing a bit of our experience, we can add to the reader's experience.

Richard Prayson, MD
Bette Kleinschmidt-DeMasters, MD
Mark Cohen, MD

Acknowledgments

Special thanks to Ms. Denise Egleton, who provided secretarial assistance for this project.

BRAIN TUMORS

Case 1: Normal Tissue

CLINICAL INFORMATION

The patient is a 28-year-old female who presents with headaches and complaints of dizziness. On imaging, subtle abnormalities are noted in the right cerebellar hemisphere. Because of persistent symptoms, a decision is made to biopsy the patient, and histologic sections are reviewed.

OPINION

Biopsies show normocellular cerebellar parenchyma. Because of the unusual orientation of the specimen, a grouping of small cells appears to be positioned in the middle of the gray matter.

We consider the biopsy as representing normal tissue and characterize it as follows: **Right Cerebellum, Biopsy—Cerebellar Tissue with No Significant Pathologic Changes**.

COMMENT

There is no definite evidence of neoplasm on the biopsy. There is no evidence of inflammation.

DISCUSSION

The usual target of a brain biopsy does not include normal tissue. Occasionally, however, the surgeon may not be on target, and the normal tissue may be inadvertently biopsied. In most instances, recognition of the tissue as normal is not problematic. On occasion, however, as a result of either the

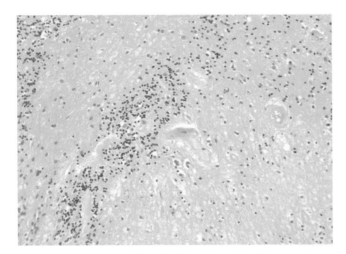

FIGURE 1.1 Section of cerebellum from this biopsy, showing a group of small, round cells from the granular cell layer, surrounded by molecular layer cortex. If one does not appreciate the unusual orientation of the section and the location of the biopsy, an erroneous diagnosis of chronic inflammation or encephalitis may be made.

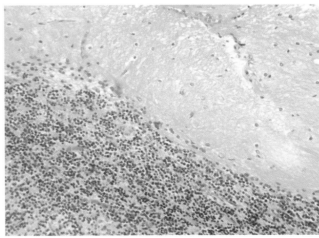

FIGURE 1.2 Normal, well-oriented cerebellum, showing the superficial molecular layer, Purkinje cell layer, and granular cell layer.

orientation of the specimen or lack of information regarding the location of the biopsy, normal tissue may mimic a tumor. This case illustrates one such example, in which failure to recognize the tissue as being from the cerebellum may result in a misinterpretation of the granular cells as lymphocytes; the result would be an erroneous diagnosis of chronic inflammation or encephalitis. Other circumstances in which normal tissue may be confused with a pathologic process include the following: (1) when

one is unsure of the exact location of the biopsy, a biopsy from the pineal gland may be misinterpreted as representing either a pineal gland tumor, such as pineocytoma or a glioma; (2) a biopsy from the subependymal zone may be interpreted as a low-grade glioma; this region frequently is mildly hypercellular in the normal state; (3) a biopsy from the pituitary neurohypophysis may resemble a low-grade astrocytoma, such as pilocytic astrocytoma, or

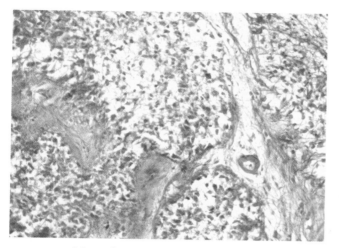

FIGURE 1.3 Normal pineal gland can mimic an anaplastic glioma.

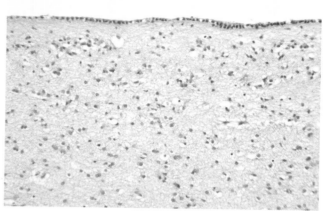

FIGURE 1.4 The subependymal zone may appear mildly hypercellular and cause confusion with a low-grade glioma.

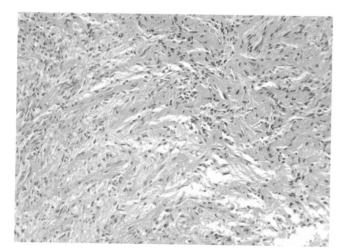

FIGURE 1.5 Pituitary neurohypophysis may resemble a low-grade astrocytoma or schwannoma.

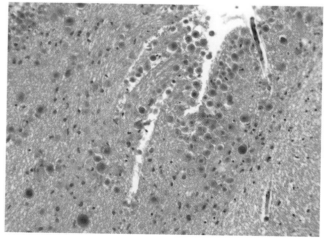

FIGURE 1.6 Corpora amylacea may resemble rounded cells at low magnification and can be confused with an oligodendroglioma.

a schwannoma; (4) the presence of numerous corpora amylacea (which may be a normal finding in a biopsy) can be misinterpreted as representing a low-grade tumor, particularly an oligodendroglioma, given the generally rounded nature of the corpora amylacea bodies.

To help avoid some of these confusions, communicating with the surgeon and knowing exactly where the biopsy is from are important.

References

1. Brat DJ. Overview of central nervous system anatomy and histology. In: Prayson RA, editor. Neuropathology. Philadelphia: Elsevier Churchill Livingstone; 2005. p. 1–36.
2. Kleinschmidt-DeMasters BK, Prayson RA. An algorithmic approach to the brain biopsy—Part 1. Arch Pathol Lab Med 2006;130:1630–8.

Case 2: Gliosis

CLINICAL INFORMATION

The patient is a 46-year-old female who presents with seizures starting seven months ago. On imaging, a low signal intensity area in the right frontal lobe, which is suspicious for a low-grade glioma, is identified. An open biopsy is performed, and diagnostic material is not obtained. The procedure is aborted early because of hemorrhage. A subsequent attempt, four months later, to reassess yields histologic sections that are reviewed.

OPINION

The second resection shows mild hypercellularity. The increased cellularity is a result of cells marked by abundant eosinophilic cytoplasm and an eccentrically placed, round-to-oval nucleus.

Occasional nuclei show small nucleoli. Mitotic figures are not observed. Malignant appearing astrocytic cells are not noted. There is no evidence of necrosis.

We consider the findings in this lesion to be consistent with a benign reactive process and characterize it as follows: **Right Frontal Lobe, Excision—Reactive Astrocytosis**.

COMMENT

There is no definite evidence of neoplasm. The changes seen in this biopsy may be related to the patient's prior surgery.

DISCUSSION

One of the most difficult differential diagnostic situations in surgical neuropathology involves the

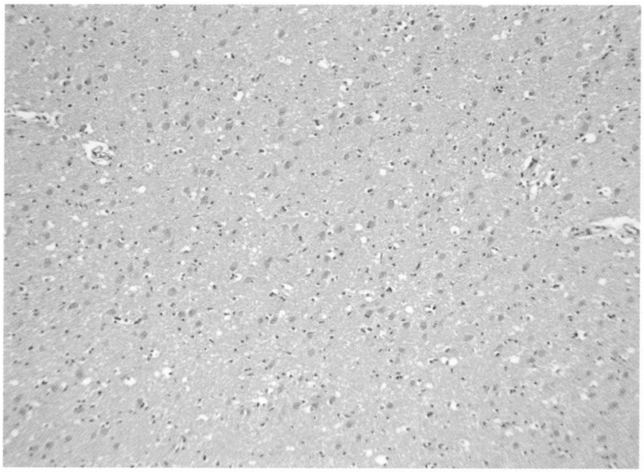

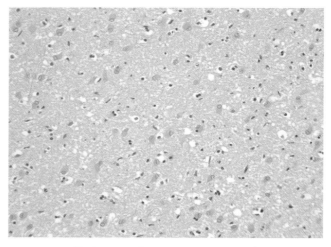

FIGURE 2.1 Low magnification view of the biopsy, showing a mild increase in cellularity. The increased cellularity appears to be relatively evenly distributed in this microscopic field, which is more consistent with reactive astrocytosis.

FIGURE 2.2 High magnification appearance, showing scattered larger cells with abundant eosinophilic cytoplasm, corresponding to reactive astrocytes.

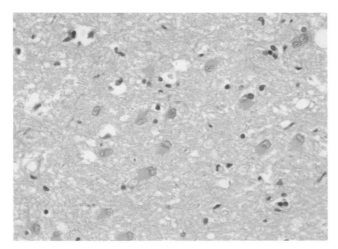

FIGURE 2.3 High magnification, showing the characteristic features of reactive astrocytes, including low nuclear-to-cytoplasmic ratio, nuclear enlargement with mild nuclear contour irregularities, and lack of nuclear hyperchromasia.

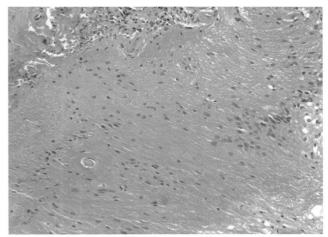

FIGURE 2.5 More dense gliosis can develop over time, adjacent to a previous surgical site or secondary to radiation therapy.

differentiation of reactive astrocytosis from low-grade glioma. It is particularly problematic because most gliomas elicit some degree of reactive astrocytosis. Reactive astrocytes are usually marked by increased eosinophilic cytoplasm and nuclear enlargement. The nuclear-to-cytoplasmic ratio is relatively low. In contrast, low-grade astrocytomas are marked by cells

with a higher nuclear-to-cytoplasmic ratio. Nuclear contour irregularities and nuclear hyperchromasia are more typically noted. An occasional mitotic figure may also be present. Additionally, reactive astrocytes are fairly evenly distributed in a microscopic field—in contrast to malignant astrocytic cells, which may show some uneven distribution of cellularity. Calcifications, microcystic degenerative changes, and satellitosis, in the form of secondary structures of Scherer, are more typically observed in gliomas than in gliosis.

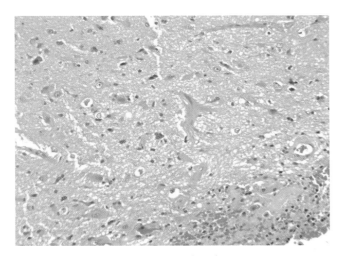

FIGURE 2.4 Prominent perivascular gliosis is present.

References

1. Burger PC, Vogel FS. Frozen section interpretation in surgical neuropathology. I. Intracranial lesions. Am J Surg Pathol 1977;1:323–47.
2. Prayson RA, Cohen ML. Gliosis. In: Practical Differential Diagnosis in Surgical Neuropathology. Totowa, NJ: Humana Press; 2000. p. 5–7.
3. Taratuto AL, Sevlever G, Piccardo P. Clues and pitfalls in stereotactic biopsy of the central nervous system. Arch Pathol Lab Med 1991;115:596–602.

Case 3: Recurrent High-Grade Glioma with Radiation Changes

CLINICAL INFORMATION

The patient is a 58-year-old male who presents with a right parietal-temporal, focally enhancing mass. The patient is biopsied, and a diagnosis of glioblastoma is made. He subsequently undergoes a course of radiotherapy. On recent follow-up imaging studies, the lesion appears to be expanding in size, and a decision to place an intraoperative chemotherapeutic agent is made. The patient subsequently undergoes partial resection of the region, and histologic sections are reviewed.

OPINION

Histologic sections show focally prominent numbers of reactive astrocytes, accompanied by perivascular chronic inflammation consisting primarily of benign-appearing lymphocytes. Several vessels show sclerotic changes, with homogeneous thickening of vessel walls. Areas of geographic necrosis, not rimmed by a pseudopalisade of atypical-appearing cells, are identified. Focal microcalcifications are observed. In areas including the frozen section slide, more prominent cellularity, marked by atypical-appearing cells and fibrosis, is seen. Occasional mitotic figures are identified in the more cellular areas. Foci of vascular proliferative changes, in some instances focally altered by fibrosis, are observed.

We consider the pathology to be that of a recurrent or residual high-grade astrocytoma (glioblastoma) with superimposed therapy effect, and we characterize it as follows: **Right Parietal-Temporal Lobe, Excision—Recurrent/Residual Glioblastoma, WHO Grade IV. Changes Consistent with Radiation Therapy Effect**.

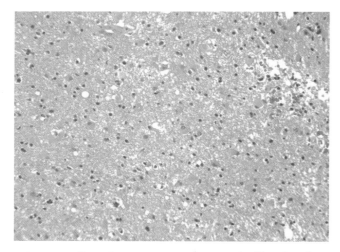

FIGURE 3.1 Reactive astrocytes, characterized by abundant eosinophilic cytoplasm and eccentrically placed, round-to-oval nuclei, are commonly seen in the setting of radiotherapy effect.

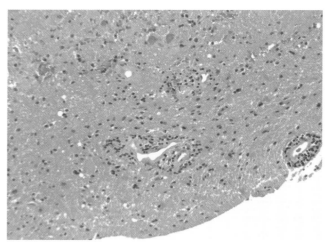

FIGURE 3.2 Focal perivascular chronic inflammation, marked by benign-appearing lymphocytes is frequently seen.

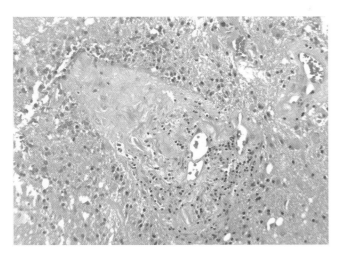

FIGURE 3.3 Vascular sclerotic changes, similar to those observed in other organ systems, can be seen in the irradiated brain.

COMMENT

Although many of the changes in the resection are secondary to radiation therapy effect, there is evidence of definitive recurrent or residual glioblastoma.

DISCUSSION

Standard treatment for high-grade astrocytoma includes radiotherapy. Radiation can cause changes in tissue that are important to recognize so that they are not confused with tumor. It is important to remember that the morphologic changes secondary to radiotherapy are typically delayed and do not manifest themselves until weeks or months after the radiation has been administered. The earliest changes include the development of edema and perivascular chronic inflammation. Reactive astrocytosis and gliosis may be focally prominent. Areas of white matter demyelination can develop. Vascular sclerotic changes can become prominent, and eventually necrosis may develop. It is common for dystrophic mineralization, often associated with zones of necrosis, to be evident. Frequently, areas of necrosis may contain macrophages. In some instances, particularly in the meninges, a prominent fibroblastic reaction may ensue. In contrast to necrosis associated with glioblastoma, a palisading of reactive astrocytes around necrotic zones is not seen.

In order to distinguish recurrent or residual glioma from radiation therapy effect, useful features to assess include the following: (1) Look for cytologic atypia. Cells with high nuclear-to-cytoplasmic ratio, irregular nuclear contours and nuclear hyperchromasia

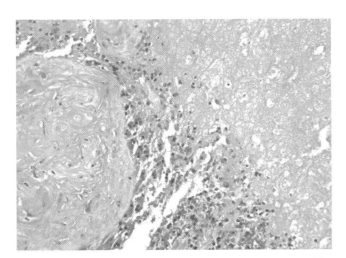

FIGURE 3.4 Sclerotic vascular changes are accompanied by a zone of geographic necrosis.

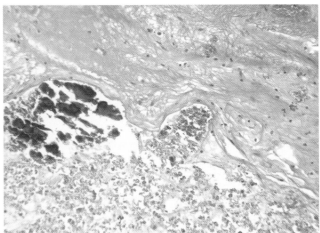

FIGURE 3.5 Focal dystrophic mineralization may develop in the irradiated brain.

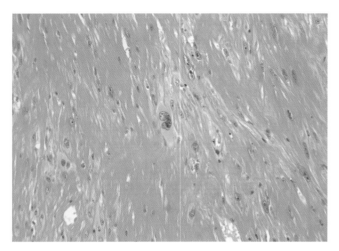

FIGURE 3.6 Fibrosis, with intervening atypical-appearing cells, is present. An occasional cell shows marked cytologic atypia, which may represent radiation-related atypia in a neoplastic astrocyte.

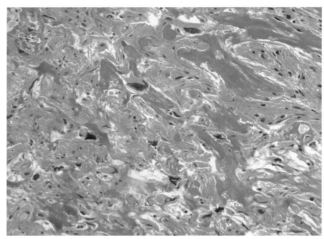

FIGURE 3.7 Scattered, bizarre-appearing astrocytic cells, in the background of dense gliosis, are indicative of irradiated, recurrent tumor.

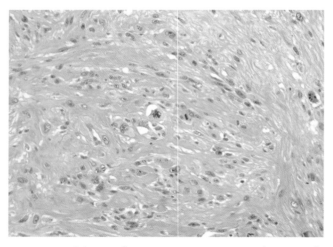

FIGURE 3.8 Mitotic figures, in association with atypical-appearing astrocytic cells, indicate recurrent or residual glioblastoma.

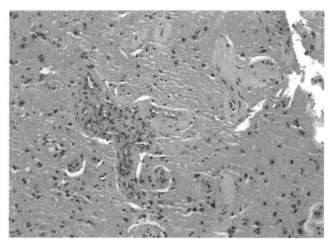

FIGURE 3.9 Vascular proliferative changes (also indicative of recurrent or residual glioblastoma) are focally altered by radiation-associated vascular sclerosis. Several adjacent smaller vessels also show vascular sclerotic changes secondary to radiation.

are generally tumor cells. Radiation may also induce cytologic atypia. In this instance, the atypical cells are often very bizarre and may be multinucleated. (2) Mitotic figures are indicative of tumor, not reactive astrocytosis or gliosis associated with radiotherapy. (3) True vascular proliferative changes are indicative of recurrent or residual tumor. The vascular changes associated with radiotherapy are primarily those of sclerosis and fibrosis of vessel walls. (4) Palisaded necrosis is a feature of glioblastoma, not radionecrosis.

In this particular case, recognition of the presence of recurrent or residual tumor at the time of intraoperative consultation is important in dictating placement of the chemotherapeutic agent into the surgical bed. Sometimes, in the setting of radiated gliomas, patients are biopsied to assess or evaluate the nature of changes observed on imaging studies, i.e., whether changes are secondary to radiation therapy effect or the tumor is resistant to radiation therapy and another treatment modality should be considered.

References

1. Burger PC, Mahaley Jr MS, Dudka L, et al. The morphologic effects of radiation administered therapeutically for intracranial gliomas: a postmortem study of 25 cases. Cancer 1979;44:1256–72.
2. Prayson RA, Cohen ML. Radiation change. In: Practical Differential Diagnosis in Surgical Neuropathology. Totowa, NJ: Humana Press; 2000. p. 27–31.

Case 4: Low-Grade Astrocytoma

CLINICAL INFORMATION

The patient is a 38-year-old female who presents with seizures. On computed tomography (CT) imaging, an ill-defined, homogeneous-appearing mass of low signal intensity is noted in the right temporal lobe. Stereotactic biopsies of the tumor are taken, and histologic sections are reviewed.

OPINION

On the frozen section slide, mildly hypercellular parenchyma is noted. Occasional atypical-appearing astrocytic cells, marked by nuclear enlargement and irregularities of nuclear contour, are identified, suggestive of an infiltrating astrocytoma. On permanent sections, hypercellularity is evident. Atypical-appearing astrocytic cells are clearly present. In focal areas, subpial aggregation of atypical astrocytic cells is noted. Mitotic figures, vascular proliferative changes, and necrosis are not seen. There is no evidence of Rosenthal fibers or granular bodies. A Ki-67 immunostain shows a labeling index of 0.4.

We consider the lesion an astrocytoma and characterize it as follows: **Right Temporal Lobe, Biopsies—Low-Grade Fibrillary Astrocytoma, WHO Grade II**.

COMMENT

The tumor has a low rate of cell proliferation (Ki-67 labeling index 0.4), consistent with a low-grade tumor. Features of higher-grade astrocytoma, including

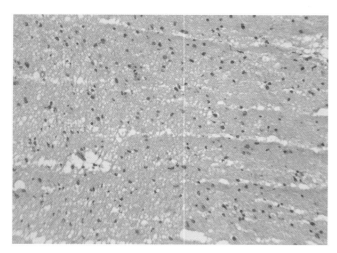

FIGURE 4.1 Low magnification appearance of the frozen section, showing a mildly hypercellular parenchyma, raising the question of a glioma versus gliosis differential diagnosis.

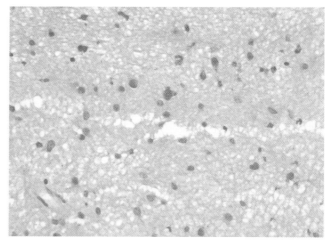

FIGURE 4.2 Hypercellular parenchyma shows scattered, atypical-appearing astrocytic cells suggestive of a low-grade astrocytoma.

mitotic activity, vascular proliferative changes, and necrosis, are not seen.

DISCUSSION

The most common primary tumor of the central nervous system is the astrocytoma; in most instances, the tumors are high-grade (glioblastoma multiforme). Astrocytomas are infiltrative lesions. Low-grade tumors usually present as low signal intensity, somewhat ill-defined lesions on imaging. Because of the widely infiltrative nature of these tumors, surgical cure is seldom realized. Microscopically, the tumors are marked by mildly hypercellular parenchyma. The increased cellularity is often not evenly distributed. Increased cellularity is a result of two components. Atypical-appearing astrocytic cells, marked by nuclear enlargement, nuclear hyperchromasia, and nuclear pleomorphism, are evident. The tumor cells may be accompanied by reactive astrocytes, which are generally characterized by increased eosinophilic cytoplasm and enlarged nuclei, with round-to-oval nuclear contours. With infiltration, the malignant tumor cells have a propensity to satellite around pre-existing structures, including neurons and blood vessels. Subpial aggregation of tumor cells, as they infiltrate toward the surface of the cortex, may also be observed. True microcystic change is a variable but useful diagnostic feature of tumor, as opposed to gliosis. Microcalcifications may be evident in approximately 15% of low-grade astrocytomas. Mitotic figures are generally difficult to identify or are evident in low numbers.

Cell proliferation markers can be helpful in differentiating between low-grade tumors and tumors that are more likely to behave in an aggressive fashion. Ki-67 is probably the most widely utilized of these immunohistochemical markers. Low-grade astrocytomas typically have low labeling indices, usually less than 3–4%. Higher labeling indices are often associated with more cellular lesions and may be indicative of a more aggressive-behaving tumor, akin to anaplastic astrocytoma or WHO grade III neoplasms. In trying to differentiate gliosis from low-grade glioma, a high labeling index is more indicative of a glioma. A low labeling index is not helpful in this differential diagnosis, because low rates of cell proliferation have been described in association with reactive astrocytosis.

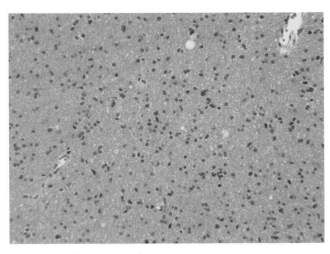

FIGURE 4.3 Low magnification appearance on permanent section is marked by increased cellularity.

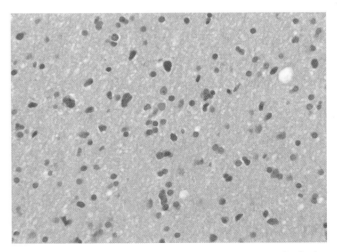

FIGURE 4.4 Atypical-appearing astrocytes, marked by nuclear enlargement, irregularities to nuclear contour, and nuclear hyperchromasia, are present.

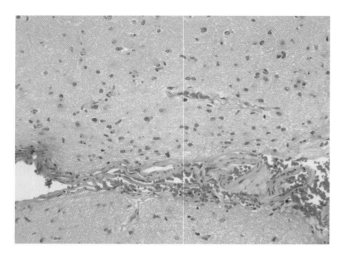

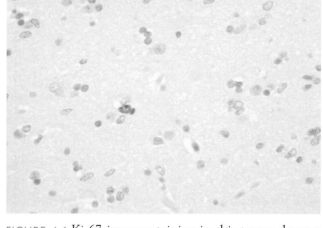

FIGURE 4.5 Subpial aggregation is present in this infiltrating, low-grade astrocytoma.

FIGURE 4.6 Ki-67 immunostaining in this tumor shows a labeling index of 0.4.

Astrocytomes are also heterogeneous lesions; different regions of the tumor may have different rates of cell proliferation. Consequently, a low labeling index may also be attributable to sampling.

References

1. Adelman LS. Grading astrocytomas. Neurosurg Clin N Am 1994;5:35–41.
2. Burger PC, Scheithauer BW. Tumors of neuroglia and choroid plexus. In: Tumours of the Central Nervous System. AFIP Atlas of Tumour Pathology Series 4. Washington DC: American Registry of Pariology 2007. p. 33–50.
3. Montine TJ, Vandersteenhoven JJ, Aguzzi A, et al. Prognostic significance of Ki-67 proliferation index in supratentorial fibrillary astrocytic neoplasms. Neurosurgery 1994;34:674–9.
4. von Deimling A, Burger PC, Nakazato Y, et al. Diffuse astrocytoma. In: Louis DN, Ohgaki H, Wiestler OD, Cavenee WK, editors. WHO Classification of Tumours of the Central Nervous System. Lyon, FR: IARC Press;2007. p. 25–9.

Case 5: Anaplastic Astrocytoma

A 51-year-old female presents with seizures and left-sided weakness. On imaging, a right frontal-parietal, ill-defined mass is noted. The patient undergoes sub-total resection of the mass, and histologic sections are reviewed.

OPINION

Histologic sections show a variably cellular lesion. The center of the lesion shows moderate hypercellularity, which trails off at the infiltrating edge of the tumor. In areas where the tumor is observed to infiltrate into the cortex, satellitosis of atypical cells around pre-existing structures, including blood vessels and neurons, is observed. Tumor cells are marked by nuclear hyperchromasia, nuclear enlargement, and irregular nuclear contours. Mitotic figures are readily identifiable. Although an increased number of blood vessels is observed in the tumor, there is no evidence of vascular proliferative changes or necrosis. Focally, the tumor appears to infiltrate into the leptomeninges. A Ki-67 immunostain was performed and a labeling index of 5.2% noted.

We consider the lesion to be an astrocytoma of intermediate grade and characterize it as follows: **Right Frontal-Parietal Lobe, Excision—Anaplastic Astrocytoma, WHO Grade III.**

COMMENT

There is no evidence of vascular proliferative changes or necrosis to indicate that the lesion represents a glioblastoma multiforme.

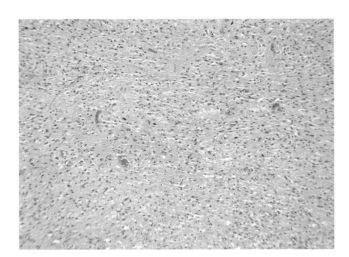

FIGURE 5.1 Low magnification appearance shows a moderately hypercellular tumor.

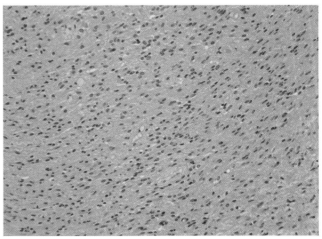

FIGURE 5.2 Higher magnification appearance shows moderate hypercellularity and clear evidence of nuclear atypia.

DISCUSSION

Anaplastic astrocytoma represents an intermediate grade lesion between the low-grade fibrillary astrocytoma (WHO grade II) and the glioblastoma multiforme (WHO grade IV). Distinction of these tumors from low-grade astrocytomas is predicated on the presence of increased cellularity, more prominent nuclear atypia, and readily identifiable mitotic activity. Distinction of this entity from glioblastoma multiforme is marked by the absence of vascular proliferative changes and/or necrosis in the anaplastic astrocytoma.

Cell proliferation markers, such as Ki-67 or MIB-1, can be useful in corroborating the diagnosis. Labeling indices typically range between 5 and 10; this is generally higher than the labeling indices

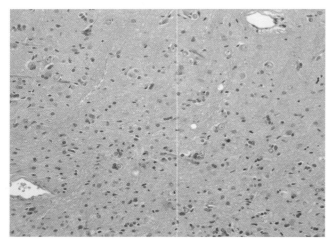

FIGURE 5.3 The infiltrating edge of the tumor has the appearance of a low-grade astrocytoma. This underscores the heterogeneity that is commonly encountered in gliomas.

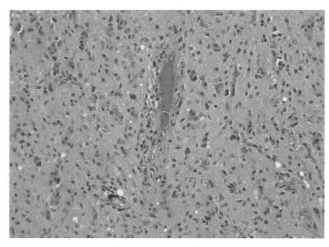

FIGURE 5.4 The infiltrating edge of tumor shows perivascular satellitosis of tumor cells around pre-existing structures, so-called secondary structures of Scherer.

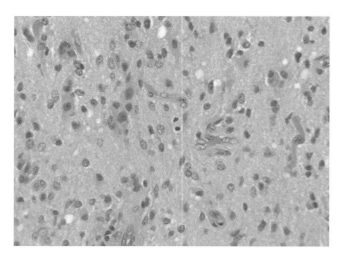

FIGURE 5.5 Mitotic figures are readily identifiable in an anaplastic astrocytoma.

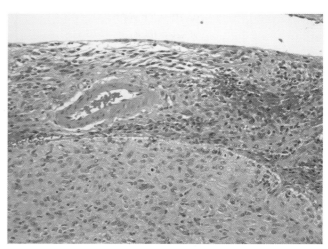

FIGURE 5.6 Focal leptomeningeal extension of the tumor does not necessarily afford a worse prognosis.

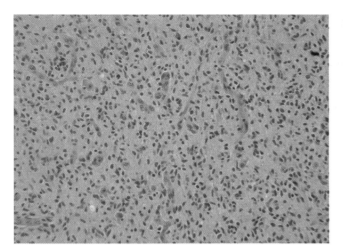

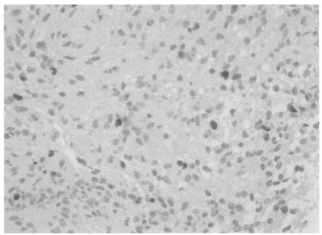

FIGURE 5.7 Although an increased number of small caliber blood vessels may be encountered in the many gliomas, this particular tumor shows no evidence of vascular proliferative changes or necrosis to warrant a WHO grade IV designation.

FIGURE 5.8 A Ki-67 labeling index of 5.2 is observed in this tumor.

observed in low-grade astrocytomas. It is important to remember, however, that these tumors are heterogeneous in nature, and labeling indices and rates of cell proliferation may vary from region to region in the tumor. Consequently, a low labeling index in an anaplastic astrocytoma may be a result of sampling.

From prognostic and treatment standpoints, distinction of anaplastic astrocytoma from low-grade astrocytoma is significant. Anaplastic astrocytomas are more often treated like high-grade astrocytomas and generally undergo a course of radiation therapy. The prognosis is intermediate between low-grade astrocytoma and the poor prognosis glioblastoma.

References

1. Burger PC, Vogel FS, Green SB, et al. Glioblastoma multiforme and anaplastic astrocytoma: pathologic criteria and prognostic implications. Cancer 1985;56:1106–11.
2. Coons SW, Johnson PC. Regional heterogeneity in the proliferative activity of human gliomas as measured by the Ki-67 labeling index. J Neuropath Exp Neurol 1993;52:609–18.
3. Kleihues P, Burger PC, Rosenblum MK, et al. Anaplastic astrocytoma. In: Louis DN, Ohgaki H, Wiestler OD, Cavenee WK, editors. WHO Classification of Tumours of the Central Nervous System. Lyon, FR: IARC Press; 2007. p. 30–2.

Case 6: Glioneuronal Tumor with Neuropil-Like Islands

CLINICAL INFORMATION

The patient is a 38-year-old female who presents with seizures and headaches. On magnetic resonance imaging (MRI) studies, a mass involving the left frontal and temporal lobes and measuring 4.2 cm in diameter is noted; there is no evidence of enhancement. The tumor is associated with prominent vasogenic edema. Histologic sections from a subtotal resection are reviewed.

OPINION

Histologic sections show an infiltrative neoplasm, marked by a proliferation of atypical-appearing astrocytic cells characterized by nuclear enlargement, nuclear hyperchromasia, and irregular nuclear contours. Rare mitotic figures are observed. There is no evidence of vascular proliferative changes or necrosis. An atypical ganglion cell component is not identified in the lesion. Scattered focally in the neoplasm are neuropil-like islands. These islands appear somewhat sharply demarcated from the background tumor and demonstrate diffuse positive staining with antibody to synaptophysin. In contrast, GFAP immunoreactivity stains the background tumor and does not stain the neuropil-like islands. The overlying cortex shows satellitosis of tumor cells around pre-existing structures (secondary structures of Scherer).

We consider the lesion to be an astrocytoma and characterize it as follows: **Left Frontal and Temporal Lobes, Subtotal Resection—Glioneuronal Tumor with Neuropil-Like Islands, WHO Grade III.**

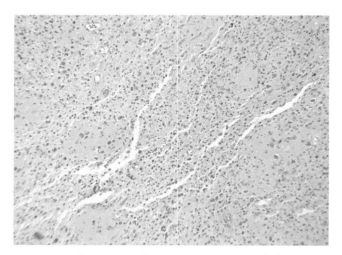

FIGURE 6.1 Low magnification appearance of the tumor shows less cellular, neuropil-like islands, arranged against the background of an infiltrating astrocytoma.

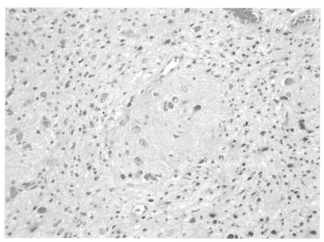

FIGURE 6.2 Higher magnification shows well-circumscribed neuropil island in the background of a fibrillary astrocytoma.

COMMENT

In the most recent WHO Classification of Tumours of the Central Nervous System, the glioneuronal tumor with neuropil-like islands is considered a variant of diffuse or fibrillary astrocytoma. The cellularity of the tumor and presence of mitotic figures in this case support a diagnosis of grade III astrocytoma.

DISCUSSION

The glioneuronal tumor with neuropil-like islands or rosetted glioneuronal tumor is a recent addition to the WHO classification of central nervous system tumors and represents a pattern of anaplastic astrocytoma. The clinical presentation overlaps with that of ordinary diffuse or fibrillary astrocytomas. The

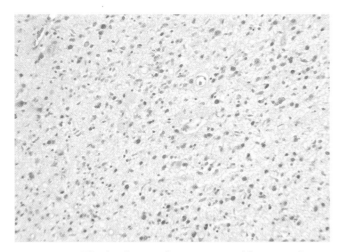

FIGURE 6.3 The background tumor resembles an ordinary anaplastic astrocytoma.

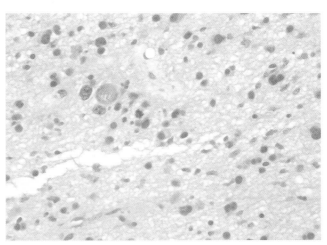

FIGURE 6.4 Occasional mitotic figures are present in this tumor.

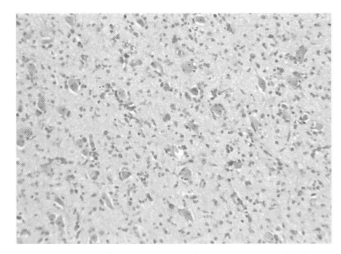

FIGURE 6.5 Satellitosis or secondary structures of Scherer are present at the infiltrating margin of the neoplasm.

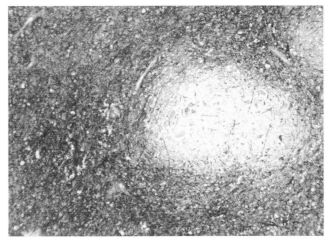

FIGURE 6.6 GFAP immunostaining shows a relative absence of staining in the neuropil-like island.

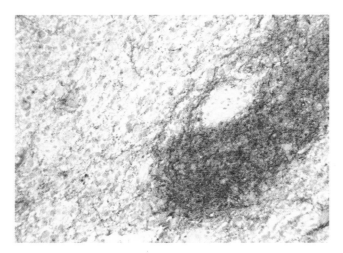

FIGURE 6.7 Prominent synaptophysin immunoreactivity is observed in the neuropil-like island.

majority of cases seem to affect adults and involve the cerebral hemispheres as nonenhancing lesions on imaging. The background of these tumors resembles an ordinary anaplastic astrocytoma, and the tumor is marked by focally prominent cellularity, readily identifiable nuclear atypia, and scattered mitotic activity. Vascular proliferative changes and necrosis are generally not observed in this tumor. A distinct morphologic feature of this lesion is the presence of fairly circumscribed neuropil-like or rosetted islands. By immunohistochemistry, these islands demonstrate immunoreactivity with neural antibodies, such as synaptophysin, and generally demonstrate a paucity of GFAP immunostaining. This is in sharp contrast to the background tumor, which is GFAP-positive and demonstrates little in the way of synaptophysin immunostaining.

These tumors are graded according to the background astrocytic component and usually represent grade II and, more commonly, grade III tumors. Their prognosis seems to correspond to the WHO grade of the tumor.

References

1. Edgar MA, Rosenblum MK. Mixed glioneuronal tumors, recently described entities. Arch Pathol Lab Med 2007;131:228–33.
2. Prayson RA, Abramovich CM. Glioneuronal tumor with neuropil-like islands. Hum Pathol 2000;31:14:35–8.
3. Teo JGC, Gultekin H, Bilsky M, Gutin P, et al. A distinctive glioneuronal tumor of the adult cerebrum with neuropil-like (including "rosetted") islands. Report of 4 cases. Am J Surg Pathol 1999;23:502–10.

Case 7: Glioblastoma Multiforme

CLINICAL INFORMATION

The patient is a 72-year-old male who presents with a focally enhancing mass in the right frontal lobe. Biopsies are taken, and histologic sections are reviewed.

OPINION

Histologic sections show a markedly cellular neoplasm with a fibrillary background, consistent with a high-grade glioma. Focal dystrophic calcification is observed. Tumor cells are marked by a high nuclear-to-cytoplasmic ratio, nuclear hyperchromasia, and irregular nuclear contour. Focally, cells assume a somewhat spindled configuration. Mitotic figures are readily observable. Focal vascular proliferative change is also noted. There is no definite evidence of necrosis in this tumor. A Ki-67 labeling index of 22.6 is noted.

We consider the lesion to be a high-grade astrocytoma and characterize it as follows: **Right Frontal Lobe, Biopsies—Glioblastoma Multiforme (or Glioblastoma), WHO Grade IV.**

COMMENT

The presence of vascular proliferative changes, even in the absence of necrosis, is sufficient for a diagnosis of glioblastoma multiforme.

DISCUSSION

Glioblastoma multiforme represents the highest grade of a diffuse fibrillary astrocytoma. These tumors are typically marked by prominent cellularity, readily discernible atypia, and prominent mitotic activity. The WHO requires either the presence of vascular proliferative changes, as observed in this

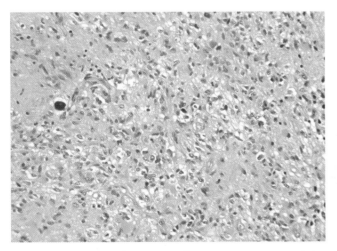

FIGURE 7.1 Intermediate magnification appearance of the tumor shows moderate hypercellularity and focal dystrophic calcification.

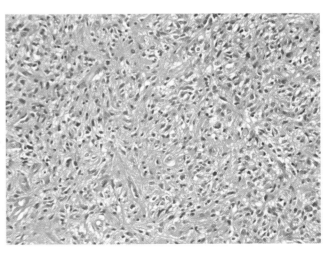

FIGURE 7.2 A moderately hypercellular tumor with a fibrillary background indicates a glial neoplasm.

tumor, or necrosis in order to make a diagnosis of glioblastoma multiforme. Older grading systems required the presence of necrosis for a diagnosis of glioblastoma. Necrosis, when present, may or may not have a pseudopalisade of tumor cells around it. Care needs to be taken in interpreting biopsies from a patient who has been previously treated with radiotherapy, because radiation can induce necrosis. The presence of nonpalisaded necrosis in the setting of prior radiation therapy should not necessarily warrant an upgrading of the tumor. Vascular proliferative changes refer to a proliferation of cells around vascular lumina. These are not tumor cells, but normal blood vessel wall constituents (i.e., endothelial cells, smooth muscle cells, fibroblasts, pericytes). An increased number of blood vessels, which is common in many gliomas, does not warrant an upgrading of the tumor.

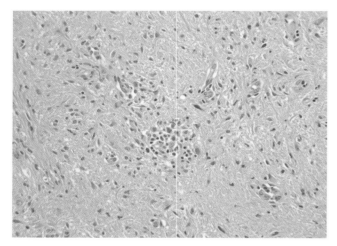

FIGURE 7.3 A focal area of the tumor with a low-grade astrocytoma appearance is seen here. This underscores the regional heterogeneity that is a characteristic feature of gliomas.

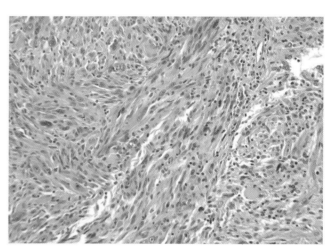

FIGURE 7.4 Focal spindled cell region in a glioblastoma is seen.

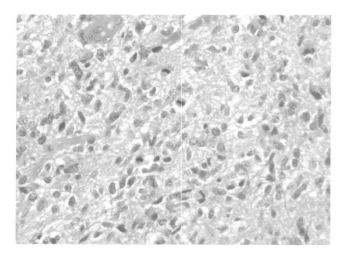

FIGURE 7.5 Readily identifiable mitotic activity is present in the tumor.

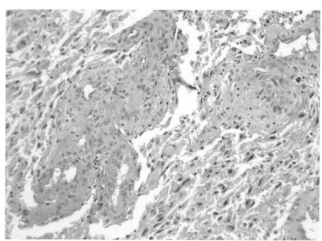

FIGURE 7.6 Focal vascular proliferative changes are present in the tumor.

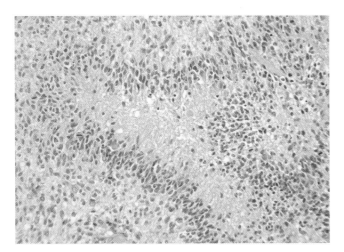

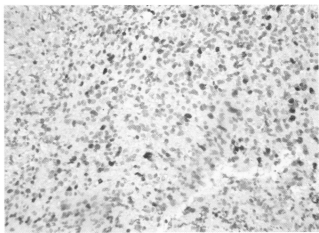

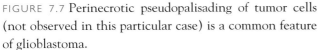

FIGURE 7.7 Perinecrotic pseudopalisading of tumor cells (not observed in this particular case) is a common feature of glioblastoma.

FIGURE 7.8 Ki-67 immunostaining demonstrates a labeling index of 22.6 in this tumor.

Particularly in the setting of biopsies, sampling of the tumor is important in arriving at the correct grade designation. Glioblastoma multiforme is a heterogeneous lesion, which may have areas resembling low-grade astrocytoma. Communication with the neurosurgeon at the time of surgery to ensure that appropriate tissue has been acquired is important.

Ki-67 labeling indices are typically high in glioblastoma and frequently exceed 10–15. Occasional tumors may have focal areas with labeling indices in excess of 50. There does not appear to be any prognostic implication of determining a Ki-67 labeling index in a glioblastoma. Prognosis is poor, even with standard treatment, which is usually radiotherapy. Most patients have a survival of 1–2 years.

References

1. Burger PC, Vogel FS, Green SB, et al. Glioblastoma multiforme and anaplastic astrocytoma: pathologic criteria and prognostic implications. Cancer 1985;56:1106–11.
2. Kleihues P, Burger PC, Aldape KD, et al. Glioblastoma. In: Louis DN, Ohgaki H, Wiestler OD, Cavenee WK, editors. WHO Classification of Tumours of the Central Nervous System. Lyon, FR: IARC Press; 2007. p. 33–47.
3. Prayson RA. Histologic classification of high-grade gliomas. In: Barnett GH, editor. High-Grade Glioma. Diagnosis and Treatment. Totowa, NJ: Humana Press;2007. p. 3–35.

Case 8: Gemistocytic Astrocytoma

The patient is a 42-year-old male who presents with right-sided weakness. On MRI imaging studies, a 3.2-cm mass involving the left frontal and parietal lobes is noted. The tumor shows no definite evidence of enhancement. Histologic sections from a subtotal resection are reviewed.

OPINION

Histologic sections show a hypercellular neoplasm, marked by a predominant population of large cells with abundant eosinophilic cytoplasm and eccentrically placed nuclei. The nuclei appear slightly irregular in shape. Intermixed with these cells are focal areas, marked by a proliferation of atypical-appearing astrocytic cells, characterized by high nucle-ar-to-cytoplasmic ratio, nuclear hyperchromasia, and irregular nuclear contour. Focal microcystic degenerative changes are observed in the tumor. A careful search reveals scattered mitotic figures. There is no definite evidence of vascular proliferative changes or necrosis. GFAP immunostaining highlights prominent immunoreactivity of both the large and small cells. Ki-67 immunostaining shows mild positivity, confined primarily to the small, atypical-appearing astrocytic cells; a labeling index of 5.6 is noted in this tumor.

We consider the lesion to be an astrocytoma with prominent numbers of gemistocytes and characterize it as follows: **Left Frontal and Parietal Lobes, Subtotal Resection—Gemistocytic Astrocytoma, WHO Grade III.**

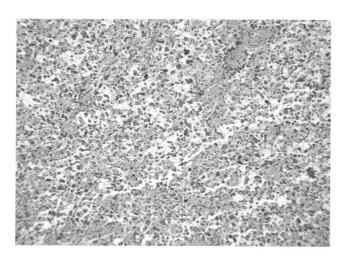

FIGURE 8.1 Low magnification appearance of the neoplasm shows hypercellularity, with clusters of larger cells.

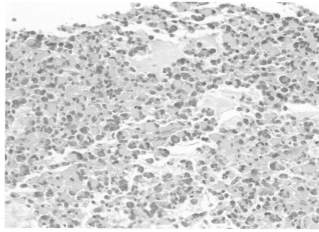

FIGURE 8.2 Microcystic degenerative changes are observed in the tumor.

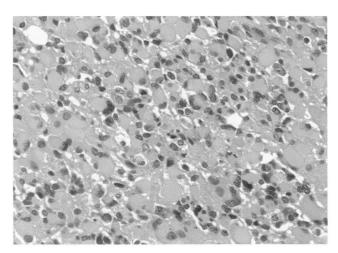

FIGURE 8.3 High magnification appearance shows a focus of confluent gemistocytes, marked by abundant eosinophilic cytoplasm and eccentrically placed, irregularly shaped nuclei.

COMMENT

The presence of mitotic figures in this tumor, in the absence of vascular proliferation and necrosis, warrants a diagnosis of a WHO grade III tumor.

DISCUSSION

A well-recognized variant of astrocytoma is marked by prominent numbers of gemistocytes. Gemistocytes are characterized by abundant eosinophilic cytoplasm and eccentrically placed, slightly irregularly shaped nuclei. Perivascular chronic inflammatory cells, in particular lymphocytes, may be focally present in these tumors.

It is well recognized that astrocytic tumors with a significant gemistocytic component tend to behave in a more aggressive fashion, although the WHO still recognizes these lesions as grade II neoplasms. Designation of a tumor as gemistocytic astrocytoma, versus an ordinary diffuse or fibrillary astrocytoma with occasional gemistocytes, is somewhat arbitrary. One study suggested a minimum 20% gemistocytic component as being clinically significant. Grading parameters that are used in evaluating diffuse fibrillary astrocytomas are also employed in evaluating gemistocytic astrocytomas. In the current case, the presence of readily identifiable mitotic activity warrants the designation of a WHO grade III neoplasm. The presence of vascular proliferative changes or necrosis in the tumor warrants the designation of a grade IV neoplasm.

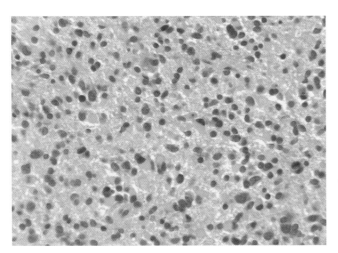

FIGURE 8.4 A focal gemistocyte-poor area, marked by a proliferation of more conventional-appearing, atypical astrocytic cells, is seen.

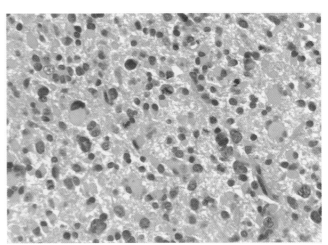

FIGURE 8.5 Mitotic activity is readily observable in this neoplasm.

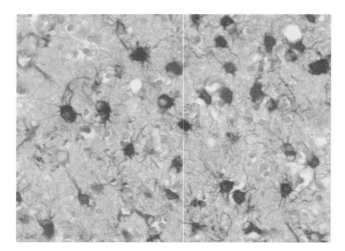

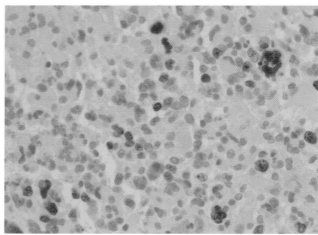

FIGURE 8.6 GFAP immunoreactivity highlights positive staining gemistocytes, underscoring their astrocytic lineage.

FIGURE 8.7 A Ki-67 labeling index of 5.6 is observed in this tumor. Ki-67 staining is typically confined to the nongemistocytic component of the tumor.

Differential diagnostic considerations include reactive astrocytosis, oligodendroglioma with minigemistocytes, and ganglioglioma. In contrast to reactive astrocytes, a gemistocytic astrocytoma should have a second population of cells that appear conventionally malignant and indicate the true nature of the lesion. Occasional oligodendrogliomas can have a prominent gemistocytic-like component. In these instances, the background of the tumor appears to be very much like an oligodendroglioma with rounded nuclei and scant cytoplasm. GFAP immunoreactivity in the gemistocytic cells in the current tumor indicates the astrocytic lineage of the cells. Occasionally, in a ganglioglioma,

some cells may assume a gemistocytic-like appearance. Immunohistochemistry can be helpful in making the distinction, in that ganglion cells stain with markers of neural differentiation, including synaptophysin.

References

1. Krouwer HGJ, Davis RL, Silver P, et al. Gemistocytic astrocytomas: a reappraisal. J Neurosurg 1991;74:399–406.
2. Tihan T, Vohra P, Berger MS, et al. Definition and diagnostic implications of gemistocytic astrocytomas: a pathological perspective. J Neurooncol 2006;76:175–83.
3. Watanabe K, Tachibana O, Yonekawa Y, et al. Role of gemistocytes in astrocytoma progression. Lab Invest 1997;76:277–84.
4. Yang HJ, Kim JE, Paek SH, et al. The significance of gemistocytes in astrocytoma. Acta Neurochir 2003;145:1097–1103.

Case 9: Granular Cell Glioblastoma

CLINICAL INFORMATION

The patient is a 59-year-old male who presents with seizures and a right temporal lobe mass on imaging studies. On imaging, the lesion shows focal enhancement. Subtotal resection of the tumor is performed, and histologic sections are reviewed.

OPINION

Sections show a moderately hypercellular neoplasm, comprised primarily of plump, eosinophilic cells. These cells are marked by abundant granular cytoplasm. Nuclei are generally eccentrically placed and round-to-oval in configuration. Occasional small nucleoli are observed. Perivascular chronic inflammation, consisting primarily of benign-appearing lymphocytes, is noted. Mitotic activity is not observed in the large granular cells. Focal areas of the tumor demonstrate necrosis. Vascular proliferative changes are noted at the parameter of the lesion. In areas of vascular proliferation, atypical-appearing astrocytic cells, with high nuclear-to-cytoplasmic ratio and an appearance more typical of a diffuse or fibrillary type astrocytoma, are identified. Several mitotic figures are observed in this region of the tumor.

We consider this lesion to be a malignant astrocytoma and characterize it as follows: **Right Temporal Lobe, Excision—Granular Cell Glioblastoma, WHO Grade IV.**

COMMENT

This neoplasm is best considered a variant of glioblastoma multiforme. The presence of granular cell differentiation does not affect the prognosis of this tumor.

FIGURE 9.1 Low magnification, showing a granular cell predominant area of the tumor.

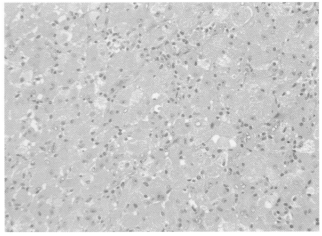

FIGURE 9.2 Higher magnification highlights the eosinophilic, granular quality to the cytoplasm of the granular cell component.

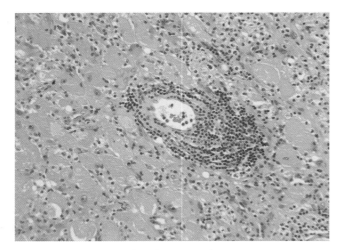

FIGURE 9.3 Perivascular chronic inflammation, consisting of benign-appearing lymphocytes, is seen in the granular cell area of the tumor.

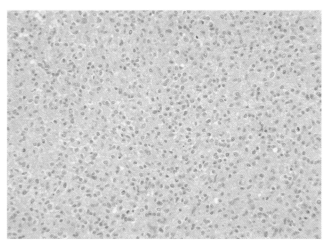

FIGURE 9.4 Areas of the tumor have the appearance of a conventional fibrillary or diffuse astrocytoma.

DISCUSSION

Rarely, glioblastoma may show evidence of granular cell differentiation. The cells in this variant are marked by abundant, eosinophilic, granular cytoplasm and resemble granular cells seen elsewhere in the body in granular cell tumors. If one searches long enough, this granular cell component is often accompanied by areas of the tumor that resemble a conventional-appearing, high-grade fibrillary or diffuse astrocytoma.

Occasionally, on intraoperative consultation, only the granular cell component of the tumor may be sampled. In such cases, the suggestion that the tumor represents part of a high-grade astrocytoma should be made. One exception to this are tumors arising in the suprasellar region; pure granular cell tumors are known to arise from the neurohypophysis of the pituitary gland and generally represent benign lesions. Ultrastructurally, the granular cells are filled with abundant, large lysosomes. Interestingly, a Ki-67 immunostain

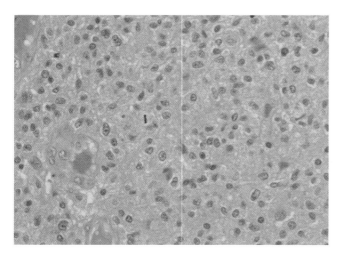

FIGURE 9.5 Mitotic figures are readily identifiable in the fibrillary astrocytoma-appearing area of the tumor.

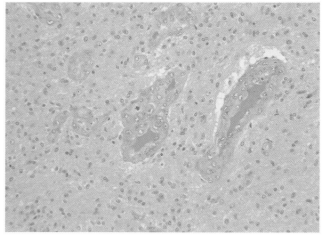

FIGURE 9.6 Vascular proliferative changes are noted in the fibrillary astrocytoma-appearing area of the tumor.

generally does not label the granular cells but highlights increased cell proliferation in the fibrillary astrocytoma-appearing component of the neoplasm. Granular cell differentiation in a glioblastoma does not appear to affect the prognosis of these lesions.

References

1. Brat DJ, Scheithauer BW, Medina-Flores R, et al. Infiltrative astrocytomas with granular cell features (granular cell astrocytomas). A study of histopathologic features, grading, and outcome. Am J Surg Pathol 2002;26:750–7.
2. Chorny JA, Evans LC, Kleinschmidt-DeMasters BK. Cerebral granular cell astrocytomas: a MIB-1, bcl-2, and telomerase study. Clin Neuropathol 2000;19:170–9.
3. Geddes JF, Thom M, Robinson SFD, et al. Granular cell change in astrocytic tumors. Am J Surg Pathol 1996;20:55–63.
4. Melaragno MJ, Prayson RA, Murphy MA, et al. Anaplastic astrocytoma with granular cell differentiation: case report and review of the literature. Hum Pathol 1993;24:805–8.

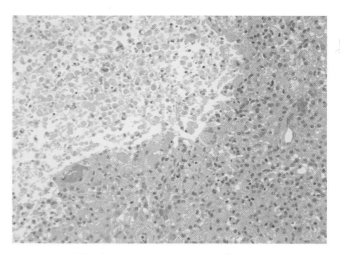

FIGURE 9.7 Focal necrosis is present in the tumor.

Case 10: Giant Cell Glioblastoma

CLINICAL INFORMATION

The patient is a 67-year-old male who presents with a left parietal lobe mass. On imaging, the lesion measures approximately 5.2 cm in greatest extent, with focal areas of enhancement. Subtotal resection of the tumor is performed, and histologic sections are reviewed.

OPINION

The histologic sections show a markedly cellular neoplasm, characterized by a large number of giant tumor cells. Many of these tumor cells are marked by prominent eosinophilic cytoplasm and large pleomorphic nuclei. Many of the cells are multinucleated, and intranuclear pseudoinclusions are frequently evident. Several of the cells show evidence of mitotic activity. Scattered cells demonstrate nuclear hyperchromasia. Occasional cells show somewhat cleared or lipidized cytoplasm. Occasional blood vessels show perivascular chronic inflammation, consisting primarily of benign-appearing lymphoid cells. Focal necrosis is observed. In many areas, the giant tumor cells are intermixed with a population of smaller cells resembling those seen in a typical diffuse or fibrillary astrocytoma. Mild vascular proliferative changes are also observed.

We consider this lesion to be a malignant astrocytoma, and we characterize it as follows: **Left Parietal Lobe, Excision—Giant Cell Glioblastoma, WHO Grade IV.**

COMMENT

This neoplasm is best considered a variant of glioblastoma. The presence of prominent numbers of giant cells in this tumor may portend a slightly better prognosis, compared with an ordinary type glioblastoma.

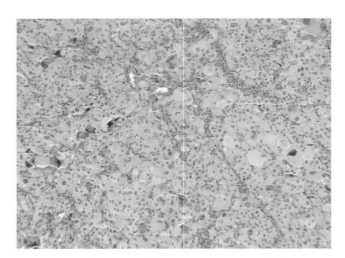

FIGURE 10.1 Low magnification appearance of the tumor shows a neoplasm marked by many giant cells.

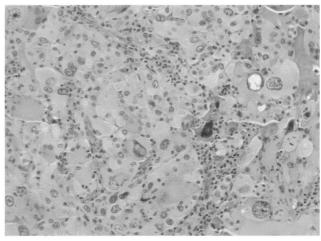

FIGURE 10.2 Many of the giant cells show nuclear pseudoinclusions (cytoplasmic invaginations).

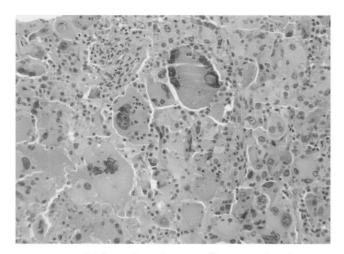

FIGURE 10.3 Multinucleated giant cells are another frequent finding.

FIGURE 10.4 Mitotic figures are observed in an occasional giant cell.

DISCUSSION

One of the histologic variants of glioblastoma is marked by the presence of giant, bizarre-appearing cells. Frequently, these cells are multinucleated. This particular variant is relatively uncommon and represents up to 5% of glioblastoma. The age distribution of this variant covers a wider range than many of the other diffuse astrocytomas and includes children. Because of an often prominent stromal reticulin network in this tumor, the lesion was historically referred to as a monstrocellular sarcoma; however, the GFAP immunoreactivity of the giant cells indicates its astrocytic lineage. p53 mutations are frequently observed in these tumors. In contrast to the small cell variant of a glioblastoma, this variant typically lacks evidence of epidermal growth factor receptor (EGFR) amplification or overexpression. The presence of prominent mitotic activity and necrosis in this tumor allow for its ready distinction from the pleomorphic xanthoastrocytoma. Ki-67 labeling indices are typically high, of the order that is usually observed in other glioblastoma

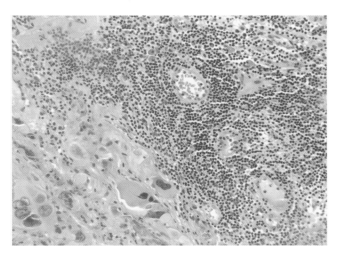

FIGURE 10.5 Focal perivascular chronic inflammation consists of benign-appearing lymphocytes.

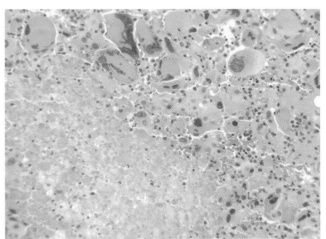

FIGURE 10.6 A focus of necrosis is seen in the tumor.

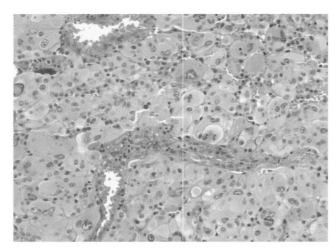

FIGURE 10.7 Vascular proliferative changes are present in the tumor.

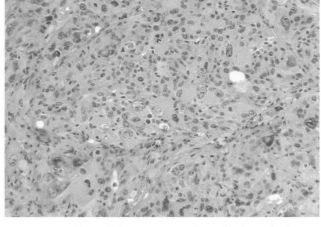

FIGURE 10.8 Part of the tumor is relatively devoid of giant cells and has an appearance similar to that of a conventional, high-grade astrocytoma.

lesions. Although most of the giant cell glioblastomas have a poor prognosis, similar to ordinary glioblastoma, there is some literature to suggest that a subset of these patients may have a somewhat better prognosis, perhaps related to the tumor's less infiltrative nature or the younger age of presentation of some patients.

References

1. Margetts JC, Kalyan R. Giant-celled glioblastoma of brain. A clinicopathological and radiological study of ten cases (including immunohistochemistry and ultrastructure). Cancer 1989;63:524–31.
2. Meyer-Puttlitz B, Hayashi Y, Waha A, et al. Molecular genetic analysis of giant cell glioblastoma. Am J Pathol 1997;151:853–7.
3. Peraud A, Watanabe K, Schwechheiner K, et al. Genetic profile of the giant cell glioblastoma. Lab Invest 1999;79: 123–9.
4. Queiroz LS, Faria AV, Zanardi VA, et al. Lipidized giant cell glioblastoma of cerebellum. Clin Neuropathol 2005;24: 262–6.

Case 11: Pleomorphic Xanthoastrocytoma

CLINICAL INFORMATION

The patient is a 20-year-old female who presents with a four-year history of seizures. On imaging, she has a partially cystic and enhancing left temporal lobe mass. The patient undergoes gross total resection of the tumor, and histologic sections are reviewed.

OPINION

Histologic sections show a tumor marked by prominent cellularity and readily apparent nuclear pleomorphism. Scattered giant cells are marked by frequent multinucleation. Intranuclear pseudoinclusions are occasionally seen in these giant cells. The amount of cytoplasm in these cells is variable and ranges from scant to prominent. Some of the cells have a light, homogeneous, eosinophilic cytoplasm, whereas others show lipidization. Dystrophic calcification is present. Perivascular chronic inflammation, consisting primarily of benign-appearing lymphocytes, is also saliently noted. Mitotic figures are absent. There is no evidence of necrosis. Focal microcystic degenerative changes are observed in the tumor. Also of note is the sharp interface between the tumor and adjacent cortex. Reticulin staining highlights increased reticulin deposition between cells and small groups of cells. A Ki-67 labeling index of 3.2 is noted.

We consider this lesion to be a low-grade astrocytic neoplasm and characterize it as follows: **Left Temporal Lobe, Excision—Pleomorphic Xanthoastrocytoma, WHO Grade II.**

FIGURE 11.1 Low magnification view, showing the relatively discrete interface between the tumor and the adjacent parenchyma.

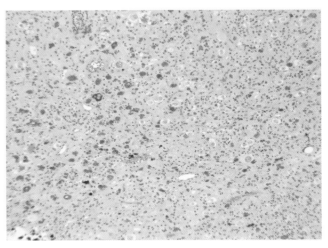

FIGURE 11.2 The marked cellularity and degree of nuclear pleomorphism are worrisome features when first looking at this tumor.

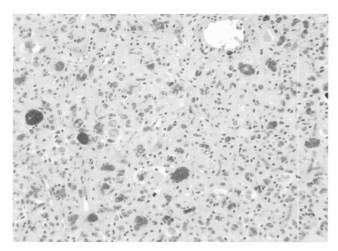

FIGURE 11.3 Scattered multinucleated giant cells, some with nuclear pseudoinclusions, are present.

COMMENT

The absence of prominent mitotic activity and necrosis supports a diagnosis of pleomorphic xanthoastrocytoma.

DISCUSSION

The pleomorphic xanthoastrocytoma is an important tumor to distinguish from a glioblastoma because of its significantly better prognosis. These tumors typically present in children and young adults, often with a

history of intractable seizures. The vast majority of these tumors arise either in the temporal or parietal lobes and are superficially based. On imaging studies, they frequently are cystic, with enhancing mural nodules. The superficial location also contrasts with typical glioblastoma, which is a white matter-based tumor in many cases. On first inspection, these tumors appear to be worrisome, given the degree of cellularity and pleomorphism of the cells. Many of the cells show features similar to that of the giant cell glioblastoma. However, in contrast to the glioblastoma, the pleomorphic xanthoastrocytoma generally demonstrates little or any mitotic figures and no necrosis. Reticulin staining may be prominently observed in this tumor. Perivascular chronic inflammation is a fairly frequent finding. A subset of tumors may demonstrate calcification. Many of the large, bizarre-appearing cells demonstrate GFAP immunoreactivity. It is not unusual to find occasional cells in these tumors demonstrating evidence of neural differentiation by immunohistochemistry (synaptophysin-positive). These tumors are generally considered low-grade (WHO grade II), although a subset recurs and these tumors require follow-up. Rare cases of more aggressive behavior in these lesions have been described;

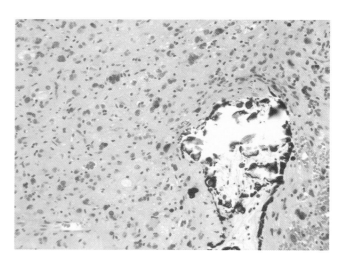

FIGURE 11.4 Large astrocytic cells with lipidized cytoplasm are seen.

FIGURE 11.5 Focal dystrophic calcification is present.

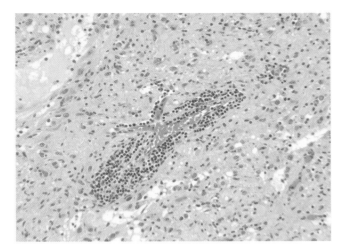

FIGURE 11.6 Perivascular chronic inflammation is a frequent finding.

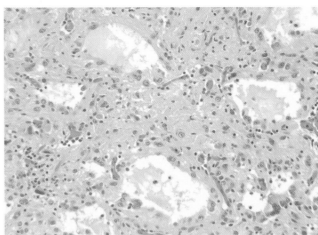

FIGURE 11.7 A focal area of microcystic degeneration is evident.

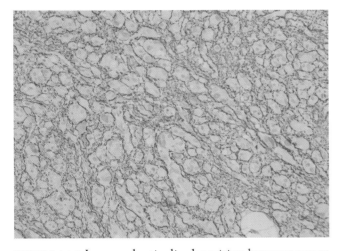

FIGURE 11.8 Increased reticulin deposition between tumor cells is evident.

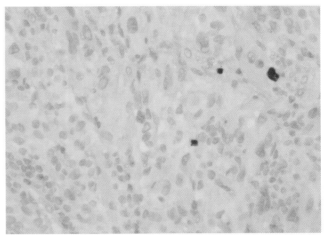

FIGURE 11.9 A low Ki-67 labeling index of 3.2 is present in this tumor.

this is often associated with worrisome histologic features, including the presence of increased mitotic activity and/or necrosis. These later tumors are designated as anaplastic pleomorphic xanthoastrocytoma and represent WHO grade III neoplasms.

References

1. Giannini C, Scheihauer BW, Burger PC, et al. Pleomorphic xanthoastrocytoma. What do we really know about it? Cancer 1999;85:2033–45.

2. Kepes JJ. Pleomorphic xanthoastrocytoma: the birth of a diagnosis and a concept. Brain Pathol 1993;3:269–74.

3. Kepes JJ, Rubinstein LJ, Eng LW. Pleomorphic xanthoastrocytoma: a distinctive meningocerebral glioma of young subjects with relatively favorable prognosis. A study of 12 cases. Cancer 1979;44:1839–52.

4. Prayson RA, Morris III, HH. Anaplastic pleomorphic xanthoastrocytoma. Arch Pathol Lab Med 1998;122:1082–6.

Case 12: Gliosarcoma

CLINICAL INFORMATION

The patient is a 58-year-old male who presents with seizures. On MRI imaging studies, a 5.6-cm mass, involving the right frontal and parietal lobes and focally crossing the corpus callosum to involve the contralateral side, is present. The tumor demonstrates focal areas of enhancement. The patient undergoes a subtotal resection, and histologic sections are reviewed.

OPINION

Histologic sections show a markedly cellular neoplasm, characterized by a proliferation of atypical-appearing cells resembling malignant astrocytes. Areas of the tumor resemble an ordinary glioblastoma multiforme; the tumor shows focal necrosis, vascular proliferative changes, and readily identifiable mitotic activity. Intermixed with the glioblastomatous-appearing areas are foci of tumor with a malignant spindle-cell appearance. The spindle cells contain atypical nuclei and demonstrate evidence of mitotic activity. Focally, malignant bone formation (osteosarcoma) is observed in the tumor. GFAP immunostaining shows positive staining, confined to the glioblastomatous-appearing areas of the tumor. Specifically, the spindle-cell areas do not stain with GFAP. Reticulin staining shows increased reticulin deposition between cells and small groups of cells in the spindle-cell regions of the tumor. Increased reticulin staining is only noted in vascular proliferative foci in the glioblastomatous component of the lesion.

We consider the lesion to be a variant of high-grade astrocytoma and characterize it as follows: **Right**

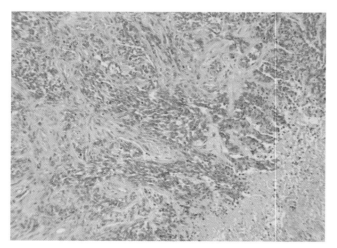

FIGURE 12.1 Low magnification appearance, highlighting a glioblastomatous-appearing region of the tumor with necrosis.

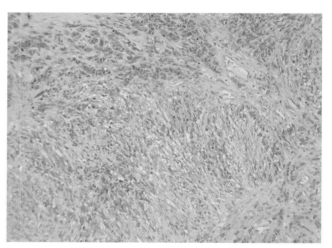

FIGURE 12.2 The glioblastomatous component is juxtaposed to a spindle-cell component in the gliosarcoma.

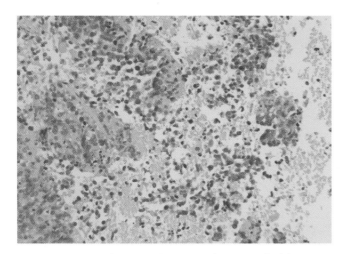

FIGURE 12.3 High magnification, showing glioblastomatous component with necrosis.

Frontal and Parietal Lobes, Subtotal Resection— Gliosarcoma, WHO Grade IV.

COMMENT

The sarcomatous component of this tumor consists of a nondescript spindle-cell proliferation, as well as an osteosarcomatous component. Increased reticulin staining highlights the spindle-cell sarcomatous component tumor. GFAP immunoreactivity highlights the glioblastomatous component of the neoplasm.

DISCUSSION

Gliosarcoma is a variant of glioblastoma, marked by a glioblastomatous component juxtaposed with a sarcomatous component. Approximately 2% of all glioblastoma multiforme are gliosarcoma type. The age of presentation, clinical presentation, and imaging findings are quite similar to those of the glioblastoma. The key to the diagnosis is recognition of the sarcomatous component. Most commonly, the sarcomatous component resembles either fibrosarcoma or malignant fibrous histiocytoma. A combination of GFAP and reticulin staining can be useful in delineating this component. The sarcomatous component is generally GFAP-negative and reticulin-rich. The only increased reticulin staining usually observed in a glioblastoma resides in areas of vascular proliferative change. In occasional glioblastoma, particularly those growing up near the surface of the brain, the tumor cells can assume a spindle configuration and resemble the gliosarcoma lesion. The spindle-cell glioblastoma shows a paucity of reticulin and evidence of GFAP immunoreactivity in the spindle-cell component. Sarcoma represents the other main differential diagnostic consideration. Sarcomas are GFAP-negative tumors.

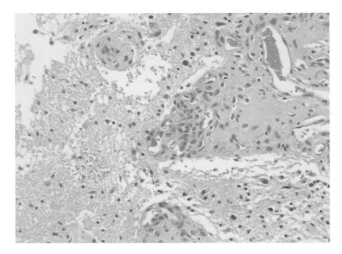

FIGURE 12.4 Vascular proliferative changes are present in the gliosarcoma.

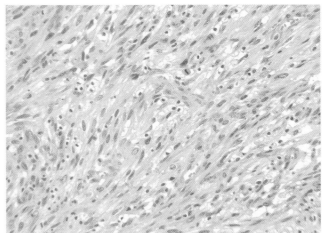

FIGURE 12.5 The sarcomatous component is seen here, with readily identifiable mitotic activity in a gliosarcoma.

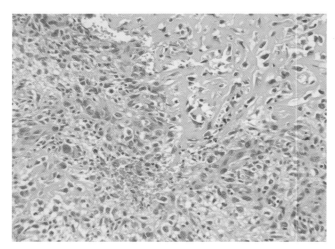

FIGURE 12.6 Focal osteosarcomatous differentiation is present in this tumor.

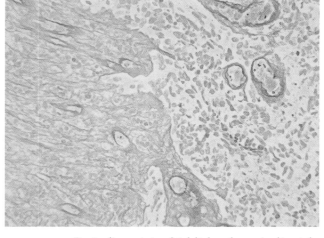

FIGURE 12.7 Reticulin staining highlights the reticulin-rich, sarcomatous component of the gliosarcoma.

The current thinking suggests that the sarcomatous component represents a form of mesenchymal differentiation in a glioblastoma. A number of studies have shown similar genetic alterations in both the glioblastomatous and sarcomatous components of the tumor. Recognition of the gliosarcoma pattern does not appear to have any significant clinical or prognostic significance and, unfortunately, shares the same dismal prognosis that marks ordinary glioblastoma multiforme.

References

1. Beirnat W, Aguzzi A, Sure U, et al. Identical mutations of the p53 tumor suppressor gene in the gliomatous and sarcomatous components of gliosarcomas suggest a common origin from glial cells. J Neuropathol Exp Neurol 1995;54:651–6.
2. Meis JM, Ho KL, Nelson JS. Gliosarcoma: a histologic and immunohistochemical reaffirmation. Mod Pathol 1990; 3:19–24.
3. Sreenan JJ, Prayson RA. Gliosarcoma. A study of 13 tumors, including p53 and CD34 immunohistochemistry. Arch Pathol Lab Med 1997;121:129–33.

Case 13: Small Cell Glioblastoma

CLINICAL INFORMATION

The patient is a 62-year-old male with a 20-pack-year history of smoking who presents with an enhancing mass in the right frontal lobe. A biopsy of the tumor is performed, and histologic sections are reviewed.

OPINION

Sections show a markedly cellular neoplasm, characterized by a monomorphous proliferation of small cells with a high nuclear-to-cytoplasm ratio. Prominent mitotic activity and focal vascular proliferative changes are observed. Individual cell necrosis and a focus of geographic necrosis are also present. Immunohistochemical staining of the tumor shows focal positive immunoreactivity, with antibodies to GFAP and EGFR. The tumor did not stain with antibodies to CD45RB (CLA) or cytokeratin CAM5.2.

We consider the lesion to be a malignant astrocytoma and characterize it as follows: **Right Frontal Lobe, Biopsy—Small Cell Glioblastoma, WHO Grade IV.**

COMMENT

This neoplasm represents a variant of glioblastoma multiforme. The small cell change in glioblastoma does not affect the prognosis.

DISCUSSION

In glioblastoma predominantly composed of small cells, the designation of small cell glioblastoma is appropriate. These tumors appear monomorphic, with slightly elongated nuclei and prominent mitotic activity. The presence of vascular proliferation and/or

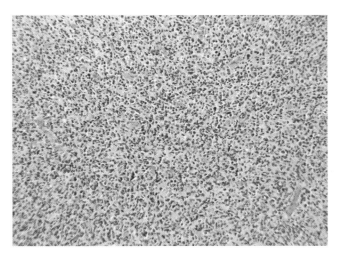

FIGURE 13.1 Low magnification appearance of the tumor, showing a markedly hypercellularity neoplasm.

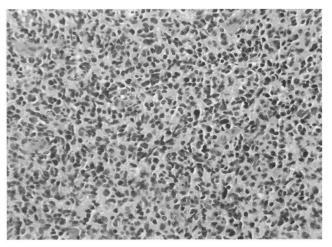

FIGURE 13.2 Higher magnification highlights the relative monotonous appearance of the cells and the high nuclear-to-cytoplasmic ratio.

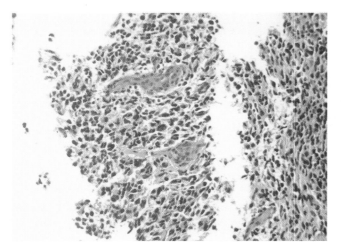

FIGURE 13.3 Focal vascular proliferative change is present.

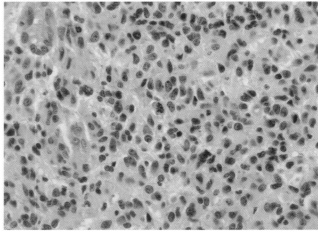

FIGURE 13.4 Mitotic figures are readily identified in the tumor.

necrosis is definitional of glioblastoma. Biopsies are particularly challenging to evaluate because of the sometimes homogeneous appearance of this tumor. The differential diagnosis may include other small cell neoplasms that may be found in older adults in the brain, including diffuse large cell lymphoma, metastatic small cell carcinoma, and anaplastic oligodendroglioma. Immunohistochemistry may be helpful in sorting out this differential diagnosis in cases where morphologic clues are absent. A diagnosis of

lymphoma is excluded with CD45RB immunostaining. The lack of cytokeratin CAM5.2 immunoreactivity and the focal GFAP staining (which, at times, may be sparse in this variant) argues against a metastatic small cell carcinoma. Increased overexpression or amplification of EGFR is a frequent finding in the small cell glioblastoma and uncommon in an anaplastic oligodendroglioma.

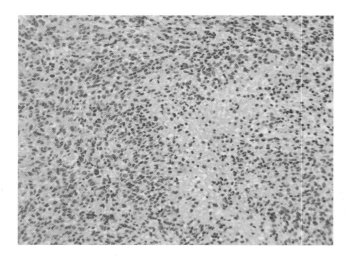

FIGURE 13.5 Focal necrosis is present.

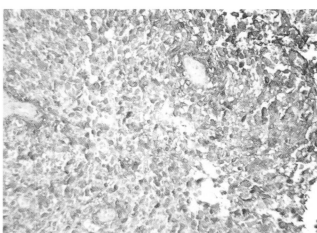

FIGURE 13.6 GFAP immunoreactivity is present and expected with a glioblastoma.

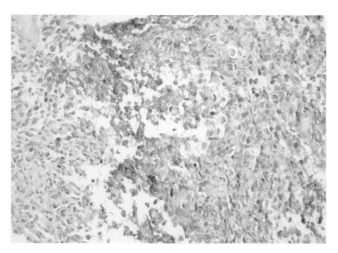

FIGURE 13.7 EGFR overexpression, as evidenced by immunohistochemistry.

References

1. Burger PC, Pearl DK, Aldape K, et al. Small cell architecture—a histological equivalent of EGFR amplification in glioblastoma multiforme? J Neuropathol Exp Neurol 2001;60:1099–1104.
2. Perry A, Aldape KD, George DH, et al. Small cell astrocytoma: an aggressive variant that is clinicopathologically and genetically distinct from anaplastic oligodendroglioma. Cancer 2004;101:2318–26.

Case 14: Epithelioid Glioblastoma

CLINICAL INFORMATION

The patient is a 72-year-old female who presents with headaches and persistent nausea. On MRI studies, she is noted to have a gadolinium-enhancing, right frontal-temporal mass with marked peritumoral edema. Biopsies of the mass are taken, and histologic sections reviewed.

OPINION

Histologic sections show a markedly cellular neoplasm, characterized by a proliferation of generally rounded cells. The cells show a moderate amount of cytoplasm, nuclear irregularities, and prominent nucleolation. Readily identifiable mitotic activity is observed in the tumor. Focal necrosis, accompanied by vascular proliferative changes, is also seen. Given the differential diagnosis of this lesion with a metastatic non-small cell carcinoma, a combination of cytokeratin markers and GFAP are evaluated. The tumor demonstrates diffuse positive staining, with antibody to GFAP. Scattered cytokeratin AE1/3 immunoreactivity is observed. The tumor did not stain with antibody to cytokeratin CAM5.2. The tumor also fails to demonstrate immunoreactivity with antibodies to Melan-A and HMB 45.

We consider the lesion to be a high-grade astrocytoma and characterize it as follows: **Right Frontal-Temporal Lobes, Biopsies—Epithelioid Glioblastoma, WHO Grade IV.**

COMMENT

The tumor demonstrates diffuse positive staining with antibody to GFAP and an absence of staining with melanoma markers and cytokeratin CAM5.2. Cytokeratin AE1/3 staining may represent cross

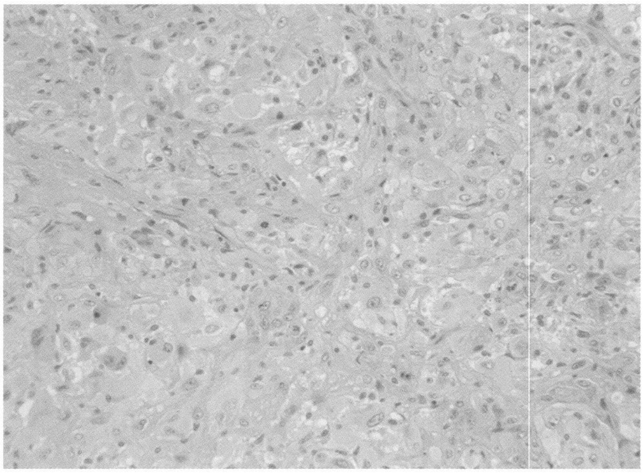

FIGURE 14.1 This epithelioid glioblastoma is marked by rounded cells with discernible cytoplasm and prominent nucleolation.

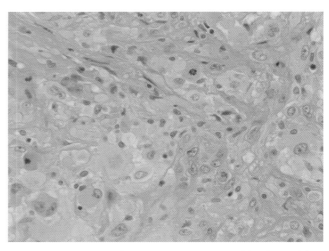

FIGURE 14.2 Increased mitotic figures are readily observable.

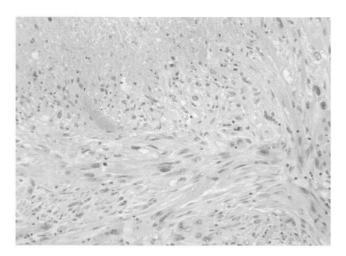

FIGURE 14.3 Focal necrosis is seen in this tumor.

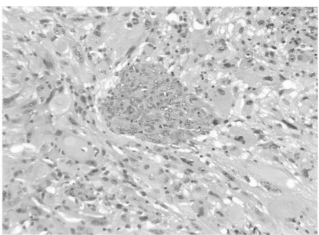

FIGURE 14.4 Vascular proliferative changes are present.

immunoreactivity. The presence of vascular proliferative changes and necrosis warrant a diagnosis of a grade IV astrocytoma.

DISCUSSION

Glioblastoma multiforme can assume an epithelioid appearance. In some instances, this takes the form of cells with lipidized cytoplasm. In these cases, differentiating the tumor from metastatic clear cell carcinoma (such as renal cell carcinoma

or adrenocortical carcinoma) or pleomorphic xanthoastrocytoma is of consideration. In contrast to the pleomorphic xanthoastrocytoma, the epithelioid glioblastoma demonstrates features typical of glioblastoma, including vascular proliferative changes, necrosis, and prominent mitotic activity.

In other instances, the cells have more eosinophilic cytoplasm and, with the presence of prominent nucleolation, can resemble either metastatic non-small

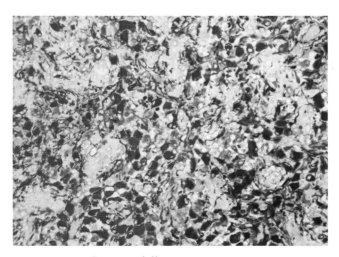

FIGURE 14.5 Strong diffuse positive immunostaining with antibody to GFAP is observed in this epithelioid glioblastoma.

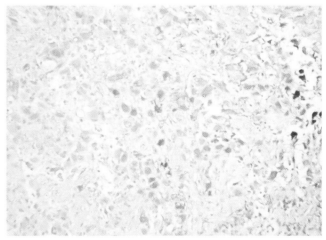

FIGURE 14.6 Scattered cytokeratin AE1/3 immunoreactivity can be observed in glioblastoma multiforme and represents cross immunoreactivity. The tumor did not stain with cytokeratin CAM5.2 antibody.

cell carcinoma or, occasionally, malignant melanoma. In such cases, immunohistochemistry can be helpful in uncovering the true lineage of the tumor, if there are no morphologic clues in the neoplasm; i.e., an area of lower-grade tumor resembling astrocytoma is not evident. Glioblastoma stains with antibodies to GFAP and S-100 protein. In differentiating glioblastoma from melanoma, which can also stain with S-100 protein, additional melanoma markers, such as Melan-A and HMB 45, can be useful. In differentiating carcinoma from glioblastoma, a combination of GFAP with cytokeratin markers is helpful. One needs to be careful which cytokeratin marker one employs. It is well known that cytokeratins AE1/3 can cross immunoreact with the intermediate molecular weight glial filaments of a glioblastoma (as in the current case) and result in positive staining. Use of other keratin markers, such as CAM5.2, may be more helpful in this situation.

This variant of glioblastoma has a similar prognosis to an ordinary glioblastoma multiforme.

References

1. Kepes JJ. Astrocytomas: old and newly recognized variants, their spectrum of morphology and antigen expression. Can J Neurol Sci 1987;14:109–21.
2. Mueller W, Lass U, Herms J, Kuchelmeister, et al. Clinical analysis in glioblastoma with epithelial differentiation. Brain Pathol 2001;11:39–43.
3. Rosenblum MK, Erlandson RA, Budzilovich GN. The lipid-rich epithelioid glioblastoma. Am J Surg Pathol 1991;15:925–34.

Case 15: Gliomatosis Cerebri

CLINICAL INFORMATION

The patient is a 42-year-old male who presents with seizures and increased lethargy. On MRI imaging, bilateral, multilobe, increased signal intensity is observed on T2-weighted images. Two biopsies, one from the right frontal and the other from the corpus callosum, are taken, and histologic sections are reviewed.

OPINION

Both biopsies show hypercellular parenchyma, marked by a proliferation of spindled cells. The cells are marked by nuclear enlargement and hyperchromasia. These cells are GFAP-positive and CD68-negative. The frontal lobe biopsy shows more cellularity, and a rare mitotic figure is observed. Vascular proliferation and necrosis are not present.

We consider the lesion to be an astrocytoma and characterize it as follows: **Right Frontal Lobe and Corpus Callosum, Biopsies—Gliomatosis Cerebri, WHO Grade III.**

COMMENT

Given the apparent widespread distribution of the lesion on imaging, the neoplasm represents a diffuse astrocytoma or gliomatosis cerebri.

DISCUSSION

Gliomatosis cerebri is a diagnosis used to describe a diffuse glioma. The tumor often shows extensive infiltration on imaging studies, usually with bilateral cerebral involvement. Involvement may extend to the brainstem and cerebellum. Often, a few biopsies are taken to confirm that the process represents a glioma.

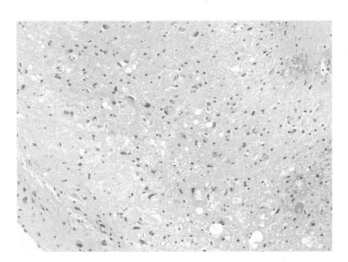

FIGURE 15.1 Lower magnification appearance of the corpus callosum biopsy, showing mild hypercellularity.

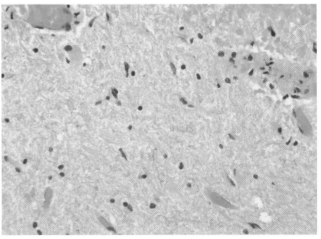

FIGURE 15.2 High magnification, showing occasional atypical spindled cells, consistent with infiltrating astrocytoma.

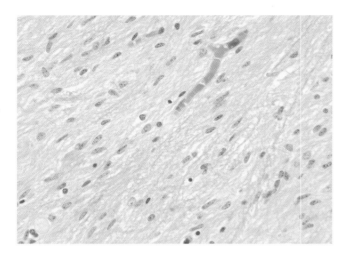

FIGURE 15.3 Another area from the corpus callosum biopsy, showing an increased number of spindled cells.

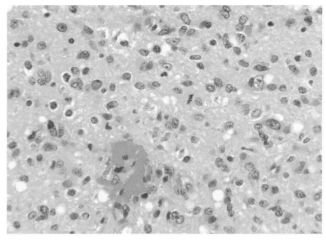

FIGURE 15.4 The frontal lobe biopsy shows more in the way of cellularity, and a rare mitotic figure is present.

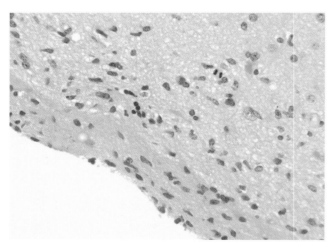

FIGURE 15.5 Subpial aggregation of spindled tumor cells is present in the frontal lobe biopsy.

The diagnosis is usually made by correlating the biopsy results with the imaging findings. Morphologically, the glioma component may resemble an astrocytoma, oligodendroglioma, or mixed glioma. Although much of the tumor may appear low-grade, foci of higher-grade tumor may be present. Because tumor cells may be spindled, distinction of this entity from a pathologic process marked by prominent microglial cell proliferation may be challenging. Immunohistochemistry can be helpful in these circumstances, with a combination of GFAP and CD68 staining; this allows for the assessment of the lineage of the spindled cells. Prognosis corresponds to a WHO grade III neoplasm.

References

1. Jennings MT, Frenchman M, Shahab T, et al. Gliomatosis cerebri presenting as intractable epilepsy during early childhood. J Child Neurol 1995;10:37–45.
2. Kros JM, Zheng P, Dinjens WNM, et al. Genetic aberrations in gliomatosis cerebri support monoclonal tumorigenesis. J Neuropathol Exp Neurol 2002;61:806–14.
3. Mawrin C. Molecular genetic alterations in gliomatosis cerebri: what can we learn about the origin and course of the disease? Acta Neuropathol 2005;110:527–36.

Case 16: Pilocytic Astrocytoma

CLINICAL INFORMATION

The patient is a 3-year-old male who presents with a history of dysconjugate gaze since infancy. A minor accident with a toy prompts an emergency department visit and, after physical examination, imaging studies are obtained. A mass is identified in the midline of the cerebellum. A decision is made to resect the lesion, and histologic sections are reviewed.

OPINION

Biopsies show a moderately hypercellular glial tumor that, in most areas, forms a solid mass but, at the edges, shows individual cell infiltration of cerebellar parenchyma. Adjacent cerebellar folia demonstrate neuronal loss and gliosis as a result of compression from the long-standing, low-grade tumor. The tumor is biphasic and composed of zones of compact, highly fibrillated astrocytes, alternating with loose-textured microcystic areas containing cells with short, multipolar processes. The tumor is focally calcified and extends into leptomeninges.

We consider the pathology to be that of a low-grade astrocytoma and characterize it as follows: **Midline Cerebellum, Excision—Pilocytic Astrocytoma, WHO Grade I.**

COMMENT

There are no high-grade features in this neoplasm. Extension into the leptomeninges is a common finding in pilocytic astrocytoma, especially in cases involving cerebellum or optic nerve, and does not

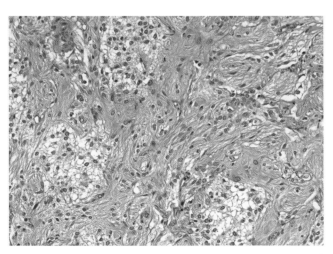

FIGURE 16.1 Section showing a biphasic tumor, composed of compact, eosinophilic areas of highly fibrillary astrocytes, alternating with looser microcystic areas.

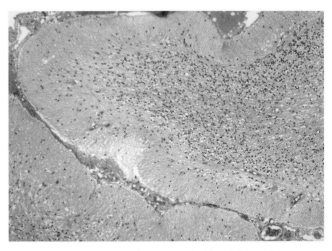

FIGURE 16.2 Non-neoplastic cerebellar folia, adjacent to the tumor, show atrophy from compression by this long-standing, low-grade tumor; there has been loss of both Purkinje cell and granule cell neurons.

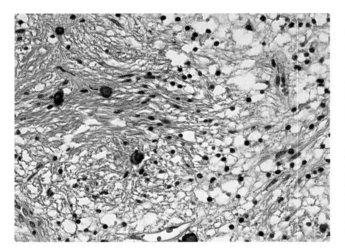

FIGURE 16.3 High magnification illustrates the coarse, "hair-like" piloid, bipolar cell processes in the denser areas of tumor.

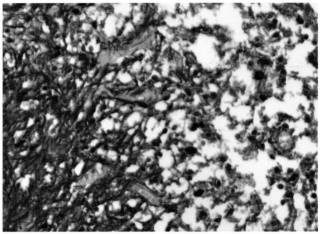

FIGURE 16.4 Dense, pilocytic areas of tumor manifest strong GFAP immunoreactivity.

indicate aggressive or malignant behavior, nor does it predict eventual cerebrospinal fluid spread. Similarly, although most of the tumor is discrete and cohesive, infiltrating cells at the edge of a pilocytic astrocytoma do not predict recurrence or affect prognosis.

DISCUSSION

Pilocytic astrocytoma is an important variant of astrocytoma, to distinguish from diffuse infiltrating high-

er-grade astrocytomas, because pilocytic astrocytoma has a much better prognosis. Pilocytic astrocytoma can be seen in both adults and children, but it is the most common glioma in children. Characteristic anatomic locations for this tumor include cerebellum, optic nerve, thalamus, basal ganglia, cerebellum, brainstem (dorsally as an exophytic lesion), and spinal cord. Tumor location influences prognosis; hypothalamic and brainstem sites usually preclude total removal, and

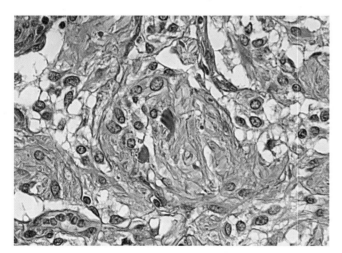

FIGURE 16.5 Dense, compact areas contain variable numbers of eosinophilic, sausage-shaped Rosenthal fibers.

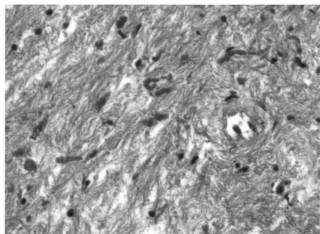

FIGURE 16.6 Rosenthal fibers should be distinguished from erythrocytes in tissue and can be highlighted by trichrome stain.

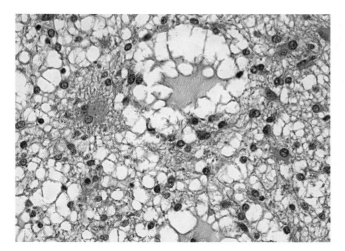

FIGURE 16.7 Looser, microcystic areas often contain pools of pale, eosinophilic mucin; nearby astrocytes manifest short, multipolar processes rather than coarse pilocytic features.

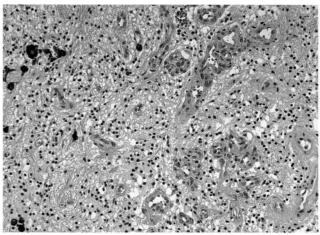

FIGURE 16.8 Calcifications are an infrequent finding in pilocytic astrocytomas.

tumor can eventually, after years or decades, cause patient demise because of compromise of critical brain functions. Nevertheless, in many instances, even with known residual tumor, growth can be absent, and tumor may even regress. Progression to higher grades (i.e., malignant transformation) almost never occurs unless the patient has received radiotherapy.

Histologically, diagnosis rests on identifying a biphasic tumor, with the dense compact areas containing coarsely fibrillar astrocytes with bipolar, "hair-like" processes that are strongly immunoreactive for GFAP. Rosenthal fibers (amorphous, sausage-shaped, eosinophilic structures that are easily seen on hematoxylin and eosin stain) are more frequent in compact areas, but they may be very irregular in distribution and are not absolutely required for the

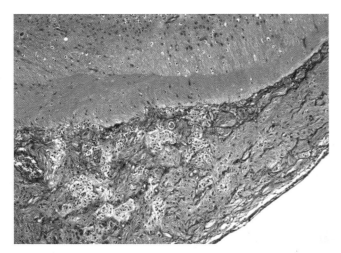

FIGURE 16.9 Extension of pilocytic astrocytoma to leptomeninges is common and does not indicate aggressive tumor or foreshadow cerebrospinal fluid metastases.

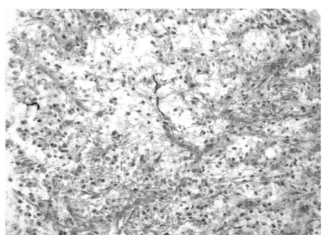

FIGURE 16.10 Pilocytic astrocytomas grow as relatively solid tumor masses and thus envelope few neurofilament-positive axons except near the edge of the tumor.

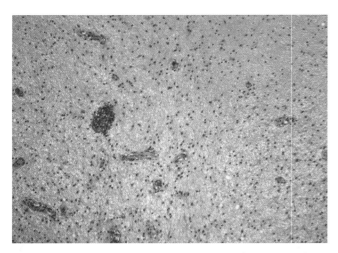

FIGURE 16.11 Pilocytic astrocytoma may show an infiltrative margin; this also does not have prognostic significance, but tumor in this area cannot be distinguished from diffuse astrocytoma.

diagnosis. Eosinophilic granular bodies (EGBs), which are composed of proteinaceous material, can also be found in some pilocytic astrocytomas and are highlighted by periodic acid Schiff stain. Neither Rosenthal fibers nor EGBs are specific to pilocytic astrocytoma, or even to neoplastic conditions, but both tend to be seen in low-grade tumors (i.e., WHO grades I and II), such as ganglioglioma, pilocytic astrocytoma, pleomorphic xanthoastrocytoma, and subependymoma, when they do occur in glial neoplasms.

Looser microcystic areas in pilocytic astrocytomas may show small cysts, filled with pools of pale, eosinophilic mucin. Astrocytes in these areas have short, blunted cell processes and stain considerably less well with GFAP. More solid growth of pilocytic astrocytoma displaces normal brain tissue, leading to few anti-neurofilament-positive axons within the tumor, compared to diffuse astrocytomas, which tend to infiltrate between axons and preserve them deep within the infiltrating tumor mass. Mitoses are infrequent in pilocytic astrocytomas but can occasionally be seen. MIB-1 cell cycle labeling index is usually less than 4%.

Abundant vasculature is characteristic of pilocytic astrocytoma. Both hyalinized and "glomeruloid" vessels can be seen, with the latter accounting for the enhancement seen preoperatively on neuroimaging studies. Glomeruloid vessels often are arranged in chains near the edge of macroscopic cysts, or in clusters, and should not prompt the pathologist to overgrade the tumor. Calcifications are relatively infrequent in pilocytic astrocytoma but are thought to be a "regressive" change, as is the occasional finding of necrosis. Degenerative features include nuclear hyperchromatism, pleomorphism, and nuclear pseudoinclusions and also do not affect prognosis.

References

1. Kleinschmidt-DeMasters BK, Prayson RA. An algorithmic approach to the brain biopsy—Part 1. Arch Pathol Lab Med 2006;130:1630–8.
2. Perry, A. Glial and glioneuronal tumors. In: Prayson RA, editor. Neuropathology. Philadelphia, PA: Elsevier Churchill Livingstone;2005. p. 434–8.
3. Scheithauer BW, Hawkins C, Tihan T, et al. Pilocytic astrocytoma. In: Louis DN, Ohgaki H, Wiestler OD, Cavenee WK, editors. WHO Classification of Tumours of the Central Nervous System. Lyon, FR: IARC Press;2007. p. 14–21.

Case 17: Pilomyxoid Astrocytoma

CLINICAL INFORMATION

The patient is a 6-month-old male who presents with failure to thrive and abnormal head shape. On imaging, a heterogeneously enhancing, hypothalamic-chiasmatic mass is identified. Subtotal resection is performed, and histologic sections are reviewed.

OPINION

The tumor is a mildly hypercellular, monomorphic lesion, with clustering of tumor cells around blood vessels ("angiocentric" tumor cell arrangement). Unlike pilocytic astrocytomas, no biphasic pattern, coarsely fibrillated "piloid" astrocytes, Rosenthal fibers, or eosinophilic granular bodies are identified in this relatively monotonous neoplasm. Tumor cells have small, bland, round-to-oval nuclei and wispy, delicate, eosinophilic cytoplasm. Mitotic figures are variably observed but are few in this case. There is no necrosis.

We consider the findings in this lesion to be those of a low-grade glioma and characterize it as follows: **Hypothalamic/Optic Chiasm, Excision— Pilomyxoid Astrocytoma, WHO Grade II.**

COMMENT

The bland cytological appearance of the lesion, coupled with mild hypercellularity and absence of mitoses or necrosis, belies the often aggressive nature of this tumor.

DISCUSSION

Pilomyxoid astrocytoma is a relatively newly described tumor, which is a variant of a pilocytic

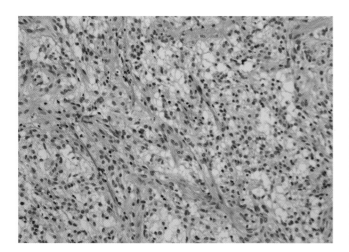

FIGURE 17.1 Low magnification view of the biopsy, showing a mildly hypercellular neoplasm with a monomorphic population of delicate wispy cells; note absence of Rosenthal fibers or eosinophilic granular bodies.

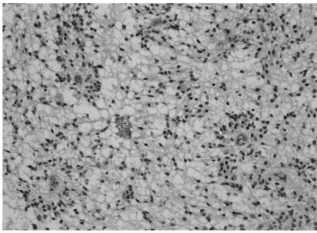

FIGURE 17.2 Some regions of tumor manifest prominent angiocentricity of tumor cells.

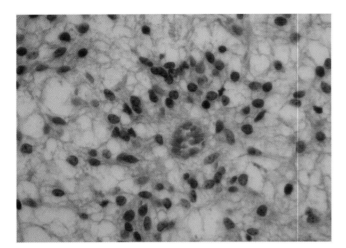

FIGURE 17.3 High magnification, showing the characteristic features of tumor cells, including low nuclear-to-cytoplasmic ratio, bland nuclear features, delicate wispy eosinophilic cytoplasm, and absence of mitoses.

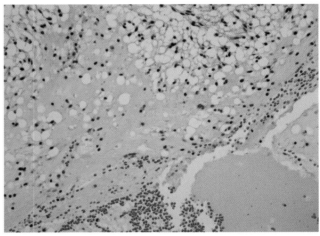

FIGURE 17.4 Mucin background is variably present in pilomyxoid astrocytoma but may be prominent in some examples.

astrocytoma but has been assigned a WHO grade of II (rather than a grade of I, as for pilocytic astrocytoma), to reflect the more aggressive biological course of pilomyxoid compared to pilocytic astrocytoma. Pilomyxoid astrocytomas may manifest local recurrence, as well as cerebrospinal fluid metastases, and patients can succumb to locally destructive effects

of tumor on the hypothalamus. The typical patient is less than 2 years of age, with a median age of 10 months. The hypothalamic-chiasmatic region is the most common location, although bona fide examples have been described in sites frequented by pilocytic astrocytoma, including cerebellum, brainstem, and spinal cord. Occasional pilomyxoid astrocytomas evolve into typical pilocytic astrocytomas over time,

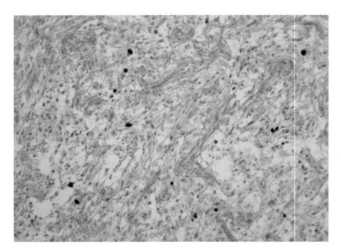

FIGURE 17.5 MIB-1 is variable and cannot be used to distinguish most cases of pilomyxoid from pilocytic astrocytoma.

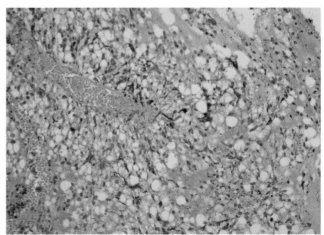

FIGURE 17.6 GFAP highlights delicate wispy cytoplasm in tumor cells, contrasting with the more coarsely pilocytic cytoplasm in pilocytic astrocytoma.

suggesting a common origin for these two tumors. Unfortunately, this does not happen for all patients with pilomyxoid astrocytoma and, indeed, this child succumbed 6 months after his diagnosis.

Histologically, the tumor is only moderately hypercellular and usually does not show necrosis. Often, pilomyxoid astrocytoma does not demonstrate any higher mitotic rate than ordinary pilocytic astrocytoma. The diagnosis of pilomyxoid astrocytoma is made easier if the MIB-1 rate is high, but the range of labeling index is quite broad, from 2–20%, and overlaps at the lower end with pilocytic astrocytoma. Hence, correct diagnosis requires recognition of the architectural pattern, including angiocentricity of tumor cells, monomorphic appearance, mucin pools, and absence of Rosenthal fibers. Immunostaining of

pilocytic astrocytoma with GFAP often shows thinner and more delicate, wispy tumor cell processes in tumor cells than those seen in coarsely fibrillated pilocytic astrocytoma. Very focal areas, with pilomyxoid-like histology within an otherwise ordinary pilocytic astrocytoma, should not prompt this diagnosis.

References

1. Komakula ST, Fenton LZ, Kleinschmidt-DeMasters BK, et al. Pilomyxoid astrocytoma: neuroimaging with clinicopathologic correlates in 4 cases followed over time. J Pediatr Hematol Oncol 2007;29:465–70.
2. Scheithauer BW, Hawkins C, Tihan T, et al. Pilocytic astrocytoma. In: Louis DN, Ohgaki H, Wiestler OD, Cavenee WK, editors. WHO Classification of Tumours of the Central Nervous System. Lyon, FR: IARC Press; 2007. p. 20–21.
3. Tihan T, Fisher PG, Kepner JL, et al. Pediatric astrocytomas with monomorphous pilomyxoid features and a less favorable outcome. J Neuropathol Exp Neurol 1999;58:1061–8.

Case 18: Subependymal Giant Cell Astrocytoma

CLINICAL INFORMATION

The patient is a 12-year-old male who presents with history of seizures and skin lesions in the nasolabial fold region. On physical exam, he is also noted to have periungual fibroma on the third digit of the right hand and pitting in the dental enamel of several of his teeth. On imaging, a large, contrast-enhancing, lateral ventricular mass is identified. The lesion is resected, and histologic sections are reviewed.

OPINION

Histologic sections show a mass marked by a proliferation of large cells with abundant eosinophilic cytoplasm and eccentrically placed nuclei with prominent nucleoli. Occasionally, these cells appear to be arranged around blood vessels. Focally, perivascular sclerosis is observed. Vascular proliferative changes,

prominent mitotic activity, and necrosis are not observed. Microcalcifications are present. In areas, the tumor cells assume a more spindled appearance. A Ki-67 labeling index of 0.8 is observed in the tumor.

We consider the lesion to be a low-grade astrocytic neoplasm and characterize it as follows: **Lateral Ventricle, Excision—Subependymal Giant Cell Astrocytoma, WHO Grade I.**

COMMENT

The clinical findings, in this patient, along with the diagnosis of subependymal giant cell astrocytoma, suggest that the patient may have tuberous sclerosis.

DISCUSSION

Subependymal giant cell astrocytomas (SEGA) represent low-grade, well-demarcated, predominantly intraventricular tumors. There is a well-known association

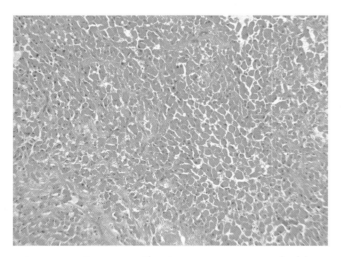

FIGURE 18.1 Low magnification, appearance marked by a sheetlike proliferation of large cells.

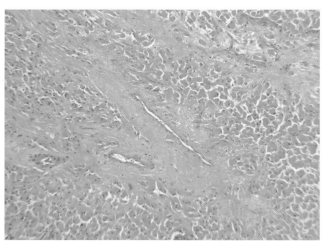

FIGURE 18.2 Foci of perivascular sclerosis are present.

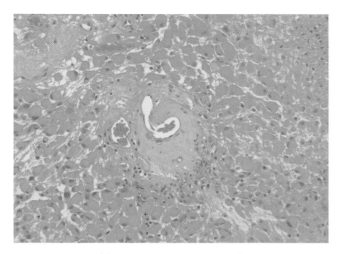

FIGURE 18.3 Mild perivascular chronic inflammation, associated with perivascular sclerosis.

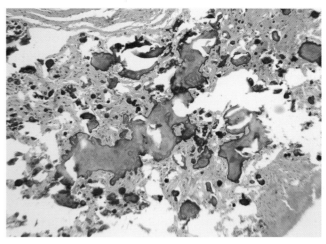

FIGURE 18.4 Focal microcalcifications are present in the tumor.

of this tumor with tuberous sclerosis, although the tumor may be encountered outside the setting of tuberous sclerosis. It is thought that SEGAs evolve from enlargement of hamartomatous subependymal nodules, which are commonly encountered in the lateral ventricular walls in patients with tuberous sclerosis. On imaging, they are contrast-enhancing and may show variable evidence of calcification.

Histologically, the SEGA, as its name suggests, is marked by a proliferation of large astrocytic cells, with abundant eosinophilic cytoplasm and eccentrically placed nuclei with prominent nucleoli. GFAP immunoreactivity confirms the astrocytic nature of these cells. This component is usually admixed with a spindle-cell component. Evidence of higher-grade tumor, such as necrosis, vascular proliferative changes, and mitotic activity, is unusual in these tumors. Cell proliferation markers indicate a very low rate of cell proliferation, as in the current case.

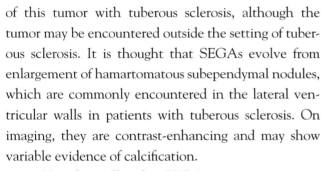

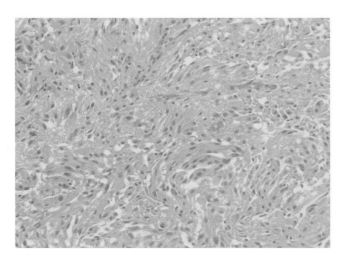

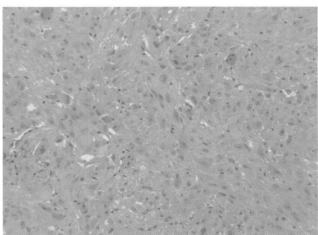

FIGURE 18.6 Higher magnification appearance of the large, rounded astrocytic cells, with abundant eosinophilic cytoplasm and large nuclei with prominent nucleoli.

FIGURE 18.5 The spindle-cell region of the tumor.

The importance of the diagnosis lies in recognizing the association with tuberous sclerosis. The tumor is considered benign and potentially curable with surgical excision. Many people have viewed the tumor more as a hamartoma than as a true malignancy. Differential diagnostic considerations include distinguishing this tumor from a gemistocytic astrocytoma, neuronal tumor, such as gangliocytoma or ganglioglioma, and glioblastoma. Gemistocytic astrocytomas are generally not intraventricular lesions and are more infiltrative by nature. Mitotic activity and increased rates of cell proliferation are more commonly encountered in the gemistocytic astrocytoma. The large cells, with prominently nucleolated nuclei, may ostensibly resemble neuronal cells and suggest ganglioglioma in the differential diagnosis. Immunohistochemistry, in such cases, can be useful in delineating the glial nature of the large cells. Glioblastoma multiforme involving the ventricle demonstrate evidence of necrosis and/or vascular proliferative changes, usually accompanied by readily identifiable mitotic activity. Although the intraventricular location of the SEGA may also raise ependymomas as a differential diagnostic possibility, the astrocytic cells in SEGA are generally much larger than the cells observed in an ependymoma; prominent nucleolation is also an unusual finding in ependymoma.

References

1. Gyure KA, Prayson RA. Subependymal giant cell astrocytoma: a clinicopathologic study with HMB45 and MIB-1 immunohistochemical analysis. Mod Pathol 1997;10:313–17.
2. Kim SK, Wang KC, Cho BK, et al. Biological behavior and tumorigenesis of subependymal giant cell astrocytomas. J Neurooncol 2001;52:217–25.
3. Lopes MB, Altermatt HJ, Scheithauer BW, et al. Immunohistochemical characterization of subependymal giant cell astrocytomas. Acta Neuropathol (Berl) 1996;91:368–75.
4. Shepherd CW, Scheithauer BW, Gomez MR, et al. Subependymal giant cell astrocytoma: a clinical, pathological, and flow cytometric study. Neurosurgery 1991;28:864–8.

Case 19: Low-Grade Oligodendroglioma

CLINICAL INFORMATION

The patient is a 32-year-old male who presents with focal left-sided arm weakness and a right frontal-parietal lobe mass. On MRI studies, a hypointense lesion on T1-weighted images, measuring approximately 3.2 cm, is observed. T2-weighted images show a well-demarcated lesion with little edema. Histologic sections from a subtotal resection are reviewed.

OPINION

Histologic sections show an infiltrative neoplasm, marked by mild hypercellularity, most pronounced in the white matter. The tumor cells are characterized by a generally round nuclear shape, a vesicular chromatin pattern, an absence of prominent nucleolation, and scant cytoplasm. Focally, pericellular clearing is observed in a subpopulation of these cells. An arcuate capillary vascular pattern is observed in the background of the tumor. Focal microcystic changes are also present. Tumor cells show a propensity to satellite around neurons and blood vessels as they infiltrate the cortex. Focal aggregation of tumor cells underneath the pial surface is also present. Focal dystrophic calcification is observed in the neoplasm. Only rare mitotic figures are noted. Vascular proliferative changes and necrosis are not seen. A Ki-67 labeling index of 3.2 is noted. Evidence of allelic loss on chromosomes 1p and 19q is observed using fluorescent in situ hybridization (FISH) analysis.

We consider the lesion to be an oligodendroglioma and characterize it as follows: **Right Frontal-Parietal Lobes, Subtotal Resection—Low-Grade Oligodendroglioma, WHO Grade II.**

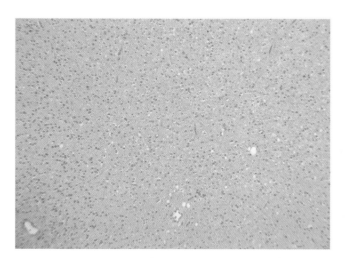

FIGURE 19.1 Low magnification appearance of the tumor, showing a mildly hypercellular white matter.

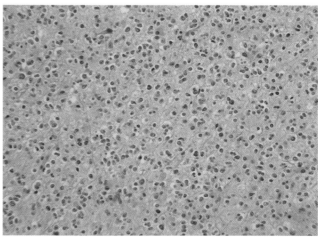

FIGURE 19.2 Pericellular clearing or "fried egg" appearance of tumor cells is present in this low-grade oligodendroglioma.

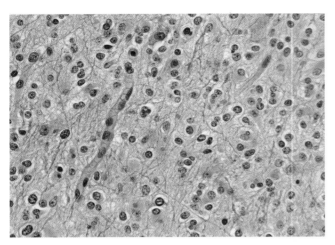

FIGURE 19.3 High magnification appearance of the tumor, showing a monomorphic population of cells with rounded nuclei and a background arcuate capillary vascular pattern.

COMMENT

The tumor demonstrates mild nuclear pleomorphism and rare mitotic figures. Vascular proliferative changes and necrosis are not observed. These findings, in conjunction with a relatively low Ki-67 labeling index, are consistent with a low-grade oligodendroglioma.

DISCUSSION

Low-grade oligodendrogliomas are much less common than their astrocytoma counterparts, comprising approximately 5–6% of all gliomas. The clinical presentation of these tumors overlaps with that of their fibrillary astrocytoma counterparts. Similar to astrocytomas, these tumors typically arise in the white matter of the cerebral hemispheres, with the frontal lobe being the most common location. Imaging studies often show a fairly well-circumscribed tumor with minimal edema. Evidence of calcifications and hemorrhage are common in these neoplasms. Despite their apparent circumscription on imaging studies, these tumors microscopically are infiltrative by nature, and it is not unusual for tumor cells to extend into the cortex and aggregate under the subpial surface. Morphologically, these tumors can be distinguished from astrocytomas because of their generally round nuclear contour and their overall monotony. They typically lack the hyperchromasia that is more commonly encountered in astrocytic tumors. The presence of calcifications, although quite common in oligodendrogliomas, can be observed in astrocytomas. Pericellular clearing, or

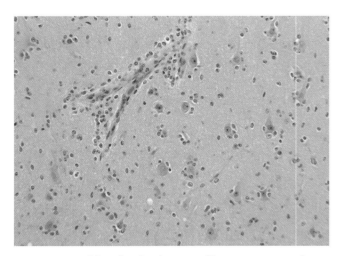

FIGURE 19.4 Oligodendroglioma infiltrating cortex, showing satellitosis of tumor cells around pre-existing neurons and blood vessels.

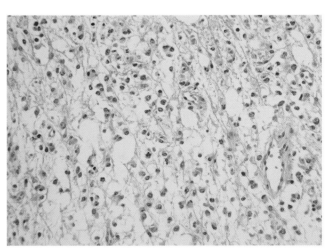

FIGURE 19.5 Focal microcystic degenerative change is present in this tumor.

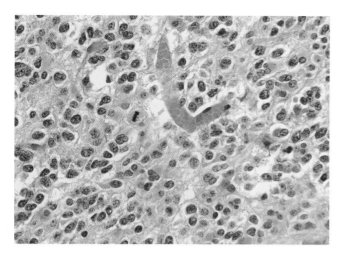

FIGURE 19.6 A rare mitotic figure is observed in this tumor. Rare mitotic figures are not sufficient to warrant upgrading the tumor.

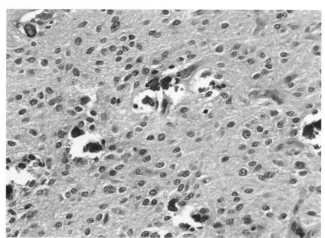

FIGURE 19.7 Focal dystrophic mineralization is seen.

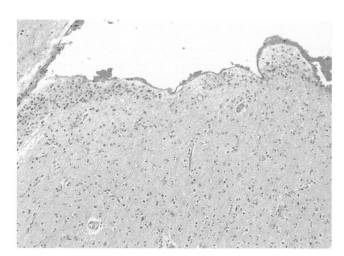

FIGURE 19.8 Subpial aggregation of tumor cells is noted.

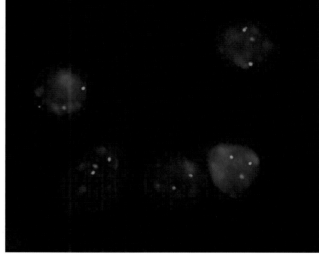

FIGURE 19.9 In situ hybridization study (FISH), showing evidence of loss on chromosome 1p in a low-grade oligodendroglioma.

the "fried egg" appearance, is also a somewhat characteristic feature of these tumors, but it represents an artifact of delayed formalin fixation. Therefore, the "fried egg" change is not evident at frozen section or in tissue that has been promptly fixed. The prominent arcuate capillary network is also a salient feature of these process-poor tumors.

Unfortunately, there is a lack of specific immunomarkers for oligodendroglial tumors. Prolifera-tion markers, such as Ki-67, demonstrate indices in the low-grade tumors that are comparable to those observed with the grade II astrocytomas. The majority of low-grade oligodendrogliomas demonstrate large deletions on chromosomes 1p and 19q. The presence of these findings has been correlated, particularly in the higher-grade oligodendrogliomas, with better prognosis and chemoresponsiveness. Other tumors that morphologically may consist of rounded cells with pericellular clearing, such as central neurocytoma and dysembryoplastic neuroepithelial tumors, generally lack the large chromosomal deletions that mark oligodendrogliomas.

The importance of distinguishing this tumor from an astrocytoma lies in the treatment approach and, ultimately, in the prognosis. The majority of oligodendrogliomas are chemoresponsive, and a trial of chemotherapy is warranted in the majority of cases. Grade for grade, oligodendrogliomas have a significantly better prognosis than astrocytomas.

References

1. Burger PC, Rawlings CE, Cox EB, et al. Clinicopathologic correlations in the oligodendroglioma. Cancer 1987;59:1345–52.
2. Coons SW, Johnson PC, Pearl DK. The prognostic significance of Ki-67 labeling indices for oligodendrogliomas. Neurosurgery 1997;41:878–84; discussion 884–5.
3. Mork SJ, Halvorsen TB, Lindegaard KF, et al. Oligodendroglioma. Histologic evaluation and prognosis. J Neuropathol Exp Neurol 1986; 45:65–78.
4. Reifenberger G, Kros JM, Louis DN, et al. Oligodendroglioma. In: Louis DN, Oghaki H, Wiestler OD, Cavenec WK, editors. WHO classification of tumours of the central nervous system. Lyon, FR: IARC Press, 2007.
5. Wiestler OD, Cavenee W, eds. WHO classification of tumours of the central nervous system. Lyon, FR: IARC Press; 2007. pp 54–9.

Case 20: Anaplastic Oligodendroglioma

The patient is a 49-year-old female who presents with seizures and a contrast-enhancing mass on CT imaging involving the left frontal lobe. She undergoes subtotal resection of the mass, and histologic sections are reviewed.

OPINION

Histologic sections show an infiltrative neoplasm, marked by focally prominent cellularity. On frozen section, although cells appear somewhat pleomorphic, there is a monotony to the pleomorphism. Occasional mitotic figures are noted, and, on permanent sections, mitotic activity as high as 7 mitotic figures (MF) per 10 high-power fields (HPF) is noted. Focal vascular proliferative changes are present.

Necrosis is not identified. The background of the tumor is marked by a prominence of small capillary blood vessels. A lower-grade-appearing area of the tumor is evident at the periphery, which shows an infiltrating neoplasm, marked by cells with generally rounded nuclear contours, scant cytoplasm, and pericellular clearing. Focally, cells with increased eosinophilic cytoplasm and eccentrically placed nuclei, resembling minigemistocytes, are present. A Ki-67 labeling index in excess of 25 is focally noted.

We consider the lesion to be an oligodendroglioma and characterize it as follows: **Left Frontal Lobe, Subtotal Resection—Anaplastic Oligodendroglioma, WHO Grade III.**

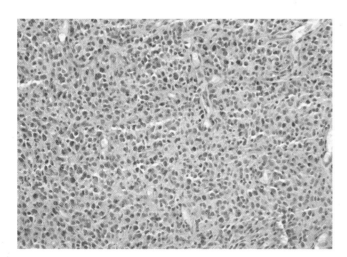

FIGURE 20.1 Intermediate magnification appearance of frozen section, showing an increased cellularity lesion, marked by monotonous atypia and an occasional mitotic figure.

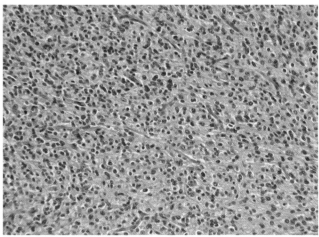

FIGURE 20.2 A cellular focus of the tumor is illustrated with mild nuclear atypia and arcuate capillary vascular pattern.

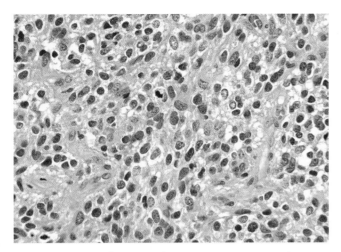

FIGURE 20.3 High magnification appearance, showing moderate nuclear pleomorphism and readily identifiable mitotic activity.

COMMENT

The degree of cellularity, presence of prominent mitotic activity, and vascular proliferative changes warrant a diagnosis of anaplastic oligodendroglioma. The Ki-67 labeling index is consistent with this diagnosis.

DISCUSSION

The monotony of cells on frozen section is suggestive of the diagnosis. In the vast majority of cases,

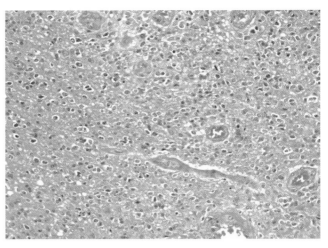

FIGURE 20.4 A focal area around the edge of the tumor shows an appearance resembling a low-grade oligodendroglioma, with pericellular clearing, or "fried-egg" change, which is an artifact of delayed formalin fixation.

differentiating a high-grade astrocytoma from a high-grade oligodendroglioma, in the context of intraoperative consultation, is not critical. Because of the differences in prognosis and treatment approach, however, accurate classification of the tumor for purposes of final diagnosis is significant.

Morphologically, distinction of high-grade oligodendroglioma from low-grade oligodendroglioma is

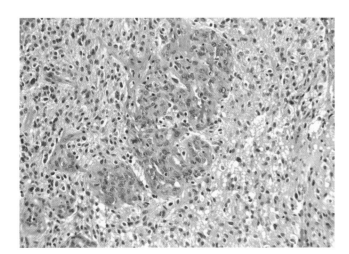

FIGURE 20.5 Vascular proliferative changes are focally present.

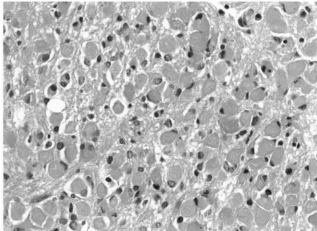

FIGURE 20.6 Minigemistocytic cells are marked by increased cytoplasm and eccentrically placed nuclei.

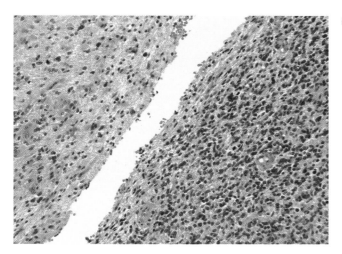

FIGURE 20.7 The interface is present between a lower-grade-appearing area of the tumor on the left and a more cellular, higher-grade-appearing area of the tumor on the right.

somewhat subjective. In general, the parameters that are used to grade astrocytomas (cellularity and atypia, increased mitotic activity, vascular proliferative changes, and necrosis) are also evaluated in grading oligodendroglial neoplasms. Oligodendrogliomas have only two grade designations, compared with the three-tiered grading system for fibrillary astrocytomas. In general, anaplastic oligodendroglioma are more cellular and pleomorphic than low-grade tumors, with increased mitotic activity (generally in excess of 5–6 MF per 10 HPF) and may variably demonstrate other worrisome morphologic features, including vascular proliferation and/or necrosis. The presence of minigemistocytes may cause confusion with an astrocytoma; these cells are acceptable within the context of oligodendroglioma and do not afford any particular prognosis when present. Occasional tumors may have small hypercellular nodules or foci within an otherwise low-grade-appearing tumor. The significance of these small foci is uncertain. Similar to astrocytomas, the Ki-67 labeling indices roughly correlate with tumor grade, with higher-grade tumors generally having higher labeling indices.

The major differential diagnostic consideration is high-grade astrocytoma. On purely morphologic grounds, this may, at times, be difficult. As in the current case, a lower-grade-appearing area of the tumor at the perimeter presents a clue as to the proper diagnosis. Immunohistochemistry is generally of little avail in distinguishing these two tumor types. Molecular genetic alterations can be helpful in this instance. Large deletions on chromosomes 1p and 19q have been well established to be associated with the oligodendroglioma phenotype. Smaller deletions on one or both chromosomes may be occasionally encountered in glioblastoma. However, it is important to remember that these chromosomal alterations may not always be present. Genetic alterations more commonly encountered in glioblastomas, including losses on chromosome 10q, p53 mutations, and EGFR amplification or overexpression, are not commonly observed in anaplastic oligodendrogliomas.

Despite the high-grade designation, many of these tumors are remarkably responsive to chemotherapy and radiotherapy. Assessment of chromosome 1p/19q status in these tumors can be helpful in predicting which tumors are more likely to respond to treatment and, ultimately, allow for a longer survival.

References

1. Cairncross JG, Ueki K, Zlatescu MC, et al. Specific genetic predictors of chemotherapeutic response and survival in patients with anaplastic oligodendrogliomas. J Natl Cancer Inst 1998;90:1473–9.
2. Coons SW, Johnson PC, Pearl DK. The prognostic significance of Ki-67 labeling indices for oligodendrogliomas. Neurosurgery 1997;41:878-84; discussion 884–5.
3. Giannini C, Scheithauer BW, Weaver AL, et al. Oligodendrogliomas: reproducibility and prognostic value of histologic diagnosis and grading. J Neuropathol Exp Neurol 2001;60:248–62.
4. Ino Y, Betensky RA, Zlatescu MC, et al. Molecular subtypes of anaplastic oligodendroglioma: implications for patient management at diagnosis. Clin Cancer Res 2001;7:839–45.
5. Miller CR, Dunham CP, Scheithauer BW, et al. Significance of necrosis in grading of anaplastic oligodendroglial tumors: a clinicopathological and genetic study of 916 high-grade gliomas. J Clin Oncol 2006;24:5419–26.

Case 21: Low-Grade Oligoastrocytoma (Low-Grade Mixed Glioma)

CLINICAL INFORMATION

The patient is a 38-year-old male who presents with seizures and a right frontal-temporal lobe mass on imaging. A subtotal resection of the lesion is performed, and histologic sections are reviewed.

OPINION

Approximately 60% of the lesion is marked by a mild hypercellularity and a proliferation of cells with rounded nuclear contour and pericellular clearing, resembling a low-grade oligodendroglioma. Mitotic figures, vascular proliferative changes, necrosis, and calcifications are not observed. Approximately 20–25% of the tumor shows areas resembling low-grade fibrillary astrocytoma, marked by a proliferation of more elongated nuclei and high nuclear-to-cytoplasmic ratio. Again, mitotic figures, vascular proliferative changes, and necrosis are not identified in these later areas. The remainder of the tumor consists of a mixture of the two aforementioned cell types. A Ki-67 labeling index of 2.8 is noted.

We consider the lesion to be a low-grade glioma and characterize it is as follows: **Right Frontal-Temporal Lobes, Subtotal Resection—Low-Grade Oligoastrocytoma (Low-Grade Mixed Glioma), WHO Grade II.**

COMMENT

The tumor consists of geographically distinct areas resembling low-grade oligodendroglioma and low-grade astrocytoma. Mitotic activity, vascular proliferative changes, and necrosis are not observed. The low Ki-67 labeling index is consistent with a low-grade neoplasm.

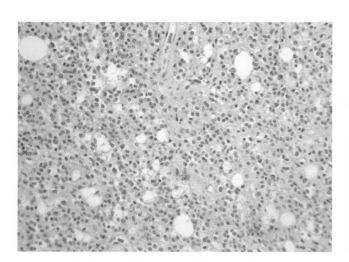

FIGURE 21.1 Intermediate magnification, showing an area of the tumor resembling a low-grade oligodendroglioma.

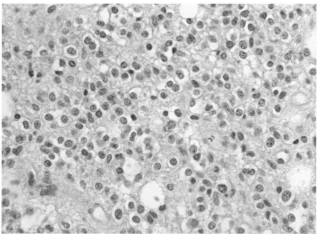

FIGURE 21.2 High magnification area of tumor resembling oligodendroglioma with generally rounded nuclei.

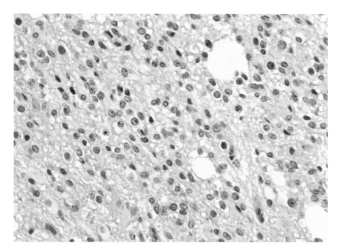

FIGURE 21.3 Small areas of the tumor show an admixture of oligodendroglioma and astrocytoma type cells.

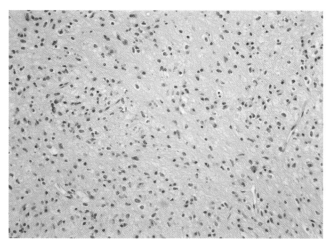

FIGURE 21.4 Intermediate magnification of an area of the tumor resembling a low-grade fibrillary astrocytoma.

DISCUSSION

The clinical and imaging features of so-called oligoastrocytoma, or mixed glioma, overlap with those of pure oligodendroglioma and pure fibrillary astrocytoma. The pathologic criteria for the diagnosis of oligoastrocytoma remain somewhat nebulous. Most pathologists require geographically distinct areas of astrocytoma and oligodendroglioma in order to render the diagnosis. The percentages of the minor component of tumor are not clearly delineated; percentages of the minor component in the literature range from 20–35%. Particularly challenging are tumors in which there appears to be an admixture of cell types in the same area. It is well recognized that, within tumors that are generally considered pure oligodendrogliomas or pure fibrillary astrocytomas, there may be a small population of cells that phenotypically resemble the other tumor type intermixed in the neoplasm. There is some literature to suggest that evaluation of mixed gliomas for deletions on chromosomes 1p and 19q can provide some guidance in terms of eventual prognosis and treatment; those tumors that demonstrate large deletions tend to behave more like oligodendrogliomas.

The histologic parameters used to grade oligodendrogliomas and astrocytomas, including cellularity, mitotic activity, vascular proliferative changes, and necrosis, are also used to assign grade in mixed gliomas. Cell proliferation indices generally show lower labeling indices in low-grade tumors, compared with higher-grade neoplasms. Because of the issues of problems with the definition of entity and the lack of uniform approach in terms of diagnosis

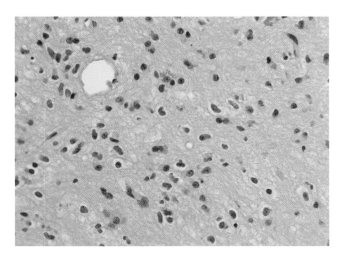

FIGURE 21.5 High magnification of an astrocytoma-like area of the tumor is marked by cells with more elongated nuclei.

of these tumors, it is difficult to ascertain from the literature what the true natural behavior of these tumors is. Their prognosis has generally been thought to be intermediate between pure astrocytomas and oligodendrogliomas.

References

1. Beckmann MJ, Prayson RA. A clinicopathologic study of 30 cases of oligoastrocytoma including p53 immunohistochemistry. Pathology 1997;29:159–64.

2. Fuller CE, Schmidt RE, Roth KA, et al. Clinical utility of fluorescence in situ hybridization (FISH) in morphologically ambiguous gliomas with hybrid oligodendroglial/astrocytic features. J Neuropathol Exp Neurol 2003;62:1118–28.

3. Hart MN, Petito CK, Earle KM. Mixed gliomas. Cancer 1974;33:134–40.

4. Jaskolsky D, Zawieski M, Papierz W, et al. Mixed gliomas. Their clinical course and results of surgery. Zentralbl Neurochir 1987;48:120–3.

5. Kraus JA, Koopmann J, Kaskel P, et al. Shared allelic losses on chromosomes 1p and 19q suggest a common origin of oligodendroglioma and oligoastrocytoma. J Neuropathol Exp Neurol 1995;54:91–5.

Case 22: Anaplastic Oligoastrocytoma (Anaplastic Mixed Glioma)

CLINICAL INFORMATION

A 52-year-old female presents with right-sided weakness. On imaging studies, a focally enhancing tumor in the left frontal-parietal lobes is noted on MRI studies. Subtotal resection of the lesion is performed, and histologic sections are reviewed.

OPINION

Histologic sections show a glioma, marked by geographically distinct areas resembling oligodendroglioma and astrocytoma. The astrocytoma areas are marked by mild nuclear pleomorphism, focal vascular proliferative changes, and identifiable mitotic activity. There is no evidence of necrosis. Areas around the periphery of the lesion show low-grade tumor resembling both oligodendroglioma and astrocytoma.

We consider the lesion to be a high-grade glioma and characterize it as follows: **Left Frontal-Parietal Region, Subtotal Resection—Anaplastic Oligoastrocytoma (Anaplastic Mixed Glioma), WHO Grade III.**

COMMENT

The tumor is marked by geographically distinct areas resembling astrocytoma and oligodendroglioma. Moderate nuclear atypia, readily identifiable mitotic activity, and vascular proliferative changes are consistent with the diagnosis of anaplastic oligoastrocytoma. There is no evidence of necrosis.

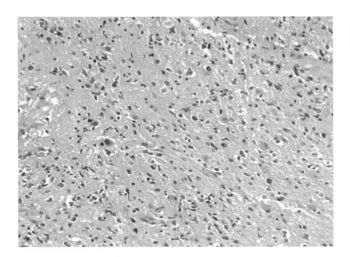

FIGURE 22.1 Focal areas of the tumor, particularly at the periphery, resemble a low-grade astrocytoma.

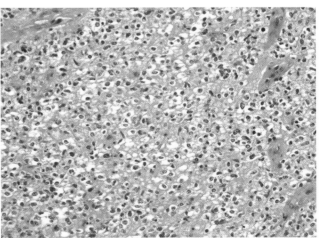

FIGURE 22.2 Other areas of the neoplasm look like low-grade oligodendroglioma.

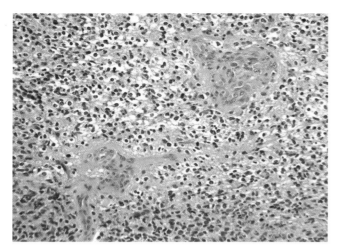

FIGURE 22.3 Focal vascular proliferative changes are present in the tumor.

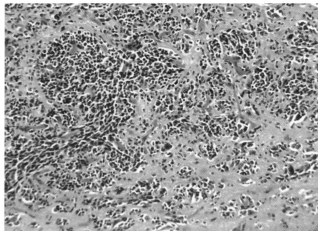

FIGURE 22.4 A cellular focus of tumor is situated in the cortex.

DISCUSSION

The diagnosis of anaplastic oligoastrocytoma is particularly challenging. In addition to the definitional issues for mixed glioma discussed in Case 21, the degree of atypia and pleomorphism in these tumors make distinction from high-grade oligodendroglioma and glioblastoma multiforme, at times, challenging. The key to the diagnosis lies in the recognition of distinct areas of oligodendroglioma and astrocytoma.

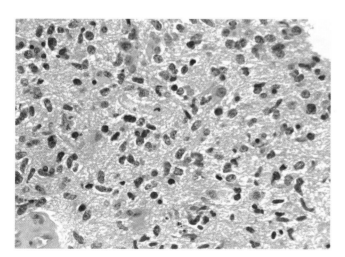

FIGURE 22.5 Mitotic figures are readily identifiable in the tumor.

Particularly helpful in this case is the presence of lower-grade, more readily recognizable phenotypes of both glioma types in the tumor. Similar to low-grade oligoastrocytomas, the status of chromosomes 1p and 19q serves as an important prognosticating factor.

Historically, a subset of these tumors demonstrated areas of necrosis. In the most recent update in the WHO classification of brain tumors, anaplastic oligoastrocytomas with necrosis are classified as glioblastoma with oligodendroglioma component, despite the fact that this particular lesion carries a better prognosis than ordinary glioblastoma.

References

1. Eoli M, Bissola L, Bruzzone MG, et al. Reclassification of oligoastrocytomas by loss of heterozygosity studies. Int J Cancer 2006;119:84–90.
2. Mueller W, Hartmann C, Hoffmann A, et al. Genetic signature of oligoastrocytomas correlates with tumor location and denotes distinct molecular subsets. Am J Pathol 2002;161:313–19.
3. Shaw EG, Scheithauer BW, O'Fallon JR, et al. Mixed oligoastrocytomas: a survival and prognostic factor analysis. Neurosurgery 1994;34:577–82.

Case 23: Glioblastoma with Oligodendroglioma Component

CLINICAL INFORMATION

The patient is a 64-year-old male who presents with headaches and seizures. On imaging, a ring-enhancing mass is located in the right temporal lobe. Biopsies of the mass are taken, and histologic sections are reviewed.

OPINION

Biopsies show a high-grade neoplasm, marked by prominent cellularity, moderate nuclear atypia, and focally prominent arcuate vascular pattern. Mitotic activity is readily observable in the tumor. Focal vascular proliferative changes are noted. Areas of the tumor resemble an oligodendroglioma with cells marked by rounded nuclear contours and pericellular clearing. Other areas of the tumor clearly resemble an astrocytoma with more elongated-appearing nuclei. Foci of necrosis, at times, rimmed by a pseudopalisade of cells and intravascular thrombi, are also present.

We consider the lesion to be a high-grade glioma and characterize it as follows: **Right Temporal Lobe, Biopsies—Glioblastoma with Oligodendroglioma Component, WHO Grade IV.**

COMMENT

The tumor is marked by geographic areas resembling high-grade oligodendroglioma and high-grade astrocytoma. In addition, focal palisaded necrosis is observed. The tumor's morphologic appearance is most consistent with a glioblastoma with oligodendroglioma component.

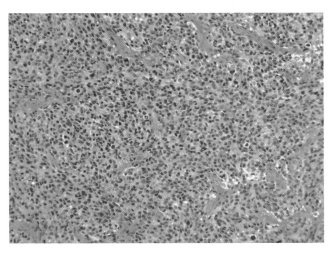

FIGURE 23.1 The tumor is markedly cellular, with moderate nuclear atypia and a focally prominent arcuate capillary vascular pattern.

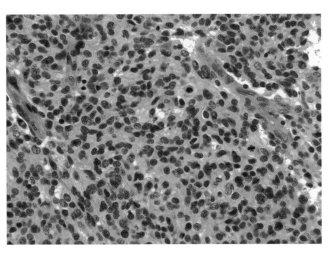

FIGURE 23.2 Mitotic figures are readily identifiable in the neoplasm.

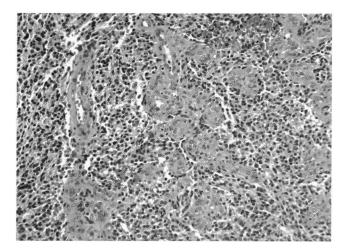

FIGURE 23.3 Vascular proliferative changes are also present in the tumor.

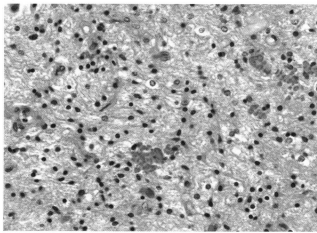

FIGURE 23.4 Areas resembling oligodendroglioma are noted in the tumor.

DISCUSSION

Glioblastoma with oligodendroglioma component is a new designation in the WHO. Historically, these tumors were classified as anaplastic oligoastrocytomas (anaplastic mixed gliomas). Recent studies have demonstrated that anaplastic mixed gliomas that demonstrate necrosis tended to behave more aggressively than anaplastic mixed gliomas without necrosis. Although this variant of glioblastoma is not felt to be quite as aggressive as the ordinary glioblastoma, the behavior of this lesion is thought to be more akin to glioblastoma than to anaplastic mixed glioma.

The challenges from a pathology standpoint are similar to those previously discussed in the prior case (Anaplastic Oligoastrocytoma).

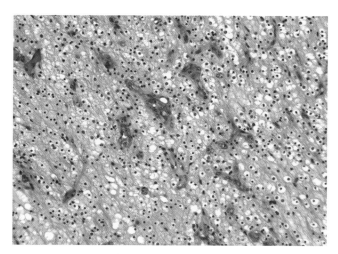

FIGURE 23.5 Vascular proliferative changes are observable in the oligodendroglioma-like areas of the tumor.

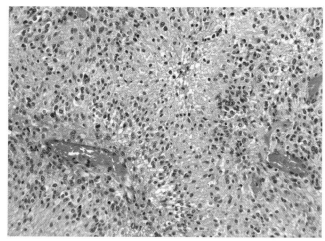

FIGURE 23.6 Palisaded necrosis is present in the neoplasm, consistent with a high-grade glioma.

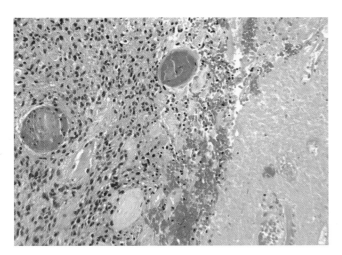

FIGURE 23.7 More elongated nuclear features, suggestive of an astrocytoma phenotype, are seen, associated with focal geographic necrosis and intravascular thrombi adjacent to the necrosis.

References

1. He J, Mokhtari K, Sanson M, et al. Glioblastomas with an oligodendroglial component: a pathological and molecular study. J Neuropathol Exp Neurol 2001;60:863–71.
2. Homme T, Fukushina T, Vaccarella S, et al. Correlation among pathology, genotype and patient outcomes in glioblastoma. J Neuropathol Exp Neurol 2006;65:846–54.
3. Kraus JA, Lamszus K, Glesmann N, et al. Molecular genetic alterations in glioblastomas with oligodendroglial component. Acta Neuropathol 2001;101:311–20.

CLINICAL INFORMATION

The patient is a 48-year-old male who presents with headaches. Work-up includes a MRI scan, which reveals a sharply demarcated, non-contrast-enhancing mass in the left lateral ventricle, measuring 2.5 cm in greatest dimension. A decision is made to excise the lesion, and histological sections are reviewed.

OPINION

Biopsies show a hypocellular neoplasm, with a nodular or lobular overall architectural pattern and multifocal calcifications. Extensive microcystic change is present, but no necrosis is seen. The tumor is composed of clusters of small, cytologically bland, and monotonous cells, embedded in a densely eosinophilic fibrillar background. Cellular areas alternate with anuclear eosinophilic zones. Vessels are focally hyalinized, but perivascular pseudorosettes are poorly developed, and mitotic activity is absent.

We consider the tumor to be a low-grade neoplasm and characterize it as follows: **Left Lateral Ventricle, Excision—Subependymoma, WHO Grade I.**

COMMENT

Microcystic change is often most prominent in lateral ventricle examples of subependymoma.

DISCUSSION

Subependymomas occur most frequently in the fourth ventricle, followed by the lateral ventricle. Less common supratentorial sites include the third

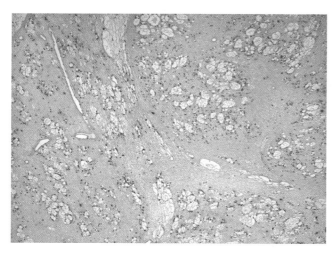

FIGURE 24.1 Low-power magnification illustrates the nodular or lobular architectural pattern of this tumor, which was attached to the wall of the lateral ventricle, but sharply demarcated from the adjacent subependymal brain tissue.

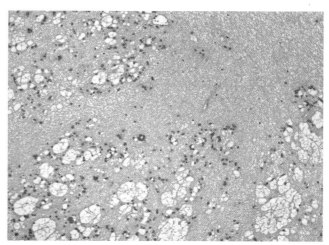

FIGURE 24.2 Clusters of bland monotonous cells alternate with anuclear zones composed of eosinophilic matrix.

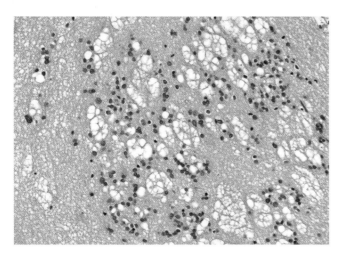

FIGURE 24.3 Microcysts contain basophilic mucin and are particularly conspicuous in this lateral ventricle example of subependymoma.

ventricle and septum pellucidum. In the spinal cord, subependymomas are most frequent in the cervical and cervico-thoracic levels.

Subependymomas are usually sharply demarcated, lobular masses, with varying amounts of calcification, vascular hyalinization, and sometimes even vascular proliferation and thrombosis. They may show recent or remote hemorrhage. Necrosis

and mitoses are usually absent. The striking pattern on low-power magnification is that of clusters of monotonous cells, alternating with anuclear areas composed of dense eosinophilic fibrillar matrix. Microcysts are usually most conspicuous in lateral ventricular examples and may be absent at other sites. True perivascular pseudorosettes can be discerned in some examples, but, in others, the observer must utilize their imagination.

Cytologically, the tumor cells are monotonous, with bland, round nuclei containing small nucleoli. In some examples, tumor cells show considerable nuclear pleomorphism, but this does not influence prognosis. Cytoplasm is coarsely fibrillar and strongly immunoreactive for GFAP. The microcysts contain faintly basophilic mucin. Mitoses are infrequent, and MIB-1 labeling indices are less than 1–2.

It is important to distinguish subependymomas from ependymomas because of their considerably better outcome. Surgical removal is curative. Neoplasms with mixed ependymoma and subependymoma features also occur, but they should be graded according to the ependymoma component, which is usually WHO grade II.

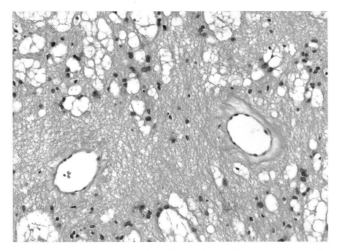

FIGURE 24.4 Vessels are focally hyalinized, and tumor cells occasionally orient around the vessels, but perpendicularly oriented cell processes and fully developed perivascular pseudorosettes may be infrequent to absent.

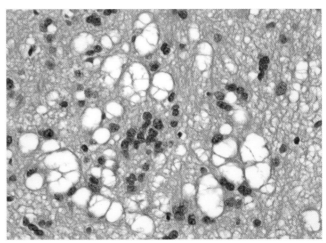

FIGURE 24.5 High power magnification shows the round nuclei, with small nucleoli and minimal hyperchromatism. Note the absence of mitotic activity.

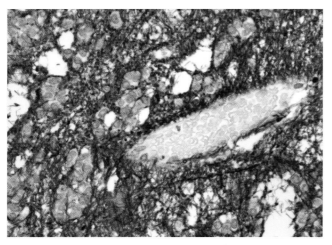

FIGURE 24.6 Strong immunoreactivity for GFAP is consistently identified, although the GFAP may fail to disclose perpendicularly oriented fibrillary cell processes around blood vessels.

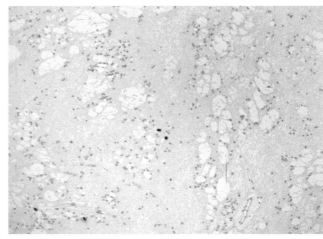

FIGURE 24.7 The MIB-1 rate is low, usually less than 1.

References

1. McLendon RE, Schiffer D, Rosenblum MK, et al. Subependymoma. In: Louis DN, Ohgaki H, Wiestler OD, Cavenee WK, editors. WHO Classification of Tumours of the Central Nervous System. Lyon, FR: IARC Press; 2007. p. 70–71.

2. Perry, A. Glial and glioneuronal tumors. In: Prayson RA, editor. Neuropathology. Philadelphia, PA: Elsevier Churchill Livingstone; 2005. p. 476–7.

3. Prayson RA, Suh JH. Subependymomas: clinicopathologic study of 14 tumors, including comparative MIB-1 immunohistochemical analysis with other ependymal neoplasms. Arch Pathol Lab Med 1999;123:306–9.

Case 25: Myxopapillary Ependymoma

CLINICAL INFORMATION

The patient is a 16-year-old female who presents with leg pain. Work-up includes an MRI scan, which reveals a sharply demarcated, intradural mass, 3.4 × 1.6 cm, lying just below the level of the conus medullaris and attached to the filum terminale. The decision is made to resect the lesion, and histological sections are reviewed.

OPINION

Biopsies show a papillary neoplasm, composed of elongate cells that are radially arrayed around fibrovascular cores. There is abundant interspersed myxoid matrix, both between individual tumor cells and around blood vessels, as well as pooled in microcysts. Mitotic activity is very low, and necrosis is absent.

We consider the tumor to be a low-grade gliol neoplasm and characterize it as follows: **Filum Terminale, Excision—Myxopapillary Ependymoma, WHO Grade I.**

COMMENT

Myxopapillary ependymoma is almost confined to the conus medullaris-cauda equina-filum terminale region.

DISCUSSION

Myxopapillary ependymomas display several different patterns, depending on how intact the perivascular pseudorosettes are in the tumor. In this example, perpendicularly oriented delicate glial processes are still easily identified around blood vessels. However, in

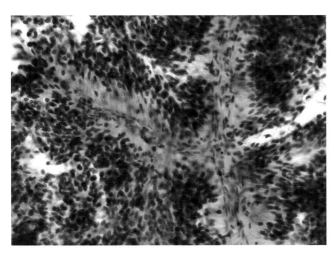

FIGURE 25.1 Intraoperative touch preparation shows the monotonous tumor cells and a well-developed perivascular pseudorosette.

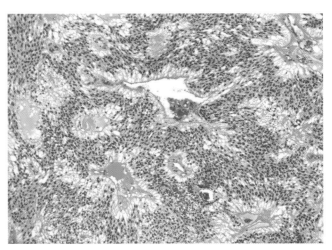

FIGURE 25.2 Low power magnification illustrates the radial arrangement of perivascular cells, as well as mucin lying between perpendicular cellular processes, seen here as relatively clear, vacuolated spaces.

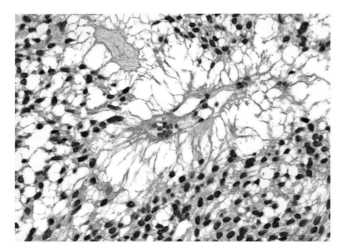

FIGURE 25.3 Higher-power view shows the absence of mitotic activity, as well as the elongate, tapering, eosinophilic fibrillary glial processes.

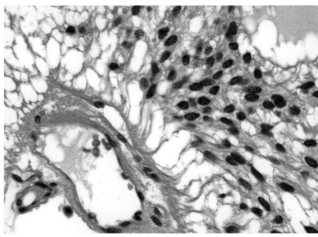

FIGURE 25.4 Note the bland oval nuclei, with delicately stippled chromatin pattern.

other examples of myxopapillary ependymoma, the glial cell processes are obliterated by the massive accumulation of mucin, leaving few visible blood vessels in the center of an epithelial-like circle of cells. Tumors with more mucin and fewer visible perivascular cell processes are easily misinterpreted by the unwary as metastatic adenocarcinoma. Extremely large amounts of mucin in tumors may also raise consideration of chordoma or myxoid chrondrosarcoma. Neither metastatic papillary adenocarcinoma nor most chordomas have strong diffuse immunoreactivity for GFAP. However, myxopapillary ependymomas, chordomas, and myxoid chondrosarcomas share immunoreactivity for S-100 protein, and both chordoma and metastatic papillary adenocarcinoma usually express cytokeratins. Myxopapillary ependymomas, like almost all ependymomas, show immunostaining for GFAP, S-100, and vimentin, but not for cytokeratin.

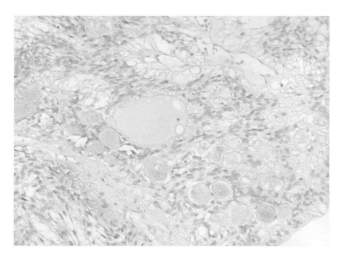

FIGURE 25.5 Alcian-blue at pH 2.5 highlights the mucin between cell processes, as well as in microcyst pools.

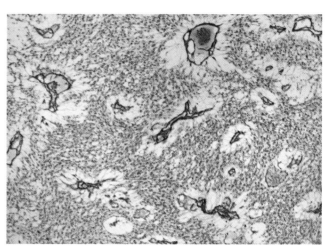

FIGURE 25.6 Reticulin is seen only around blood vessels and not between individual tumor cells, as would be seen with schwannoma.

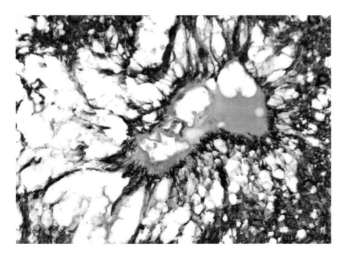

FIGURE 25.7 Strong immunoreactivity for GFAP highlights the perpendicularly oriented fibrillary cell processes around blood vessels.

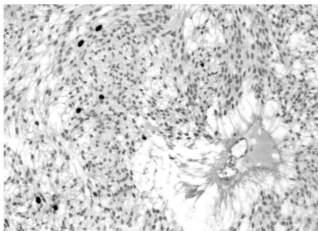

FIGURE 25.8 The MIB-1 rate is low, usually less than 1.

The mucin is typically positive on staining with Alcian-blue. Mitoses are rare, and MIB-1 labeling is very low. Myxopapillary ependymomas are WHO grade I, with high-grade variants virtually unknown. Prognosis is most favorable with complete surgical resection, which is usually achievable, with well-demarcated examples confined to the intradural space.

References

1. McLendon RE, Rosenblum MK, Schiffer D, et al. Myxopapillary ependymoma. In: Louis DN, Ohgaki H, Wiestler OD, Cavenee WK, editors. WHO Classification of Tumours of the Central Nervous System. Lyon, FR: IARC Press; 2007. p. 72–3.
2. Perry A. Glial and glioneuronal tumors. In: Prayson RA, editor. Neuropathology. Philadelphia, PA: Elsevier Churchill Livingstone; 2005. p. 476–7.

Case 26: Ependymoma

CLINICAL INFORMATION

The patient is a 63-year-old male who presents with headache, nausea, and dizziness. Work-up includes an MRI scan, which reveals a large, well-circumscribed mass with heterogeneous contrast enhancement, filling the fourth ventricle. The decision is made to resect the lesion, and histological sections are reviewed.

OPINION

Biopsies show a moderately cellular neoplasm, with multifocal calcifications, but no necrosis. At low-power magnification, perivascular pseudorosettes (defined as an eosinophilic, cell-process-rich collar of perpendicularly oriented glial cells surrounding a central blood vessel) are easily identified. Vessels are hyalinized, and mitotic activity is present only at low levels.

We consider the tumor to be an ependymoma and characterize it as follows: **Fourth Ventricle, Excision—Ependymoma, WHO Grade II.**

COMMENT

Ependymomas occur anywhere along the ventricular system, as well as occasionally in extraventricular sites. The fourth ventricle and cervico-thoracic spinal cord are the most common locations for ependymomas, and these two sites are equally affected in adults. Most pediatric patients develop infratentorial tumors.

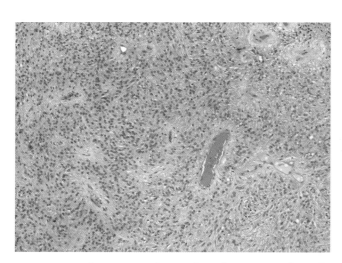

FIGURE 26.1 Low-power inspection shows a moderately cellular tumor, with a "pattern" consisting of prominent eosinophilic collars surrounding blood vessels.

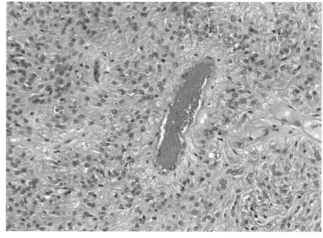

FIGURE 26.2 Higher power confirms that these eosinophilic collars are composed of perpendicularly oriented, coarsely fibrillar cell processes of the tumor cells, not hyalinized blood vessels. Note the nuclear monotony and absence of mitotic activity.

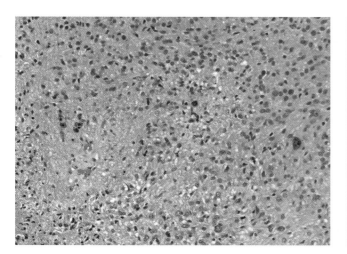

FIGURE 26.3 Focal hemosiderin pigment, caused by intra-tumoral hemorrhage and occasional enlarged nuclei, can be seen in some cases but does not affect prognosis or grading.

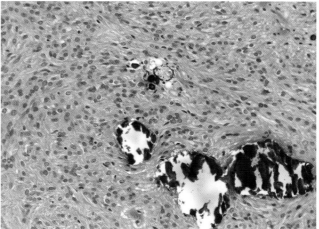

FIGURE 26.4 Calcifications are variable and considered "regressive" features.

DISCUSSION

Ependymomas are usually well-demarcated tumors that, in some instances, are quite bulky. Posterior fossa examples can fill the fourth ventricle, exuding out of the foramina of Luschka or Magendie. Obstruction of cerebrospinal fluid pathways causes hydrocephalus, with resultant headache, nausea, vomiting, and dizziness. Examples in the spinal cord present with motor and sensory deficits and may involve multiple intramedullary spinal cord segments. Some spinal cord ependymomas

are further associated with a cystic syrinx that increases the length of cord involvement. Uncommon supratentorial ependymomas may manifest with seizures.

The diagnosis of ependymoma rests on recognizing a specific pattern at low-power magnification—a feature that usually differentiates an ependymoma from a diffuse astrocytoma that tends to be patternless. The most common pattern in ependymomas is the formation within the tumor of perivascular pseudorosettes, distinguishable on low power as eosinophilic collars

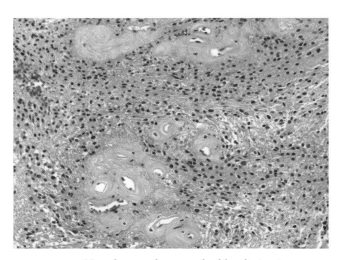

FIGURE 26.5 Vessels may show marked hyalinization.

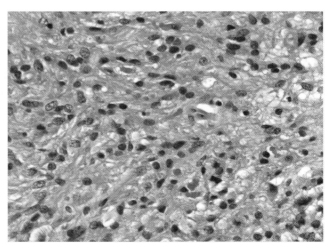

FIGURE 26.6 High-power magnification illustrates the stippled or speckled chromatin pattern of the round-to-oval tumor cell nuclei, as well as the delicate nucleoli.

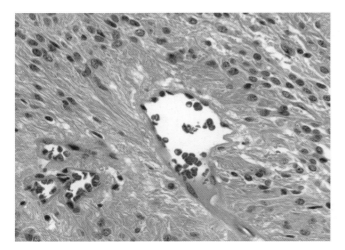

FIGURE 26.7 The coarse nature of the fibrillar tumor cell processes in perivascular pseudorosettes is typical of ependymomas and contrasts with the delicate, indistinct nature of cell processes in neurocytomas.

surrounding blood vessels. Usually, these are present in multiple areas of a true ependymoma. Closer inspection at high power reveals these eosinophilic collars to be composed of perpendicularly oriented coarse glial processes. Perivascular pseudorosettes should not be confused with the eosinophilic, extensively hyalinized vasculature seen in other types of gliomas.

Less commonly, the ependymoma contains true ependymal canals with a central lumen; these

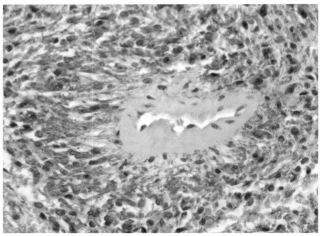

FIGURE 26.8 GFAP immunostaining is usually positive in perivascular pseudorosettes and can highlight the perpendicular arrangement of the glial processes.

are seldom isolated features and usually occur in conjunction with pseudorosettes elsewhere in the tumor. Usually, true rosettes are also best appreciated at low-power magnification but, rarely, the lumen of the central canal can be quite small and recognizable only on higher-power magnification.

The last pattern to recognize at both low- and high-power magnification that should prompt consideration of ependymoma is that of monotony in nuclear size, shape, and chromatin pattern.

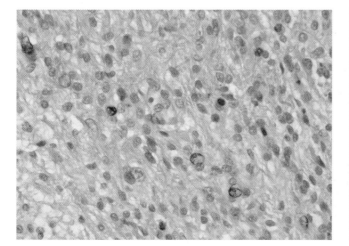

FIGURE 26.9 Ring-like and dot-like immunoreactivity for EMA can be very helpful features.

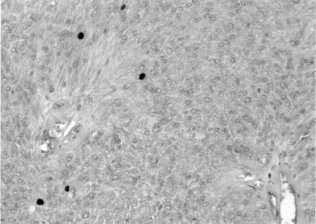

FIGURE 26.10 Mitoses are few in number in grade II ependymomas, and the MIB-1 index is typically less than 4.

Ependymomas are composed of cells with round-to-oval nuclei, "salt and pepper" speckled chromatin, and small nucleoli. Appreciation of these features can be particularly critical in small tissue samples (such as from spinal cord) or in ependymomas with relatively few or poorly developed pseudorosettes.

In some instances, immunohistochemistry or electron microscopy is necessary to resolve the diagnosis of ependymoma. Almost all ependymomas are positive for GFAP, but the strongest reaction is in the "glial" portions of the tumor, i.e., especially in the perivascular pseudorosettes. True ependymal canals often are GFAP-negative. Ependymomas are also immunoreactive for S-100 protein and vimentin, but neither of these helps distinguish them from various types of gliomas. Dot-like and ring-like immunoreactivity for epithelial membrane antigen (EMA) is slightly more specific but has been seen in other types of gliomas. Ultimately, in difficult cases, electron microscopy may be necessary to establish ependymal features.

Once the categorization of the tumor as ependymoma is established, grading becomes the next issue. Ependymomas do not generally show as tight a correlation between histological features and prognosis as do diffuse astrocytomas. In one study, "the conclusions are as follows: (1) histologic appearance and MIB-1 indices were not reliably predictive of tumor behavior, probably due in part to tumor heterogeneity; (2) tumors with two or more of the following features: identifiable mitotic figures, hypercellularity, vascular proliferation, and necrosis were more likely to behave in an aggressive manner; and (3) elevated MIB-1 labeling indices (≥ 4.0 in this study) were encountered in a higher percentage of fatal and recurrent tumors than in nonfatal or nonrecurrent tumors."

References

1. McLendon RE, Wiestler OD, Kros JM, et al. Ependymoma. In: Louis DN, Ohgaki H, Wiestler OD, Cavenee WK, editors. WHO Classification of Tumours of the Central Nervous System. Lyon, FR: IARC Press; 2007. p. 74–8.
2. Perry A. Glial and glioneuronal tumors. In: Prayson RA, editor. Neuropathology. Philadelphia, PA: Elsevier Churchill Livingstone; 2005. 468–76.
3. Prayson RA. Clinicopathologic study of 61 patients with ependymoma including MIB-1 immunohistochemistry. Annals Diagn Pathol 1999;3:11–18.

Case 27: Anaplastic Ependymoma

CLINICAL INFORMATION

The patient is a 12-year-old male who presents with headaches, nausea, and dizziness that has developed over a relatively short time. Work-up includes an MRI scan, which reveals a large, well-circumscribed mass with heterogeneous contrast enhancement, filling the fourth ventricle. The decision is made to resect the lesion, and histological sections are reviewed.

OPINION

Biopsies show a hypercellular neoplasm with microvascular proliferation, but no necrosis. At low-power magnification, much of the tumor is composed of patternless sheets of small tumor cells. However, perivascular pseudorosettes (defined as an eosinophilic, cell-process-rich collar of perpendicularly oriented glial cells surrounding a central blood vessel) can be focally identified. Where they are present, the pseudorosettes tend to be narrow and are less conspicuous than in lower-grade ependymomas. Mitotic activity is brisk.

We consider the tumor to be a high-grade ependymoma and characterize it as follows: **Fourth Ventricle, Excision—Anaplastic Ependymoma, WHO Grade III.**

COMMENT

Although ependymomas of lower grade can involve supratentorial, infratentorial, and spinal cord sites, most anaplastic ependymomas are found in either the

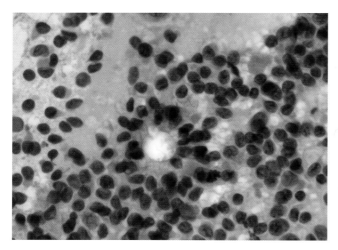

FIGURE 27.1 Intraoperative touch preparation shows a monotonous population of small cells with oval hyperchromatic nuclei and small amounts of eosinophilic cytoplasm; a small true ependymal rosette establishes the diagnosis of an ependymal tumor.

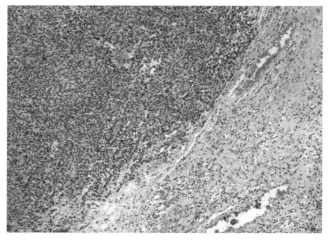

FIGURE 27.2 This patternless, anaplastic ependymoma is composed of small monotonous cells and shows sharp demarcation from adjacent brain tissue.

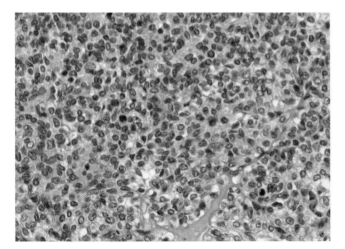

FIGURE 27.3 Hypercellularity and mitotic activity are present; necrosis and microvascular proliferation may be seen in anaplastic ependymoma but are not required for diagnosis.

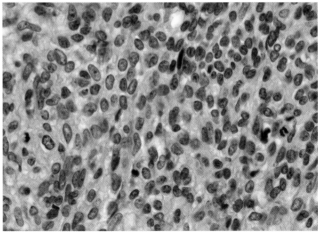

FIGURE 27.4 At least three mitotic figures are recognizable in this one high-power microscopic field alone; note the oval nuclei, small nucleoli, and less homogeneous and hyperchromatic features than usually seen in medulloblastoma.

fourth ventricle or supratentorial areas. Most anaplastic ependymomas occur in children. Spinal cord ependymomas of adults are rarely anaplastic.

DISCUSSION

Anaplastic ependymomas are defined in the 2007 World Health Organization classification system as "a malignant glioma of ependymal differentiation with accelerated growth and unfavorable clinical outcome, particularly in children; histologically characterized by high mitotic activity, often accompanied by microvascular proliferation and pseudopalisading necrosis." Anaplastic ependymoma is a WHO grade III neoplasm. The exact number of mitoses necessary to qualify as "brisk" is not specified, but the accompanying high cell density is an equally helpful feature in making the diagnosis.

Like lower-grade ependymomas, anaplastic ependymomas tend to be well demarcated from the surrounding brain, rather than diffusely infiltrative. In some anaplastic ependymomas, the patternless, sheetlike architecture places primitive neuroectodermal tumor or medulloblastoma in the differential

diagnosis. Hence, the diagnosis of anaplastic ependymoma rests on recognition of "ependymal differentiation" in the tumor.

Usually, ependymal differentiation in anaplastic ependymomas is evidenced by perivascular pseudorosettes, although these are often narrower than in lower-grade ependymomas. They may also be less frequent or more irregular in distribution. Small, true ependymal rosettes can sometimes also be seen, but conspicuous large ependymal canals are uncommon.

Almost all anaplastic ependymomas are positive for GFAP, but the strongest reaction is in the more "glial" and less "epithelial" portions of the tumor, i.e., in the processes forming the perivascular pseudorosettes. GFAP expression is usually less widespread in anaplastic ependymomas than in lower-grade ependymomas. Ultimately, in difficult cases, electron microscopy may be necessary to establish ependymal features.

Grading of ependymomas has always been problematic. Ependymomas do not show as tight a correlation between histological features and prognosis as do other types of gliomas. Foci of necrosis without

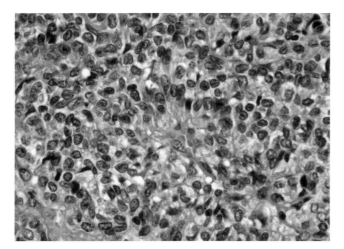

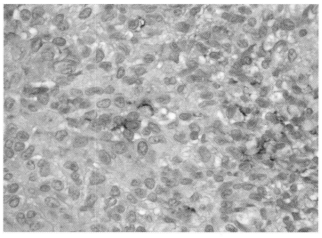

FIGURE 27.5 This example of anaplastic ependymoma had only vaguely developed perivascular pseudorosettes; the presence of tiny true ependymal rosettes was recognized on touch preparation (see Figure 27.1) and on immunostaining for epithelial membrane antigen (see Figure 27.6).

FIGURE 27.6 Immunostaining for epithelial membrane antigen highlights the microlumens of small, true ependymal rosettes in this tumor.

pseudopalisading can be seen in many grade II and III ependymomas and do not seem to influence prognosis in most studies. Sample size, differences in grading criteria used by different authors, and inclusion of adults in some studies likely confounds correlation. The role of anatomic location and its effect on the

ability to achieve gross total surgical resection also play a role in determining prognosis.

In most studies of pediatric ependymomas, patient age less than 3 years, anaplastic histopathologic features, incomplete tumor resection, and evidence of cerebrospinal fluid dissemination are adverse prognostic factors. In a recent retrospective study of prognostic factors in 96 cases of ependymoma—with the study confined to posterior fossa examples in

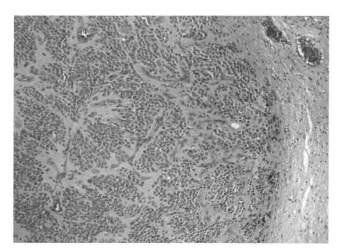

FIGURE 27.7 A second example of anaplastic ependymoma in a different patient also shows sharp demarcation from adjacent brain but, in this case, perivascular pseudorosettes make the tumor easy to categorize as ependymal.

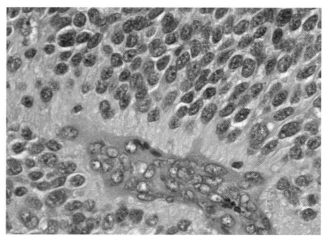

FIGURE 27.8 Microvascular proliferation, but not necrosis, was present in this second example of anaplastic ependymoma.

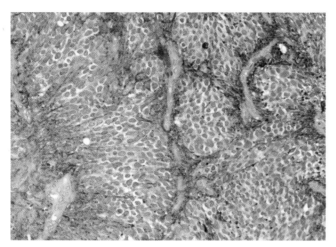

FIGURE 27.9 GFAP immunostaining highlights the cell processes forming the pseudorosettes; note the paucity of GFAP immunoreactivity in the other cells in this anaplastic ependymoma.

children—"overall survival significantly correlated with extent of resection and age, but not with histological grade" (Tihan et al.). This poor correlation with outcome was evident, despite the fact that strict histological criteria were utilized in this study to define anaplastic ependymoma (i.e., at least two of the four following features: true microvascular proliferation, palisading necrosis, mitotic rate greater than 10 per 10 HPFs, and marked hypercellularity with nuclear pleomorphism or hyperchromasia) versus grade II ependymoma (i.e., all four of the following features: perivascular pseudorosettes, uniform nuclear morphology [with focal nuclear pleomorphism allowed], mitoses less than 5 per 10 HPFs [focal areas with 5–10 per 10 HPFs allowed], and no vascular endothelial proliferation).

References

1. McLendon RE, Wiestler OD, Kros JM, et al. Anaplastic ependymoma. In: Louis DN, Ohgaki H, Wiestler OD, Cavenee WK, editors. WHO Classification of Tumours of the Central Nervous System. Lyon, FR: IARC Press; 2007, p. 79–80.
2. Prayson RA. Clinicopathologic study of 61 patients with ependymoma including MIB-1 immunohistochemistry. Ann Diag Pathol 1999;3:11–18.
3. Tihan T, Zhou T, Holmes E, et al. The prognostic value of histological grading of posterior fossa ependymomas in children: a Children's Oncology Group study and a review of prognostic factors. Mod Pathol 2008;21:165–77.

Case 28: Tanycytic Ependymoma

CLINICAL INFORMATION

The patient is a 71-year-old female who presents with initial onset of symptoms approximately 2 years prior. She describes pain in the right axilla, radiating to the anterior chest and right arm, associated with right lower extremity numbness and left buttock and leg pain. She was initially treated for presumed left sciatica. Symptoms progressed, and she ultimately develops a T4 sensory level, which prompts MRI of the thoracic spine. This demonstrates an expansile, intradural intramedullary spinal cord tumor, extending from C7 to T5, with contrast enhancement. The decision is made to resect the mass, and histological sections are reviewed.

OPINION

The specimen shows a moderately cellular tumor, composed of fascicles of cytologically uniform cells. Perivascular pseudorosettes are poorly developed, and ependymal rosettes are absent. The tumor also lacks Antoni A and B alternating dense and loose areas, as might be seen with schwannoma. Calcifications, microcysts, necrosis, and mitotic activity are all absent. Tumor cell nuclei exhibit salt-and-pepper speckling, relative nuclear monotony, and spindly eosinophilic cytoplasm.

We consider the tumor to be an ependymoma variant and characterize it as follows: **Spinal Cord C7-T5, Excision—Tanycytic Ependymoma, WHO Grade II.**

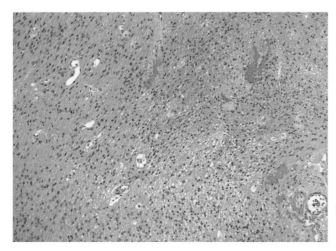

FIGURE 28.1 Low-power magnification illustrates a tumor composed of cells loosely arranged in fascicles. Note the absence of biphasic pattern, perivascular pseudorosettes, calcifications, microcysts, or necrosis in this tumor.

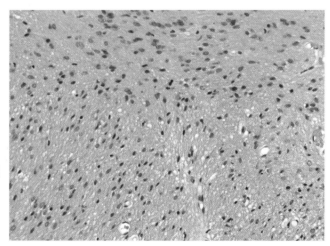

FIGURE 28.2 The tumor is composed of relatively monomorphic cells with wispy eosinophilic bipolar cytoplasm.

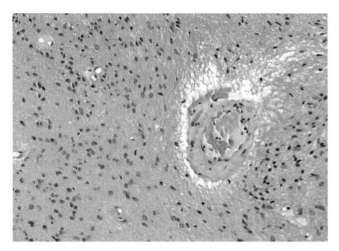

FIGURE 28.3 Blood vessels often show hyalinization, similar to that seen with other ependymoma variants.

COMMENT

Tanycytic ependymoma most commonly occurs in the spinal cord.

DISCUSSION

Tanycytic ependymoma most closely resembles schwannoma or pilocytic astrocytoma. The tumor has a more homogeneous, less biphasic architectural pattern than either of these other two tumors. Unlike schwannoma, tanycytic ependymoma shows strong GFAP immunoreactivity and an absence of reticulin fibers between individual tumor cells. Unlike pilocytic astrocytoma, the tumor is more monomorphic and usually lacks Rosenthal fibers, eosinophilic granular bodies, abundant glomeruloid vasculature, and microcysts.

Cytological features of ependymal differentiation are maintained in tanycytic ependymoma and include salt-and-pepper speckling of chromatin, monomorphic nuclei with round-to-oval shapes, and eosinophilic fibrillary processes. Ependymal rosettes are almost always absent, and perivascular pseudorosettes are poorly formed, if present at all, in tanycytic ependymomas. Mitotic activity is generally low, and tanycytic ependymomas usually are WHO grade II. Occasional nuclear enlargement and hyperchromatism in the absence of increased mitotic rate do not negate a diagnosis of WHO grade II.

Tanycytic ependymomas show immunoreactivity for S-100 protein, vimentin, and GFAP. Absence of reticulin or immunoreactivity for collagen IV or laminin between tumor cells separates the tumor

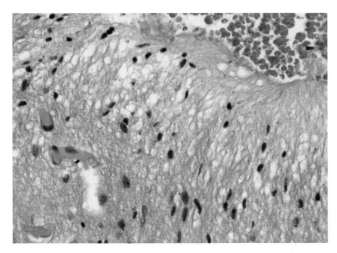

FIGURE 28.4 Close inspection may reveal vaguely developed perivascular pseudorosettes with perpendicularly oriented cell processes around vessels.

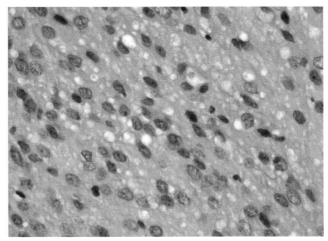

FIGURE 28.5 High-power magnification shows the round-to-oval nuclei, with small nucleoli and salt-and-pepper speckled chromatin pattern. Note the absence of mitotic activity.

from a schwannoma. Another consideration in some cases is diffuse astrocytoma of the spinal cord. GFAP does not discriminate between diffuse astrocytoma and tanycytic ependymoma, making the nuclear monotony and cytology particularly important to recognize in this ependymoma variant. Ependymomas are often suspected intraoperatively by the neurosurgeon because they tend to be more sharply demarcated from the adjacent spinal cord tissue than diffuse astrocytomas. Thus, clinicopathologic correlation should be sought by the pathologist.

On very small biopsies, it may be impossible to distinguish tanycytic ependymoma from astrocytoma without additional electron microscopic (EM) examination. Thus, in small biopsies taken from spinal cord intramedullary tumors, it is prudent to set aside a small portion of the biopsy in glutaraldehyde for elecron microscopic studies.

References

1. McLendon RE, Wiestler OD, Kros JM, et al. Anaplastic ependymoma. In: Louis DN, Ohgaki H, Wiestler OD, Cavenee WK, editors. WHO Classification of Tumours of the Central Nervous System. Lyon, FR: IARC Press; 2007, p. 74–8.
2. Perry A. Glial and glioneuronal tumors. In: Prayson RA, editor. Neuropathology. Philadelphia, PA: Elsevier Churchill Livingstone; 2005. p. 468–76.

Case 29: Clear Cell Ependymoma

CLINICAL INFORMATION

The patient is a 13-year-old male who presents with a seizure. Neuroimaging studies are performed and demonstrate a large, contrast-enhancing, well-demarcated mass located deep within the left cerebral hemisphere. Calcifications are noted in the mass. The decision is made to resect the lesion, and histological sections are reviewed.

OPINION

The specimen shows a moderately cellular tumor, punctuated by arborizing, delicate blood vessels devoid of microvascular proliferation. Perivascular pseudorosettes are manifest as eosinophilic anuclear areas around these blood vessels. Tumor cells are cytologically monotonous and contain round-to-oval nuclei and clear cytoplasm. Calcifications are present, but necrosis is absent. Scattered mitotic figures are seen, but mitotic activity is not brisk.

After immunostaining to exclude other clear cell tumor types, we diagnose this lesion as an ependymoma variant and characterize it as follows: **Left Cerebral Hemisphere, Excision—Clear Cell Ependymoma, WHO Grade II.**

COMMENT

Clear cell ependymomas most often occur in supratentorial regions of children or young adults and histologically closely simulate oligodendroglioma, neurocytoma, or hemangioblastoma.

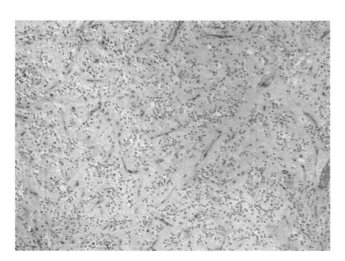

FIGURE 29.1 Low-power magnification illustrates a tumor composed of oligodendroglial-like clear cells, separated by delicate vascular septae.

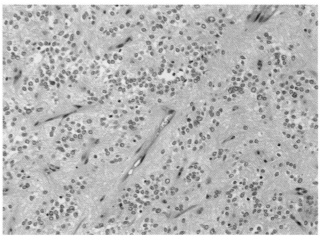

FIGURE 29.2 The tumor is composed of relatively monomorphic cells with optically clear cytoplasm. Perivascular pseudorosettes are more subtle than in other ependymoma variants.

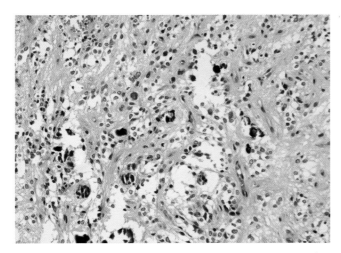

FIGURE 29.3 Microcalcifications are prominent in this example.

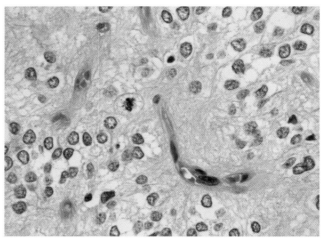

FIGURE 29.4 Close inspection on high power reveals the fibrillar cell processes.

DISCUSSION

Clear cell areas can occasionally be focally identified in otherwise typical ependymomas, but the occurrence of a pure clear cell ependymoma is uncommon. The diagnosis of clear cell ependymoma can be difficult, and immunohistochemistry or electron microscopy is often more necessary for a correct diagnosis of the clear cell variant than it is for other ependymoma subtypes.

Cytological nuclear features of ependymal differentiation are maintained in clear cell ependymoma and include salt-and-pepper speckling of chromatin and monomorphic nuclei with round-to-oval shapes. The clear cell quality of the cytoplasm mimics perinuclear halos of oligodendroglioma quite closely. Adding to the difficulty is the presence of arborizing vasculature and calcifications in both clear cell ependymoma and oligodendroglioma. The

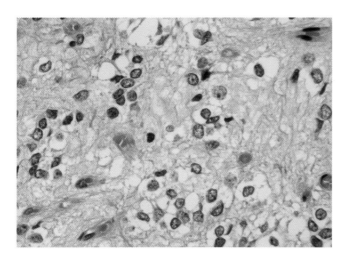

FIGURE 29.5 High-power magnification shows round-to-oval nuclei, with small nucleoli and salt-and-pepper speckled chromatin pattern.

FIGURE 29.6 Note the presence of scattered mitotic activity in this example; many clear cell ependymomas meet criteria for WHO grade III because of brisk mitotic activity.

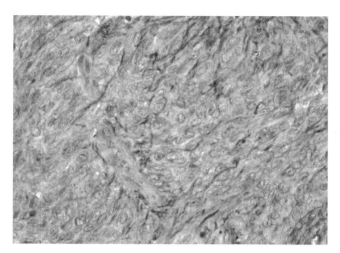

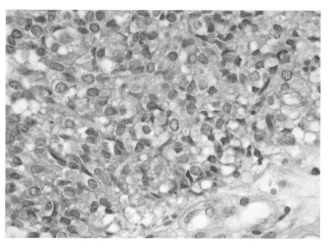

FIGURE 29.7 GFAP highlights the perivascular fibrillar cell processes and excludes consideration of hemangioblastoma.

FIGURE 29.8 EMA immunoreactivity is focally present in this example and shows a ring-like signal that highlights the surface portion of the cells forming a microlumen.

eosinophilic fibrillary processes of ependymoma are variable in number, and perivascular pseudorosettes may be poorly formed but are usually recognizable after careful scrutiny.

A feature that further aids in distinction between clear cell ependymoma and oligodendroglioma is that the former tends to be more sharply demarcated from surrounding brain tissue than oligodendrogliomas and lacks the deletions in chromosomes 1p or 19q that are present in many oligodendrogliomas.

Clear cell ependymomas show immunoreactivity for S-100 protein, vimentin, and GFAP, but the latter can be quite patchy and isolated to the few perivascular pseudorosettes that are present. Epithelial membrane antigen (EMA) immunostaining reveals the ring-like and dot-like features seen in other ependymomas but, again, the changes may be less prominent in clear cell ependymoma than in other ependymoma subtypes. Two other tumor types that enter into the differential diagnosis in clear cell ependymoma are neurocytoma and hemangioblastoma. Synaptophysin immunoreactivity is either absent entirely or very focal in clear cell ependymoma compared to neurocytoma. Immunoreactivity for GFAP and the identification of perivas-

cular pseudorosettes, even if focal, excludes consideration of hemangioblastoma.

Electron microscopic features of clear cell ependymoma are those of other ependymomas, with formation of microlumens containing microvilli and cilia. Well-developed intercellular junctions are present.

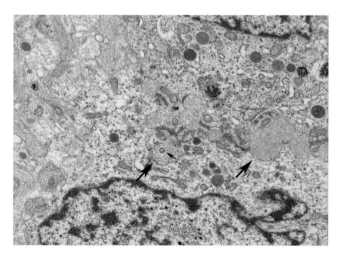

FIGURE 29.9 Electron microscopic examination of clear cell ependymoma often shows features seen in any ependymoma, with microvilli and lumen formation (large arrows), as well as cilia (small arrow). Note also the numerous intercellular junctions. (Courtesy of Gary Mierau, Ph.D.)

Clear cell ependymomas may be WHO grade II tumors but often meet criteria for WHO grade III because of significant mitotic activity. Some studies have suggested that clear cell ependymomas show a more aggressive course than other ependymoma subtypes.

References

1. Fouladi M, Helton K, Dalton J, et al. Clear cell ependymoma: a clinicopathologic analysis of 10 patients. Cancer 2003;98: 2232–44.

2. McLendon RE, Wiestler OD, Kros JM, et al. Anaplastic ependymoma. In: Louis DN, Ohgaki H, Wiestler OD, Cavenee WK, editors. WHO Classification of Tumours of the Central Nervous System. Lyon, FR: IARC Press; 2007, p. 74–8.

3. Min KW, Scheithauer BW. Clear cell ependymoma: a mimic of oligodendroglioma: clinicopathologic and ultrastructural considerations. Am J Surg Pathol 1997;21:820–6.

4. Perry A. Glial and glioneuronal tumors. In: Prayson RA, editor. Neuropathology. Philadelphia, PA: Elsevier Churchill Livingstone; 2005. p. 468–76.

Case 30: Choroid Plexus Papilloma

CLINICAL INFORMATION

The patient is a 12-year-old girl who presents with a 6- to 9-month history of "difficulty seeing the blackboard." She also reports intermittent double vision and headaches. She has recently failed a school vision screening exam. Referral to an ophthalmologist discloses 20/50 vision bilaterally and mild bilateral papilledema. MRI studies are obtained, which reveal a large, lobulated, homogeneously enhancing, fourth ventricular mass that extends through the left foramen of Luschka. Resection is undertaken, and sections are available for review.

OPINION

Sections show a highly papillary neoplasm, devoid of necrosis or brain invasion. Delicate fibrovascular connective tissue cores are covered by a single layer of monotonous epithelial cells. The columnar cells have abundant cytoplasm and generally maintain good polarity of nuclei, with nuclei located at the cell base. Mitotic activity is not identified.

We consider the pathology to be that of a choroid plexus papilloma, without atypical or malignant features, and characterize it as follows: **Fourth Ventricle, Excision—Choroid Plexus Papilloma, WHO Grade I.**

COMMENT

Choroid plexus papillomas of the fourth ventricle are found in equal proportions in children and adults. In contrast, 80% of lateral ventricular tumors occur in patients less than 20 years of age.

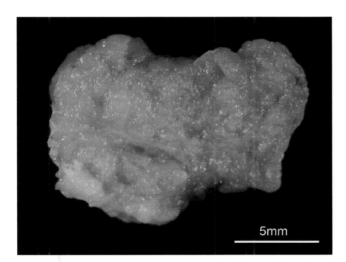

FIGURE 30.1 Gross surgical pathology specimen of a choroid plexus papilloma showing a tan-yellow tumor with a cauliflower-like appearance and bosselated surface.

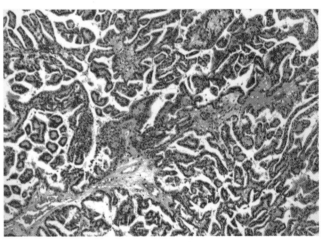

FIGURE 30.2 Low-power view of the choroid plexus papilloma shows a hyperplastic-appearing, complex papillary tumor with fibrovascular cores and no necrosis.

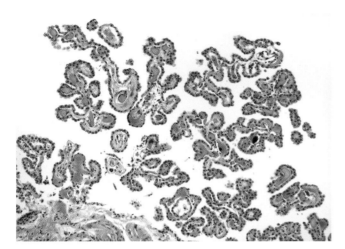

FIGURE 30.3 Normal choroid plexus, at the same magnification as Figure 30.2, for comparison, shows less complexity and hypercellularity.

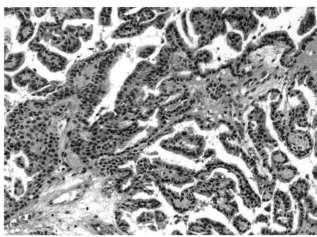

FIGURE 30.4 Medium-power view of the choroid plexus papilloma illustrates that the central fibrovascular stromal cores of the papillary tumor are covered by a single layer of crowded columnar cells.

DISCUSSION

Choroid plexus tumors are one of the few neurosurgical tumor types in which the gross examination can virtually make the diagnosis without the need for histological analysis. Macroscopically, choroid plexus papillomas are tan-yellow, soft, homogeneous masses resembling a cauliflower.

The vast majority of choroid plexus tumors are benign, WHO grade I, choroid plexus papillomas. They are relatively uncommon neoplasms but do constitute 10–20% of brain neoplasms manifesting in the first year of life. Even congenital examples have been described. The correlation between anatomic site of involvement and age of patient is striking. Tumors involving the lateral or third ventricle have a mean patient age of 1.5 years. Those in the fourth ventricle have a mean patient age of 22.5 years, and tumors occurring in the cerebello-pontine angle have a mean patient age of 35.5 years.

Histologically, choroid plexus papillomas consist of a fibrovascular core, covered by a single layer or multiple layers of cytologically bland and relatively uniform columnar-to-cuboidal epithe-lial cells. Choroid plexus papilloma resembles non-neoplastic choroid plexus, but it shows greater overall complexity and number of papillary formations. The epithelial cells in choroid plexus papilloma are more columnar and less hobnail than is normal choroid plexus epithelium, and there is more crowding of the cells. Nuclei in choroid plexus papillomas display more hyperchromasia, elongation, and stratification than in normal choroid plexus. Occasionally, choroid plexus papillomas may show oncocytic change, mucinous degeneration, calcification, ossification, or even tubular glandular architecture, none of which influence prognosis. By definition, there is neither significant mitotic activity nor severe nuclear atypia.

Choroid plexus papillomas are immunoreactive for cytokeratins and vimentin. The most common cytokeratin combination is CK7-positive and CK20-negative, but other combinations are possible. Immunostaining may involve a minority, or the majority, of the tumor cells. In a study of 35 cases, these same authors also found that 94% of choroid

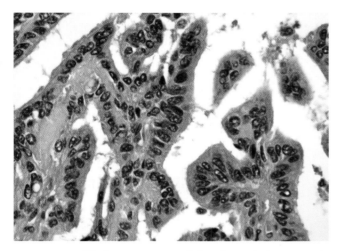

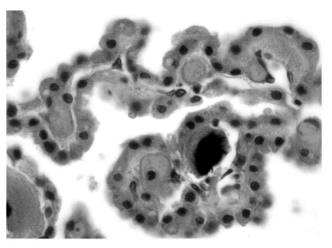

FIGURE 30.5 High-power view of the choroid plexus papilloma illustrates the mild hyperchromasia and elongation of nuclei within the columnar cells, but maintenance of basilar polarity of nuclei within the epithelium and absence of significant mitotic activity.

FIGURE 30.6 Normal choroid plexus, at the same magnification as Figure 30.5 for comparison, shows the hobnail, cuboidal epithelial cells of non-neoplastic choroid plexus. Note the basophilic calcification that typically occurs in normal choroid plexus with aging.

plexus papillomas are positive for CAM 5.2 and 69% are positive, at least focally, for GFAP.

References

1. Gyure KA, Morrison AL. Cytokeratin 7 and 20 expression in choroid plexus tumors; utility in differentiating these neoplasms from metastatic carcinomas. Mod Pathol 2000;13:638–43.

2. Paulus W, Brandner S. Choroid plexus tumors. In: Louis DN, Ohgaki H, Wiestler OD, Cavenee WK, editors. WHO Classification of Tumours of the Central Nervous System. Lyon, FR: IARC Press; 2007. p. 82–5.

3. Wolff JE, Sajedi M, Brant R, et al. Choroid plexus tumors. Br J Cancer 2002;87:1086–91.

CLINICAL INFORMATION

The patient is a 6-year-old boy who presents with 5–6 months of abnormal eye movements and visual deficits. There is also a history of difficulty walking and progressive deterioration in gross motor function. He is brought to this country from his native Ukraine for diagnosis and treatment. Neuroimaging studies reveal a large, lobulated mass in the left lateral ventricle with surrounding edema and midline shift.

OPINION

Sections show a choroid plexus papilloma with maintenance of papillary architecture, but increased mitotic activity and multifocal necrosis. Cells retain reasonable nuclear polarity, with nuclei at the base of the columnar epithelium, but crowding and elongation of the cells are noted. Mitoses number more than 2 per 10 high-power fields.

We consider this tumor to be a choroid plexus neoplasm and characterize it as follows: **Left Lateral Ventricle, Excision—Atypical Choroid Plexus Papilloma, WHO Grade II.**

COMMENT

Criteria for WHO grade II choroid plexus papilloma were recently adopted for the first time in the World Health Organization 2007 publication, WHO Classification of Tumours of the Central Nervous System.

DISCUSSION

Choroid plexus tumors are sufficiently infrequent that there had been considerable debate over the impact

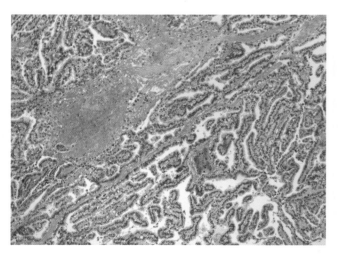

FIGURE 31.1 Low-power view shows a papillary neoplasm with zonal necrosis; this alone, however, is insufficient to diagnose WHO grade II aCPP if it occurs as an isolated feature.

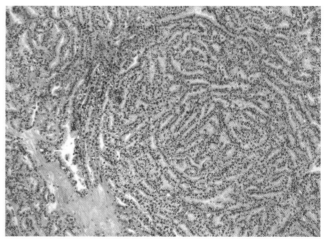

FIGURE 31.2 Areas with complex tubular and solid, less papillary, pattern can be seen, but again, this feature in isolation is insufficient to diagnose WHO grade II aCPP.

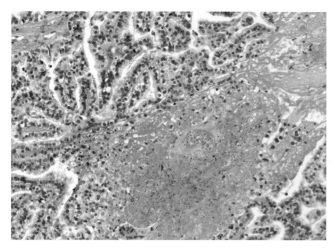

FIGURE 31.3 Necrosis in the tumor is better appreciated at higher magnification.

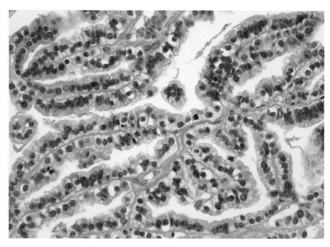

FIGURE 31.4 At least three mitoses can be seen in this single high-power microscopic field.

of various histological features on prognosis until the publication of a large study in 2006 (Jeibmann et al.). These authors collected 164 choroid plexus tumors, of which 24 showed frank signs of malignancy and were diagnosable as choroid plexus carcinoma. Of the remaining 124 assessable cases of papillomas, a high percentage [46 cases (37%)] displayed at least one of the following features: increased mitotic activity, increased cellularity, nuclear pleomorphism, blur-

ring of papillary growth pattern, or necrosis. On univariate analysis, however, only incomplete surgical resection and mitotic activity correlated with tumor recurrence. These authors proposed that the finding of increased mitotic activity (2 or more mitoses per 10 randomly selected HPFs) should allow designation as a WHO grade II tumor. This proposal was subsequently ratified in the 2007 WHO Classification System. WHO grade II "atypical" choroid plexus papilloma (aCPP) now occupies a position intermediate between the far more common choroid plexus

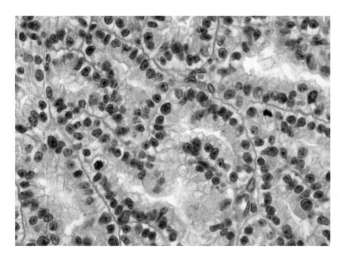

FIGURE 31.5 Mitotic activity is accompanied by a greater degree of nuclear pleomorphism, with more conspicuous nucleoli.

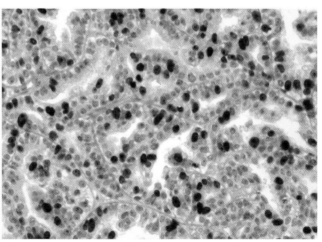

FIGURE 31.6 The MIB-1 labeling is increased in this aCPP.

papilloma, WHO grade I and the rare choroid plexus carcinoma, WHO grade III.

Indeed, it is interesting to note that after Jeibmann et al. utilized their own criteria for reclassification of choroid plexus papillomas, only 15%, not 37%, could be truly categorized as "atypical." Thus, the diagnoses of "atypical" choroid plexus papilloma or even choroid plexus "carcinoma" were likely "overcalled" in the past by some investigators, and WHO grades II and III choroid plexus tumors may be even rarer than was formerly thought. Indeed, using these newer criteria, atypical choroid plexus papillomas in the large study by Jeibmann et al. were found to actually be only about one-seventh as frequent as WHO grade I choroid plexus papillomas.

An important additional point from this study of 124 cases was the fact that, although increased mitotic activity alone correlated with a 4.9-fold higher risk of recurrence after 5 years of follow-up, "increased mitotic activity was only rarely encountered as an isolated atypical feature" in aCPP (Jeibmann et al.). Thus, the pathologist can expect to see other worrisome features in addition to ≥2 mitoses per 10 HPFs in most aCPPs. Mean MIB-1 labeling indices are often elevated for aCPP compared to CPP, but a precise discriminatory level was not established in the 2007 WHO Classification system.

References

1. Jeibmann A, Hasselblatt M, Gerss J, et al. Prognostic implications of atypical histologic features in choroid plexus papilloma. J Neuropathol Exp Neurol 2006; 65:1069–73.
2. Paulus W, Brandner S. Choroid plexus tumours. In: Louis DN, Ohgaki H, Wiestler OD, Cavenee WK, Editors. WHO Classification of Tumours of the Central Nervous System. Lyon, FR: IARC Press; 2007. p. 82–5.

Case 32: Choroid Plexus Carcinoma

CLINICAL INFORMATION

The patient is a 2-year-old child who presents with increased head circumference. Work-up reveals hydrocephalus and a large fourth ventricular mass. The decision is made to resect the lesion, and slides are available for review.

OPINION

Sections show a hypercellular neoplasm, with focal maintenance of papillary architecture, but other areas show a more patternless, sheetlike arrangement of cells with solid growth. There is increased mitotic activity, exceeding 2 per 10 high-power microscopic fields, and multifocal necrosis. Cells manifest high nuclear-to-cytoplasmic ratios, considerable nuclear pleomorphism, and only small amounts of eosinophilic cytoplasm with rounded profiles. Tumor invades the nearby cerebellum.

We consider this tumor to be a choroid plexus neoplasm and characterize it as follows: **Fourth Ventricle/Cerebellum, Excision—Choroid Plexus Carcinoma, WHO Grade III.**

COMMENT

Choroid plexus carcinomas (CPC) are rare neoplasms, and the vast majority of cases occur in very young children (median age 2–3 years), not in older children or adults. In adults with obviously malignant papillary neoplasms, metastatic carcinoma should always be the first diagnostic consideration.

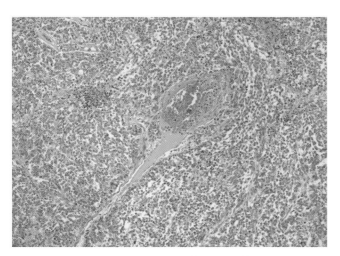

FIGURE 32.1 Low-power magnification demonstrates a hypercellular, papillary neoplasm with several small foci of necrosis.

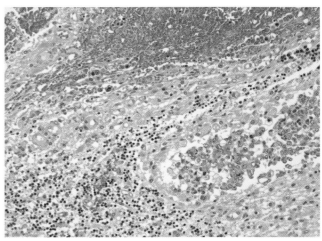

FIGURE 32.2 Tumor invades into the nearby normal cerebellum.

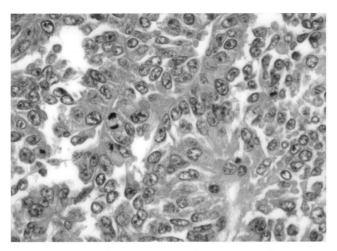

FIGURE 32.3 High-power magnification reveals mitotic activity, as well as cells with nuclear pleomorphism, high nuclear-to-cytoplasmic ratios, and prominent nucleoli.

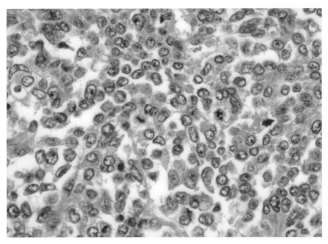

FIGURE 32.4 In other areas of the tumor, a patternless, sheetlike architecture can make distinction from atypical teratoid/rhabdoid tumor that is nearly impossible on hematoxylin and eosin light microscopy alone.

DISCUSSION

The differential diagnosis for CPC (WHO grade III) in most very young children involves separating it from lower-grade choroid plexus papillomas, especially WHO grade II, atypical choroid plexus papillomas.

Choroid plexus tumors are sufficiently infrequent that there had been considerable debate over the impact of various histological features on prognosis until the publication of a large study in 2006 (Jeibmann et al.). These authors collected 164 choroid plexus tumors, of which 24 showed frank signs of malignancy and were diagnosable as CPC, WHO grade III. Criteria utilized by these authors to diagnose CPC were the presence of four of the five following features: high cellularity, solid growth, necrosis, nuclear pleomorphism, and at least 2 mitoses per 10 randomly selected high-power microscopic fields.

It should be noted that 37% of the choroid plexus papillomas in the same series were also identified to possess at least one of these same histological features. Thus, it is important to emphasize that finding necrosis or high cellularity or nuclear pleomorphism in a choroid plexus papilloma should not prompt diagnosis of CPC. It is likely that some workers in the past overcalled choroid plexus papillomas that possessed one to three of these features as (incorrectly) a CPC.

An unresolved question is that of the importance of brain invasion in distinguishing between choroid plexus papilloma versus CPC. Too few cases with brain invasion were identified in the large series by Jeibmann et al. to assess the prognostic importance of this feature.

In some examples of CPC, the sheetlike, patternless architecture prompts diagnostic consideration of atypical teratoid/rhabdoid tumor (AT/RT), another tumor usually found in very young children less than 3 years of age. CPCs show reaction for cytokeratins, with positivity for S-100 protein and transthyretin being found less frequently than in choroid plexus papillomas. Vimentin, epithelial membrane antigen (EMA), and GFAP immunoreactivity has also been reported in some CPCs. Immunostaining for all these antibodies can also be found in AT/RT; thus, the immunohistochemistry (IHC) profile of CPC overlaps with that for AT/RT. An exception is that immunostaining for smooth muscle actin (SMA) is identified in most AT/RTs, but not in CPCs.

Further IHC distinction between CPC and AT/RT is necessary in some cases. The advent of an antibody directed toward the nuclear protein product of INI1 was reported by Judkins et al. to be valuable in this regard. Nearly all CPCs in that study showed retention of nuclear expression of INI1 protein, serving to distinguish them from histologically similar AT/RTs, which usually demonstrated nuclear loss of INI1 protein.

In the rare adult patient in whom CPC enters the differential diagnosis, immunostaining for metastatic epithelial neoplasms should be undertaken. An algorithmic approach for the workup of metastatic disease to the central nervous system has been outlined by Becher et al. This involves a "first round" of antibodies for adenocarcinoma, using CAM5.2, CK7, CK20, and thyroid transcription factor-1 (TTF-1). Depending on the outcome of these stains, metastatic epithelial tumors can be further differentiated using immunostains for GCDFP, CA125, CDX2, CD10, and estrogen receptor.

References

1. Becher MW, Abel T, Thompson RC, et al. Immunohistochemical analysis of metastatic neoplasms of the central nervous system. J Neuropathol Exp Neurol 2006;65:935–44.
2. Jeibmann A, Hasselblatt M, Gerss J, et al. Prognostic implications of atypical histologic features in choroid plexus papilloma. J Neuropathol Exp Neurol 2006;65:1069–73.
3. Judkins AR, Burger PC, Hamilton RL, et al. INI1 protein expression distinguishes atypical teratoid/rhabdoid tumor from choroid plexus carcinoma. J Neuropathol Exp Neurol 2005;64:391–7.
4. Paulus W, Brandner S. Choroid plexus tumours. In: Louis DN, Ohgaki H, Wiestler OD, Cavenee WK, Editors. WHO Classification of Tumours of the Central Nervous System. Lyon, FR: IARC Press; 2007. p. 82–5.

Case 33: Chordoid Glioma

CLINICAL INFORMATION

The patient is a 32-year-old female who presents with headaches. On imaging, she is noted to have a discrete mass lying within the third ventricle. The tumor is homogeneously contrast enhancing. The mass is excised, and histologic sections are reviewed.

OPINION

Histologic sections show a neoplasm, marked by a proliferation of epithelial cells arranged in clusters and cords. The clusters of cells are separated by a mucinous-like stroma. Focal perivascular chronic inflammation, consisting of benign-appearing lymphocytes and plasma cells, is observed. Individual tumor cells are marked by abundant eosinophilic cytoplasm. Occasional Rosenthal fibers are noted at the periphery of the lesion. Scattered eosinophilic globular bodies resembling Russell bodies are also observed. Mitotic figures are not seen in this lesion. Vascular proliferative changes and necrosis are also not observed. The tumor demonstrates diffuse positive staining with antibody to GFAP.

We consider the lesion to represent a low-grade glioma and characterize it as follows: **Third Ventricular Region, Excision—Chordoid Glioma, WHO Grade II.**

COMMENT

Chordoid gliomas are relatively rare lesions that arise in the third ventricular region. Cases that have been reported appear to behave like low-grade neoplasms.

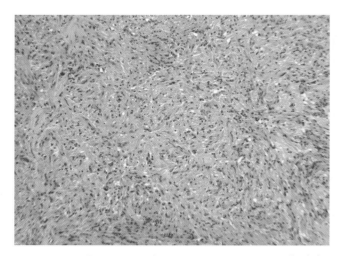

FIGURE 33.1 Low magnification appearance, marked by spindled cells arranged against a mucinous background.

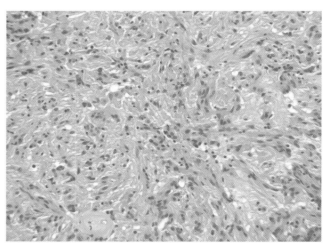

FIGURE 33.2 A mucinous background is a salient feature of the tumor.

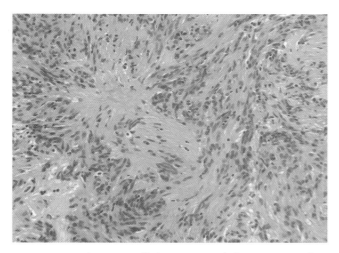

FIGURE 33.3 A more cellular region of the tumor, with a fibrillary background.

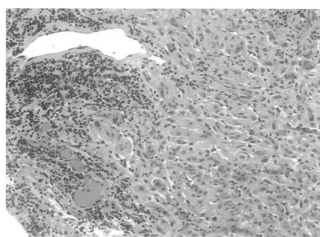

FIGURE 33.4 Focal, perivascular, chronic inflammation is present.

DISCUSSION

Chordoid gliomas are rare, slow-growing, noninvasive glial tumors that typically are situated in the suprasellar and third ventricular regions. They typically arise in adults and show a female predominance. Because of the tumor's location in the anterior portion of the third ventricle, patients with chordoid gliomas often present with symptoms related to obstructive hydrocephalus. Occasional tumors may cause endocrine hypofunctioning because of their proximity to the optic chiasm and pituitary region. On imaging, they are usually well circumscribed and uniformly contrast-enhancing.

Microscopically, the tumor is marked by clusters and cords of epithelioid cells, arranged against a mucinous background. Perivascular chronic inflammation and Russell body formations are quite common. Mitotic figures are only rarely observable. Vascular

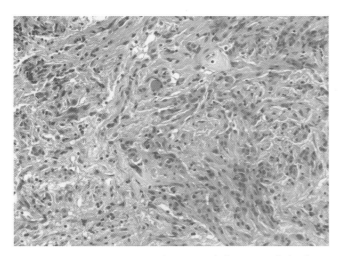

FIGURE 33.5 An occasional eosinophilic Russell body is evident.

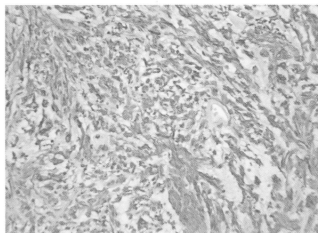

FIGURE 33.6 The tumor cells demonstrate widespread cytoplasmic staining with GFAP antibody.

proliferative changes and necrosis are not present. On immunohistochemical staining, the tumor cells stain positively with antibodies to GFAP and vimentin. Occasional positive staining with antibody to epithelial membrane antigen (EMA) has also been variably reported. Low rates of cell proliferation are evidenced by low Ki-67 and MIB-1 cell proliferative indices.

Differential diagnostic considerations, given the choroid appearance, include chordoid meningioma and chordoma. The lack of a dural or bony involvement, GFAP immunoreactivity, and physaliphorous cells (in chordoma) exclude those possibilities.

Chordoid gliomas are generally treated by surgical excision. If incompletely excised, they may recur. Postoperative complication may result by damaging adjacent structures, including the hypothalamus.

References

1. Brat DJ, Scheithauer BW, Staugaitis SM, et al. Third ventricular chordoid glioma: a distinct clinicopathologic entity. J Neuropathol Exp Neurol 2001;15:147–50.
2. Leeds NE, Lang FF, Ribalta T, et al. Origin of chordoid glioma of the third ventricle. Arch Pathol Lab Med 2006;130:625–36.
3. Reifenberger G, Weber T, Weber RG, et al. Chordoid glioma of the third ventricle: immunohistochemical and molecular genetic characterization of a novel tumor entity. Brain Pathol 1999;9:617–27.

Case 34: Angiocentric Glioma

CLINICAL INFORMATION

The patient is a 32-year-old male with a long history of drug-resistant epilepsy. An MRI scan shows a cortically based, circumscribed mass, 13 × 13 × 15 mm, in the right parietal lobe, without significant surrounding edema. After placement of intracortical electrodes, the patient undergoes resective therapy for his pharmaco-resistant epilepsy. Histologic sections corresponding to the circumscribed intracortical lesion are reviewed.

OPINION

As indicated by the neuroimaging, the abnormal cellular proliferations are identified principally within the cerebral cortex (seen as negative staining against a diffuse background of synaptophysin positivity). Solid areas, composed of fascicular arrangements of the tumor cells, give way to areas demonstrating perivascular and subpial infiltration. Perivascular tumor aggregates in many areas resemble perivascular pseudorosettes seen in classical ependymomas; in other areas, there is a more irregular arrangement of

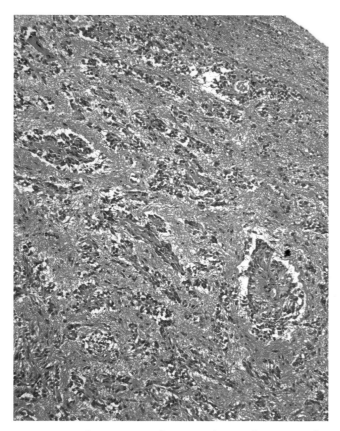

FIGURE 34.1 Low power shows preferential perivascular infiltration through the cerebral cortex.

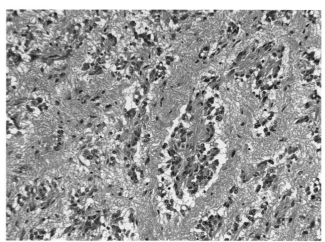

FIGURE 34.2 Despite this predilection for a perivascular aggregation, the arrangements of tumor cells with regard to the blood vessel walls are much more irregular than those seen in classical perivascular pseudorosettes of ependymal tumors.

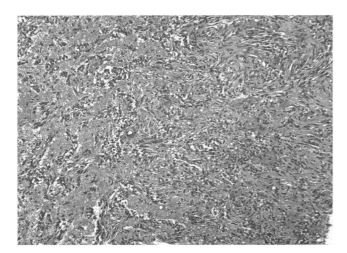

FIGURE 34.3 Perivascular infiltration merges with solid arrangements of the tumor cells, often referred to as piloid astrocytic differentiation.

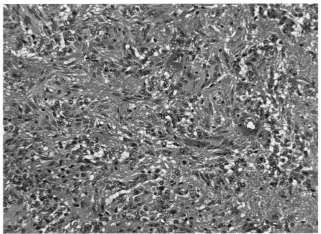

FIGURE 34.4 Higher-power view of this solid area of tumor, showing a fascicular arrangement of elongate monomorphous astrocytic cells.

tumor cells in relationship to the intracortical blood vessels. Immunohistochemical stains show strong GFAP and vimentin immunoreactivity, as well as dot-like and ring-like epithelial membrane antigen reactivity in cells forming perivascular rosettes.

We consider this cortical lesion to be representative of a low-grade tumor and characterize it as follows: **Right Parietal Lobe, Partial Removal— Angiocentric Glioma, WHO Grade I.**

DISCUSSION

In October of 2005, two separate laboratories reported series of epileptogenic/epilepsy related neoplasms referred to as "angiocentric neuroepithelial tumor" or "monomorphous angiocentric glioma," designating principally intracortical tumors demonstrating features of both infiltrating astrocytoma and ependymoma. Since then, approximately 30 tumors of this type have been reported, with all but one reporting medically resistant epilepsy, beginning in childhood. As expected, all tumors have been located within the supratentorial cerebral cortical gray matter, with variable, usually mild-to-minimal extension into the subcortical white matter. Distribution of these tumors within the cerebral cortex generally follows a mass distribution, albeit with overrepresentation of the temporal lobe and underrepresentation of the occipital lobe. Although most reported patients underwent resection during the first two decades of life, examples of angiocentric glioma have been reported in all age groups. The typical MRI appearance is that of a nonenhancing T1 hypointense/T2 hyperintense cortically based lesion. Although many of the histologic and immunohistochemical features of angiocentric glioma overlap with those of cortical ependymoma, the presence of solid fascicular areas and the inconstant orientation of tumor cells with associated blood vessels have led to the exceptions of angiocentric glioma as a distinct entity in the most recent WHO classification of central nervous system tumors. To date, recurrence of angiocentric glioma has not been reported, and the vast majority of operated patients remain seizure-free after surgery.

References

1. Lellouch-Tubiana A, Boddaert N, Bourgeois M, et al. Angiocentric neuroepithelial tumor (ANET): a new epilepsy-related clinicopathological entity with distinctive MRI. Brain Pathol 2005;15:281–6.

2. Preusser M, Hoischen A, Novak K, et al. Angiocentric glioma: report of clinicopathologic and genetic findings in 8 cases. Am J Surg Pathol 2007;31:1709–18.

3. Shakur SF, McGirt MJ, Johnson MW, et al. Angiocentric glioma: a case series. J Neurosurg Pediatr 2009;3:197–202.

4. Wang M, Tihan T, Rojiani AM, et al. Monomorphous angiocentric glioma: a distinctive epileptogenic neoplasm with features of infiltrating astrocytoma and ependymoma. J Neuropathol Exp Neurol 2005;64:875–81.

Case 35: Astroblastoma

CLINICAL INFORMATION

The patient is a 19-year-old female who presents with a seizure. A well-demarcated, noncalcified, lobulated mass with focal cystic change is noted on MRI studies. The patient undergoes gross total resection, and histologic sections are reviewed.

OPINION

Histologic sections shows proliferation of atypical-appearing glial cells, with high nuclear- to-cytoplasmic ratio and irregular nuclear contours. Prominent perivascular rosetting structures, marked by short and broad cell processes, are seen. Focal subpial aggregation of tumor cells is present. Prominent mitotic activity, vascular proliferative changes, and necrosis are not seen. A Ki-67 labeling index of less than 1 is noted. There is no evidence of true rosettes.

We consider the lesion to be a glial neoplasm and characterize it as follows: **Right Frontal Lobe, Excision—Astroblastoma.**

COMMENT

The lack of prominent mitotic activity, marked cytologic atypia, vascular proliferative changes, and necrosis, along with the low Ki-67 labeling index, support a diagnosis of low-grade or well-differentiated astroblastoma.

DISCUSSION

Astroblastomas are rare glial neoplasms that typically present in the first three decades of life. Most are located in the cerebral hemispheres and do not appear, like most ependymomas, to arise from or within the ventricles. The histologic hallmarks of this

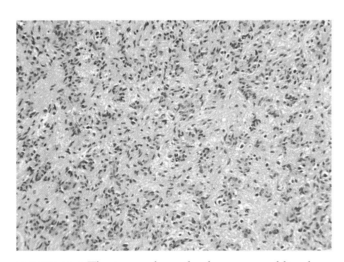

FIGURE 35.1 The tumor shows focal areas resembling low-grade astrocytoma.

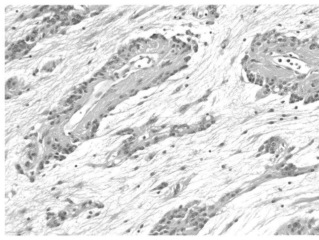

FIGURE 35.2 Intermediate magnification illustrating the appearance of astroblastomatous rosettes.

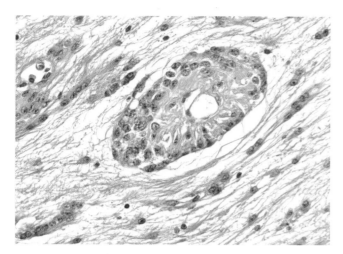

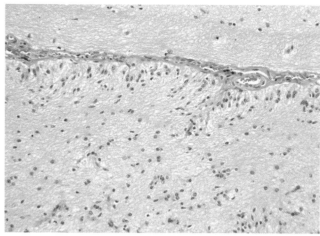

FIGURE 35.3 Higher magnification appearance of rosettes, showing broad, thickened cytoplasmic processes.

FIGURE 35.4 Focal subpial aggregation of tumor cells is evident.

tumor are its circumscription and characteristic rosetting structures. Given the salient presence of rosettes, this tumor ostensibly mimics ependymoma. Occasionally, ependymomas may arise away from the ventricular system. In general, the cytoplasmic processes of the astroblastoma cells tend to be thicker and more broad-based, rather than the narrow and tapered cell processes more typical of the ependymoma. Vascular sclerosis, which is also fairly commonly observed in astroblastoma, is a relatively uncommon feature of ependymomas. The other differential diagnostic consideration is an ordinary diffuse fibrillary astrocytoma that has some secondary structuring around blood vessels. The astrocytoma tends to be more infiltrative in nature, and the rosetting pattern not as structured as it is with the astroblastoma.

Like other gliomas, astroblastomas demonstrate S-100 and GFAP immunoreactivity. Focal membranous immunoreactivity with antibody to EMA may also be seen; however, cytokeratin immunostaining is typically not present. Ultrastructurally, astroblastoma cells usually exhibit fewer cilia and cell junctions than ependymomas.

Although there is no grade designation assigned to these tumors by the WHO, it is generally accepted that these neoplasms may have a low-grade/well-differentiated or high-grade appearance. Higher-grade tumors, in contrast to the current case, are usually marked by more prominent nuclear pleomorphism, increased mitotic activity, vascular proliferative changes, necrosis, and increased cell proliferation labeling indices. There is some suggestion in the literature that tumors with low-grade histology have a better prognosis than higher-grade neoplasms. High-grade tumors may require radiotherapy and generally allow for a poor survival.

References

1. Bonnin JM, Rubinstein LJ. Astroblastomas: a pathological study of 23 tumors with postoperative follow-up in 13 patients. Neurosurgery 1989;25:6–13.
2. Brat DJ, Hirose Y, Cohen KJ, et al. Astroblastoma. Clinicopathologic features and chromosome abnormalities defined by comparative genomic hybridization. Brain Pathol 2000;10:42–52.
3. Thiessen B, Finlay J, Kulkarni R, et al. Astroblastoma: does histology predict biologic behavior? J Neurooncol 1998;40:59–65.

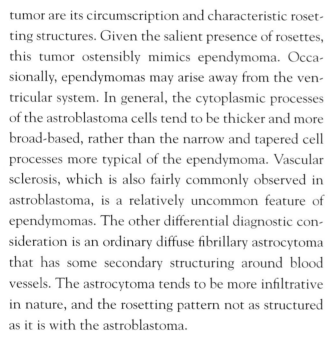

Case 36: Dysplastic Cerebellar Gangliocytoma (Lhermitte-Duclos Disease)

CLINICAL INFORMATION

The patient is an 18-year-old male who presents with dysmetria. The patient has had a history of previous seizures. Imaging studies show mild hydrocephalus and focal thickening of the cerebellar cortex, with increased signal intensity on a T2-weighted MRI study. The right cerebellar lesion is excised, and histologic sections are reviewed.

OPINION

The histologic sections show focal enlargement of the cerebellar cortex, marked by an increased number of large ganglionic cells. There appears to be a sharp interface between the lesion and the adjacent gliotic cerebellar parenchyma. The ganglionic cells are marked by eosinophilic-to-pale staining cytoplasm and an eccentrically placed nucleus with prominent nucleolus. A gliomatous component is not noted. There is no evidence of calcification. Microcystic changes are observed adjacent to the lesion.

We consider the lesion to be a low-grade ganglionic cell proliferation, and we characterize it as follows: **Right Cerebellum, Excision—Dysplastic Gangliocytoma of the Cerebellum (Lhermitte-Duclos Disease).**

COMMENT

The absence of a gliomatous component in the lesion supports the diagnosis of a pure ganglion cell mass (gangliocytoma).

DISCUSSION

Dysplastic gangliocytoma of the cerebellum is a rare disorder, well known to be associated with Cowden

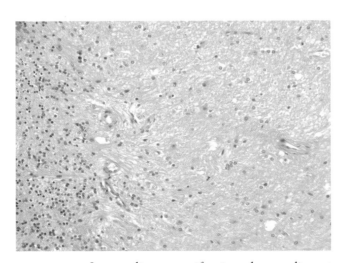

FIGURE 36.1 Intermediate magnification shows adjacent mild gliosis with preservation of the cerebellar architecture.

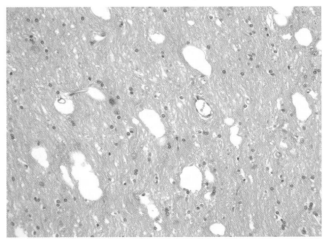

FIGURE 36.2 Focal microcystic changes and occasional reactive astrocytes are present adjacent to the lesion.

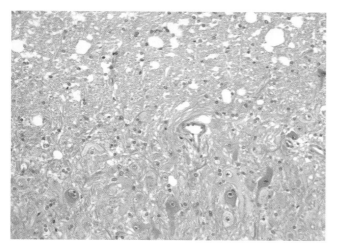

FIGURE 36.3 Intermediate magnification shows a sharp interface between the lesion and adjacent cerebellar parenchyma.

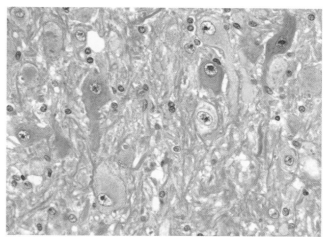

FIGURE 36.4 High magnification appearance of ganglionic cells in the lesion. Note the absence of an atypical gliomatous component in the lesion.

syndrome. It is unclear whether the gangliocytoma represents a true neoplasm or hamartoma. First described in 1920 by Lhermitte and Duclos, the entity also bears their name. Clinical presentation is usually related to signs and symptoms associated with the cerebellum. Frequent concommitent findings in the central nervous system include megalencephaly, heterotopic gray matter, hydrocephalus, seizures (noted in the current patient), and mental retardation.

Histologically, the lesion is marked by a proliferation of large ganglionic cells Although there is expansion of the cerebellum, the overall architecture is relatively preserved. Occasionally, calcification, vascular dilatation, and microcystic or vacuolar changes may be noted in association with this entity. The ganglionic cells stain with antibodies to neural markers such as synaptophysin. Cell proliferation indices generally show negligible rates of cell proliferation. A gliomatous component, typical of ganglioglioma, is distinctly absent in this lesion.

The importance of the diagnosis rests in its association with Cowden disease. Cowden syndrome is an autosomal dominant condition associated with mutations in the PTEN gene. Patients with Cowden syndrome have an increased risk of developing cancers of the breast, thyroid (medullary carcinoma), and endometrium. Cutaneous trichilemmomas are also frequently noted.

References

1. Abel TW, Baker SJ, Fraser MM, et al. Lhermitte-Duclos disease: a report of 31 cases with immunohistochemical analysis of the PTEN/AKT/mTOR pathway. J Neuropathol Exp Neurol 2005;64:341–9.

2. Milbouw G, Born JD, Martin D, et al. Clinical and radiological aspects of dysplastic gangliocytoma (Lhermitte-Duclos disease): a report of two cases with review of the literature. Neurosurgery 1988;22(Part 1):124–8.

3. Robinson S, Cohen AR. Cowden disease and Lhermitte-Duclos disease: characterization of a new phakomatosis. Neurosurgery 2000;46:371–83.

Case 37: Desmoplastic Infantile Astrocytoma/Ganglioglioma

CLINICAL INFORMATION

The patient is a 1-month-old male who presents with bulging fontanelles and lethargy. Neuroimaging studies are obtained that demonstrate a massive, multicystic, superficially located lesion in the right frontal lobe. The decision is made to resect the lesion, and histological sections are available for review.

OPINION

Biopsies show a tumor superficially located in the leptomeninges, with a sharp interface with the underlying cortex. Within the tumor, there are two different-appearing areas. The first component is a spindle-cell tumor that is accompanied by a desmoplastic (reticulin-rich) response. The cells show features of both fibroblastic-like spindle cells and more obvious glial cells with eosinophilic cytoplasm. The second population is that of poorly differentiated neuroepithelial tumor, composed of small blue cells with round, deeply basophilic nuclei and minimal cytoplasm. In some areas, these cells predominate. Few cells suggestive of neuronal cells are identified on hematoxylin and eosin, but synaptophysin immunostaining discloses immunoreactivity in the desmoplastic areas.

We consider the pathology to be that of a low-grade neoplasm, and, after immunohistochemical

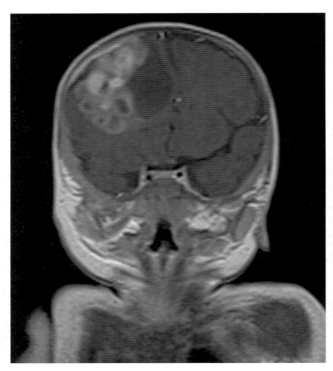

FIGURE 37.1 MRI scan, demonstrating the large multicystic tumor of the right frontal lobe that occupies a large percentage of the infant's intracranial compartment.

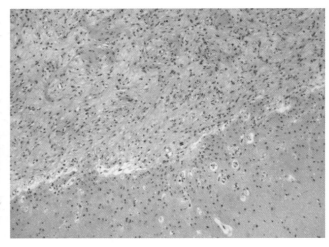

FIGURE 37.2 Low-power microscopic view shows a spindled tumor, superficially located in leptomeninges, with at least focal sharp demarcation from the underlying cerebral cortex.

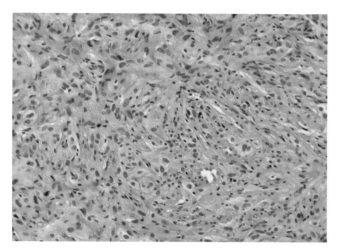

FIGURE 37.3 High-power view of the spindled portion of the tumor shows that many of the cells have obviously eosinophilic cytoplasm and glial appearance.

studies and correlation with clinical and neuroimaging features, we characterize it as follows: **Right Frontal, Excision—Desmoplastic Infantile Astrocytoma/ Ganglioglioma, WHO Grade I.**

COMMENT

Desmoplastic infantile astrocytoma/ganglioglioma (DIA/DIG) is a rare neoplasm of childhood, which almost always occurs in patients under the age of

24 months. DIA/DIG invariably arises in supratentorial areas, preferentially the frontal and parietal lobes, and often involves more than one lobe.

DISCUSSION

DIA/DIG is a diagnosis that should be rendered only after correlation between neuropathologic, clinical, and neuroimaging features of the case. Because of the often massive size of the tumor, there may be enlargement of the skull and even midline shift, features that incorrectly suggest an ominous diagnosis if the observer is unaware of the existence of this WHO grade I neoplasm.

Histologically, three components have been described. The major component is that of a leptomeningeal desmoplastic tumor, in which spindled cells with fibroblastic-like features are admixed with obvious glial cells, the latter of which are strongly GFAP-positive. Dense collagen is less frequent than abundant reticulin, and a reticulin network surrounds nearly every tumor cell, mimicking a primary mesenchymal tumor. In cases with an additional neoplastic neuronal component, immunostains for

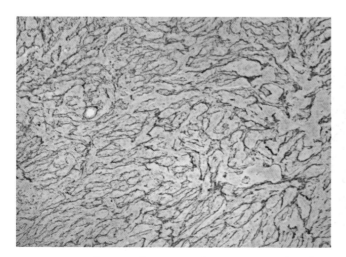

FIGURE 37.4 A reticulin stain demonstrates abundant reticulin surrounding individual tumor cells.

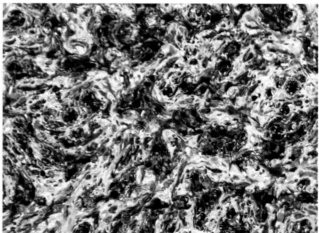

FIGURE 37.5 GFAP is strongly positive in the glial portion of the tumor, but negative in blood vessel and mesenchymal cells in the desmoplastic areas.

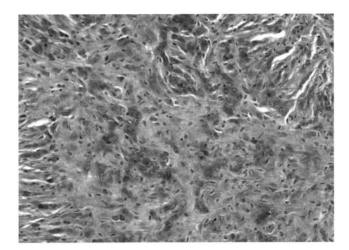

FIGURE 37.6 Synaptophysin is expressed in this same area of tumor, even in cells that lack obvious neuronal differentiation.

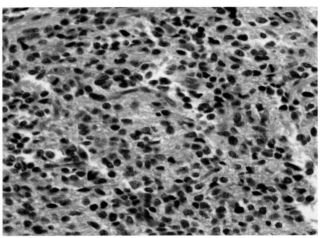

FIGURE 37.7 A small blue cell component of the tumor simulates a higher-grade lesion.

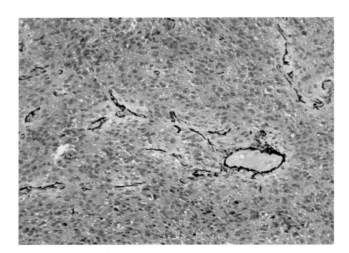

FIGURE 37.8 Small blue cell portions of the tumor usually lack reticulin fibers.

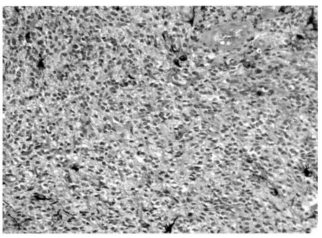

FIGURE 37.9 Little GFAP immunoreactivity is present in the small blue cell areas.

synaptophysin, neurofilament (heavy), and/or class III β-tubulin identify the neuronal population. Often, immunostaining for neuronal markers is seen, even in cells that lack obvious neuronal features on hematoxylin and eosin staining.

If these were the only features in the tumor, there would be little cause for alarm. However, by definition, these tumors also contain a poorly differentiated neuroepithelial component that mimics small blue cell tumors. These hypercellular areas of tumor are composed of small cells with rounded hyperchromatic nuclei, minimal cytoplasm, and sometimes mitotic activity. When mitotic activity is identified in the small blue cell component, it contrasts with the near-absence of mitoses in the desmoplastic astrocytic/ganglioglioma component.

A third cortical component may be seen in some tumors and is devoid of desmoplasia; that component is not evident in this case, at least in the portions of tumor that were resected.

The importance of clinicopathologic radiographic/neuroimaging correlation is that DIA/DIG is a WHO grade I tumor, whereas other small blue cell tumors of the central nervous system (medulloblastoma, central nervous system primitive neuroectodermal tumors, pineoblastomas) are WHO grade IV. Thus, there is a radical difference in therapy. Most patients do well with gross total resection alone. Even with subtotal resection, some tumors are stable or only grow slowly (although exceptional cases of DIA/DIG with a more malignant course have been documented). The diagnosis of DIA/DIG should not be made without corroborating clinical and neuroimaging features in the patient.

References

1. Brat DJ, Vandenburg SR, Figarella-Branger D, et al. Desmoplastic infantile astrocytoma and gangliglioma. In: Louis DN, Ohgaki H, Wiestler OD, Cavenee WK, Editors. WHO Classification of Tumours of the Central Nervous System. Lyon, FR: IARC Press; 2007. p. 96–8.
2. Lonnrot K, Terho M, Kahara V, et al. Desmoplastic infantile ganglioglioma: novel aspects in clinical presentation and genetics. Surg Neurol 2007;68:304–8.

Case 38: Dysembryoplastic Neuroepithelial Tumor

CLINICAL INFORMATION

The patient is a 9-year-old female who presents with chronic, pharmacologically resistant epilepsy. Electroencephalogram (EEG) studies localize the seizure activity to the left temporal lobe. T1-weighted MRI studies show a fairly well-demarcated multicystic mass involving the left temporal lobe. A gross total resection is performed, and histologic sections are reviewed.

OPINION

Histologic sections show a multinodular, microcystic neoplasm. Many of the nodules are situated in the cortex. Histologically, these nodules are comprised primarily of cells with rounded nuclear contours and scant cytoplasm, resembling oligodendrocytes. Microcystic spaces contain light eosinophilic fluid, and occasional neuronal cells are noted floating in cystic areas. There is minimal cytologic atypia identified in either component of the tumor. Focally, small gemistocytic-like cells are noted. Mitotic activity, vascular proliferative changes, and necrosis are not seen. A prominent arcuate capillary vascular pattern is present. The adjacent cortex shows architectural disorganization.

We consider the lesion to be a low-grade glioneuronal neoplasm and characterize it as follows: **Left Temporal Lobe, Excision—Dysembryoplastic Neuroepithelial Tumor, WHO Grade I.**

COMMENT

The multinodular architecture, predominant cortical location of many of the nodules, and the presence of adjacent malformation cortical development (cortical

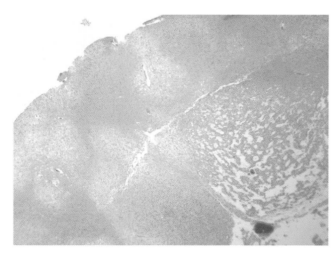

FIGURE 38.1 Low magnification appearance of the temporal lobe, showing a multinodular, cortical-based neoplasm.

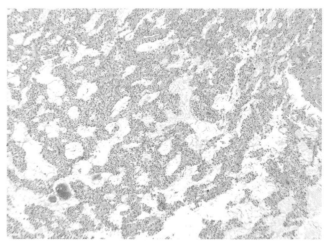

FIGURE 38.2 Microcystic change is observable in many of the nodules.

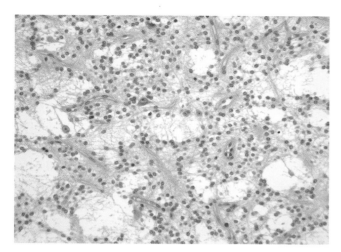

FIGURE 38.3 Higher magnification appearance of a micro-cystic area, highlighting oligodendroglial-like cells and benign-appearing neurons.

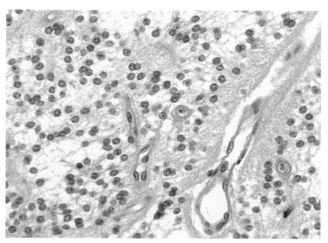

FIGURE 38.4 Cytologic atypia in the oligodendroglial-like and neuronal components of the tumor is distinctly absent.

dysplasia) support a diagnosis of dysembryoplastic neuroepithelial tumor.

DISCUSSION

The dysembryoplastic neuroepithelial tumor is a low-grade (WHO grade I) neoplasm most commonly associated with chronic epilepsy. Most patients are fairly young at the time of presentation, and the temporal lobe is the most common site of origin.

Salient histologic features of the tumor include the presence of multinodular, cortical-based foci of tumor. Tumor cells are arranged against a microcystic background, which grossly may be evident as a blister-like appearance on the surface of the involved cortex. The tumor is felt to be glioneuronal in nature and is comprised of a neuronal cell component devoid of appreciable cytologic atypia (in contrast to

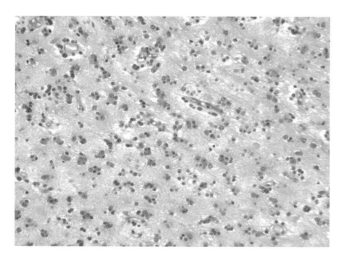

FIGURE 38.5 Focal area of minigemistocytic cells is noted in this tumor.

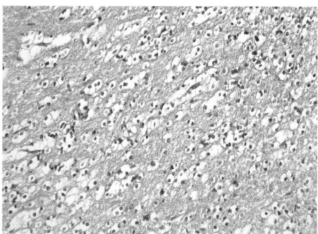

FIGURE 38.6 An area adjacent to a microcystic nodule shows oligodendroglial-like cells with pericellular clearing ("fried egg" change), reminiscent of a low-grade oligoden-droglioma.

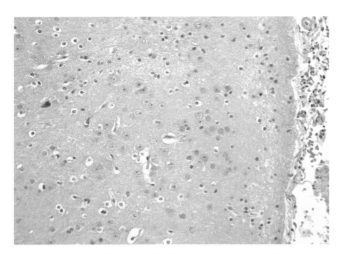

FIGURE 38.7 Architectural disorganization in the cortex adjacent to the dysembryoplastic neuroepithelial tumor, known as cortical dysplasia or malformation of cortical development, is a common finding in these tumors.

ganglioglioma). The glioma component of the lesion most closely resembles an oligodendroglioma and is comprised primarily of cells with rounded nuclear contour and scant cytoplasm. Pericellular clearing and an arcuate capillary vascular pattern may be evident. The adjacent cortex, if available for assessment, frequently demonstrates a disordered architecture, referred to as a malformation of cortical development or cortical dysplasia. The presence of this adjacent cortical dysplasia suggests that the lesion may have a malformative basis to its origin. Labeling indices, utilizing markers such as Ki-67, generally show very low rates of cell proliferation. Vascular proliferative changes and necrosis are distinctly uncommon in this tumor.

Differential diagnostic considerations usually include ganglioglioma and microcystic oligodendroglioma. Gangliogliomas, in contrast to dysembryoplastic neuroepithelial tumors, demonstrate cytologic atypia in both the neuronal as well as gliomatous components of the lesion. Most gangliogliomas are uninodular masses. Although gangliogliomas may have focal areas in which the gliomatous component

resembles an oligodendroglioma, most commonly the gliomatous component in ganglioglioma has the appearance of an astrocytoma. Distinction of a dysembryoplastic neuroepithelial tumor from a microcystic oligodendroglioma, particularly in a limited biopsy, may be virtually impossible. In smaller fragmented specimens, the ability to appreciate the multinodularity and cortical-based location of the tumor may not be possible. In such cases, evaluation of the tumor for allelic loss on chromosomes 1p and 19q may be helpful. If the tumor demonstrates evidence of large deletions on these chromosomes, the diagnosis of oligodendroglioma is favored, because such large deletions have not been described with the dysembryoplastic neuroepithelial tumor. In the setting of a tumor that does not demonstrate evidence of these deletions, the differential diagnosis still remains problematic, in that a subset of classic oligodendrogliomas may not show the chromosomal deletions. The significance of distinguishing the oligodendroglioma from dysembryoplastic neuroepithelial tumor lies in its prognosis and treatment; oligodendrogliomas have a propensity to infiltrate, recur, and progress to higher-grade lesions. Dysembryoplastic neuroepithelial tumors are theoretically curable on gross total excision.

References

1. Daumas-Duport C, Scheithauer BW, Chodkiewicz JP, et al. Dysembryoplastic neuroepithelial tumor: a surgically curable tumor of young patients with intractable partial seizures. Report of thirty-nine cases. Neurosurgery 1988;23:545–56.
2. Hirose T, Scheithauer BW, Lopes MB, et al. Dysembryoplastic neuroepithelial tumor (DNT): an immunohistochemical and ultrastructural study. J Neuropathol Exp Neurol 1994;53:184–95.
3. Prayson RA, Castilla EA, Hartke M, et al. Chromosome 1p allelic loss by fluorescence in situ hybridization is not observed in dysembryoplastic neuroepithelial tumors. Am J Clin Pathol 2002;118:512–17.
4. Prayson RA, Morris HH, Estes ML, et al. Dysembryoplastic neuroepithelial tumor: a clinicopathologic and immunohistochemical study of 11 tumors including MIB1 immunoreactivity. Clin Neuropathol 1996;15:47–53.

Case 39: Ganglioglioma

CLINICAL INFORMATION

The patient is a 7-year-old female who presents with seizures of 6.5 years duration. CT imaging shows a circumscribed, partially cystic mass, with focal calcification situated in the left temporal lobe. The mass is resected, and histologic sections are reviewed.

OPINION

Histologic sections show hypercellular parenchyma, marked by a proliferation of atypical, spindled glial cells with high nuclear-to-cytoplasmic ratio. Mitotic activity is not noted. Intermixed with the spindled cells is a second population of ganglionic type cells, with abundant eosinophilic cytoplasm and generally rounded nuclear contours with prominent nucleolation. Foci of perivascular chronic inflammation, consisting primarily of benign-appearing lymphocytes, are noted. Focal calcifications are also observed in the lesion. Vascular proliferative changes and necrosis are not seen. Focally, the mass appears to extend into the leptomeninges. Rosenthal fibers and granular bodies are not noted in this lesion.

We consider the lesion to be a glioneuronal neoplasm and characterize it as follows: **Left Temporal Lobe, Excision—Ganglioglioma, WHO Grade I.**

COMMENT

The admixture of a gliomatous component resembling a low-grade fibrillary astrocytoma with an atypical ganglion cell component is consistent with a diagnosis of ganglioglioma. Mitotic activity, necrosis, and vascular proliferative changes, suggesting a higher-grade lesion, are not observed.

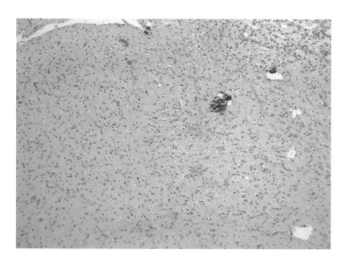

FIGURE 39.1 Low magnification appearance of the tumor, showing a moderately cellular neoplasm with focal calcification.

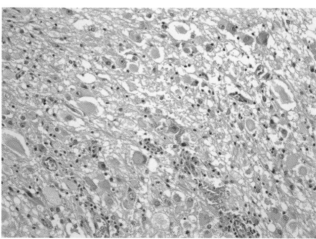

FIGURE 39.2 Atypical ganglion cells are readily identifiable in the neoplasm.

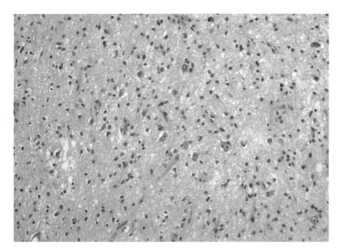

FIGURE 39.3 Cytologically atypical glial cells resembling neoplastic astrocytes are also noted in the tumor, associated with occasional ganglionic cells.

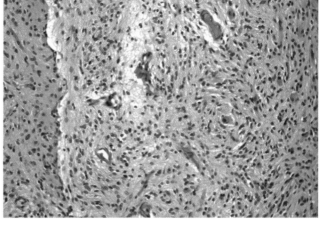

FIGURE 39.4 Tumor is seen to extend focally, to involve the leptomeningeal space to the right. Occasional ganglionic cells are present in the leptomeningeal tumor.

DISCUSSION

Gangliogliomas are a well-recognized glioneuronal neoplasm that has a peak incidence in the first few decades of life. The tumors have been variably described to arise in all areas of the brain, but they are most commonly located in the temporal lobes. In patients with temporal lobe tumors, medically intractable epilepsy is often the clinical presentation.

Tumors may present as solid or cystic masses. Requisite for a diagnosis is identification of an atypical gliomatous component, which may resemble an ordinary fibrillary astrocytoma, pilocytic astrocytoma or, less commonly, an oligodendroglioma. Admixed with the gliomatous component is an atypical ganglion cell component, marked by abnormal number

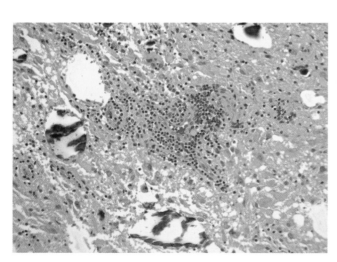

FIGURE 39.5 Foci of perivascular chronic inflammation and calcification are present.

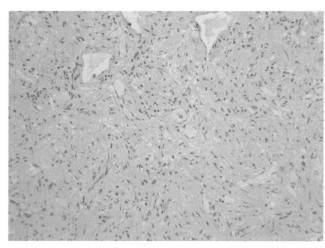

FIGURE 39.6 An area of tumor consists exclusively of spindled glial cells resembling astrocytoma. Failure of adequate sampling in such a case may result in an erroneous diagnosis of astrocytoma.

of ganglion cells, which are frequently cytologically atypical (e.g., abnormal distribution of Nissl substance, neuronal cytomegaly, multinucleation). The two components of the tumor may not be evenly admixed throughout the neoplasm, and therefore, when the diagnosis is suspected, the tumor should be well sampled in order to guarantee that both components are identified. Failure to do so may result in an erroneous diagnosis of a low-grade glioma, which carries with it a worse prognosis. Perivascular chronic inflammation and calcifications are common findings in these tumors. Occasionally, eosinophilic granular bodies or Rosenthal fibers may also be observed in the neoplasm. Like dysembryoplastic neuroepithelial tumors, the adjacent uninvolved cortex may show architectural disorganization (malformation of cortical development or cortical dysplasia). Proliferative activity, as evidenced by Ki-67 immunostaining, is generally low, frequently <1. Immunohistochemistry may be helpful in identifying the atypical ganglion cell component in some tumors. Care should be taken not to overinterpret morphologically normal,

resident neurons, entrapped by an infiltrating glioma, as an atypical ganglion cell component. As with the current case, gangliogliomas may occasionally extend to involve the leptomeninges; this has not necessarily been associated with a particularly worse prognosis.

The vast majority of gangliogliomas represent grade I neoplasms and are associated with an excellent prognosis. They generally do not require adjuvant therapy and are theoretically curable with gross total resection.

References

1. Diepholder HM, Schwechheimer K, Mohadjer M, et al. A clinicopathologic and immunomorphologic study of 13 cases of ganglioglioma. Cancer 1991;68:2192–2201.
2. Lang FF, Epstein FJ, Ransohoff J, et al. Central nervous system gangliogliomas. Part 2: Clinical outcome. J Neurosurg 1993;79:867–73.
3. Prayson RA, Khajavi K, Comair YG. Cortical architectural abnormalities and MIB1 immunoreactivity in gangliogliomas: a study of 60 patients with intracranial tumors. J Neuropathol Exp Neurol 1995;54:513–20.
4. Zentner J, Wolf HK, Ostertun B, et al. Gangliogliomas: clinical, radiological, and histopathological findings in 51 patients. J Neurol Neurosurg Psychiatry 1994;57:1497–1502.

Case 40: Anaplastic Ganglioglioma

CLINICAL INFORMATION

The patient is a 26-year-old male who presents with long history of seizures. He had a history of surgery at age 4 years, at which time a diagnosis of a ganglioglioma was made. More recently, in addition to increasing seizure frequency, he has noticed periodic severe headaches. Imaging studies shows a 3-cm mass involving the right temporal lobe. The mass is surgically excised, and histologic sections are reviewed.

OPINION

Histologic sections show a hypercellular lesion, marked by a proliferation of atypical-appearing astrocytic cells with nuclear enlargement and hyperchromasia. Intermixed with the astrocytoma-appearing areas are foci of atypical-appearing ganglionic cells, increased in number and cytologically abnormal. Focally, the astrocytoma-appearing area of the tumor shows marked cellularity, with readily identifiable mitotic activity, focal vascular proliferative changes, and even focal areas of necrosis. A Ki-67 immunostain was performed, and a labeling index of 10.8 is noted.

We consider the lesion to be a glioneuronal neoplasm and characterize it as follows: **Right Temporal Lobe, Excision—Anaplastic Ganglioglioma, WHO Grade III.**

COMMENT

The morphologic appearance of the tumor is consistent with that of a recurrent ganglioglioma. The presence of focally prominent cellularity with increased readily identifiable mitotic activity, high Ki-67 labeling index, vascular proliferative changes,

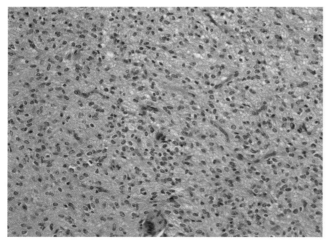

FIGURE 40.1 Intermediate magnification appearance of the tumor, showing an area resembling a low-grade fibrillary astrocytoma.

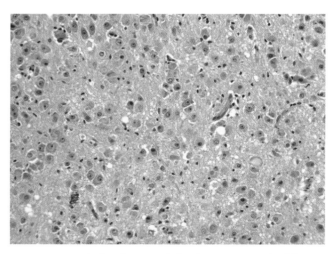

FIGURE 40.2 A focal area of the lesion is marked by an atypical ganglion cell component.

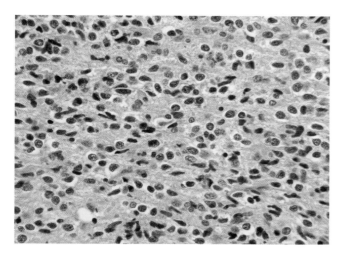

FIGURE 40.3 In areas, the gliomatous component is more cellular and marked by more nuclear pleomorphism, more akin to a higher-grade fibrillary astrocytoma.

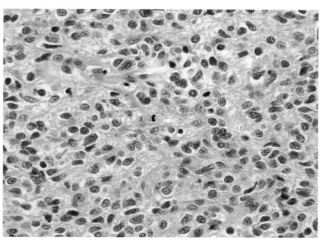

FIGURE 40.4 Mitotic figures are readily identifiable in the gliomatous component of the tumor.

and necrosis indicate a higher-grade, more aggressive-behaving tumor.

DISCUSSION

Although the vast majority of gangliogliomas are low-grade, WHO grade I neoplasms, it has been recognized that a small number of these tumors may degenerate into a higher-grade neoplasm (anaplastic ganglioglioma). Precise criteria for the diagnosis

of anaplastic ganglioglioma remain somewhat vague. In general, these tumors are marked by a morphology in the gliomatous component that resembles a malignant glioma, i.e., increased mitotic activity, vascular proliferative changes, and even necrosis. In the few cases that have been studied in the literature, these tumors also tend to demonstrate markedly increased rates of cell proliferation, as evidenced by Ki-67 or MIB-1 immunostaining. Although histologic sections from the original resection in the current case were

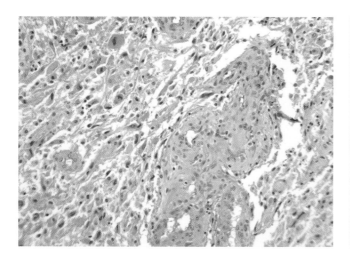

FIGURE 40.5 Focal vascular proliferative changes are also observed in the tumor.

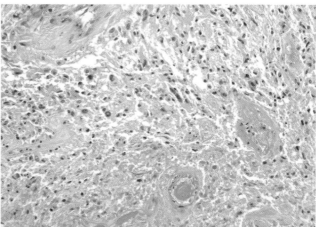

FIGURE 40.6 Geographic necrosis is present in the neoplasm.

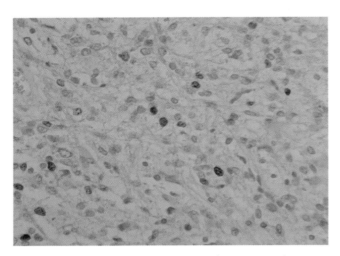

FIGURE 40.7 Ki-67 immunostaining shows more than rare positive staining cells. The tumor had a labeling index of 10.8; usual low-grade gangliogliomas have lower labeling indices, typically <1.

unavailable for examination, the prior diagnosis of ganglioglioma suggests an initial low-grade lesion. The recent increase in seizure frequency and development of headaches indicate a potential change in the status of the tumor. In terms of differential diagnosis, similar to ordinary low-grade gangliogliomas, distinction of this lesion from a high-grade glioma is important; documentation of the atypical ganglion cell component is critical to rendering the correct diagnosis.

References

1. Luyken C, Blumcke I, Fimmers R, et al. Supratentorial gangliogliomas: histopathologic grading and tumor recurrence in 184 patients with a median follow-up of 8 years. Cancer 2004;101:146–55.
2. Prayson RA, Khajavi K, Comair YG. Cortical architectural abnormalities and MIB1 immunoreactivity in gangliogliomas: a study of 60 patients with intracranial tumors. J Neuropathol Exp Neurol 1995;54:513–20.
3. Suzuki H, Otsuki T, Iwasaki Y, et al. Anaplastic ganglioglioma with sarcomatous component: an immunohistochemical study and molecular analysis of p53 tumor suppressor gene. Neuropathology 2002;22:40–7.

Case 41: Papillary Glioneuronal Tumor

CLINICAL INFORMATION

The patient is a 36-year-old male who presents with a 3-month history of recurrent headaches and new onset seizures. Imaging studies show a right temporal lobe mass with focal enhancement and cystic change. The lesion is resected, and histologic sections are reviewed.

OPINION

Histologic sections show a neoplasm marked by a focal papillary architectural pattern. The centers of the papillae are formed by vessels that are variably sclerotic. Surrounding the vessels are rounded cells with a small amount of clear-to-eosinophilic cytoplasm. Intermixed between the papillary structures are a population of cells with generally rounded nuclei and scant cytoplasm. Hemosiderin-laden macrophages, indicative of prior hemorrhage, are observed. On immunohistochemical staining, the cells lining the papillae demonstrate positive immunoreactivity with antibody to GFAP. Focally, collections of cells situated between the papillae demonstrate synaptophysin immunoreactivity.

We consider the lesion to be a glioneuronal tumor and characterize it as follows: **Right Temporal Lobe, Excision—Papillary Glioneuronal Tumor, WHO Grade I.**

COMMENT

The presence of GFAP- and synaptophysin-positive staining of subpopulations of cells in the tumor support a diagnosis of glioneuronal neoplasm.

DISCUSSION

Papillary glioneuronal tumors are a relatively recently described entity. Most of the tumors described have

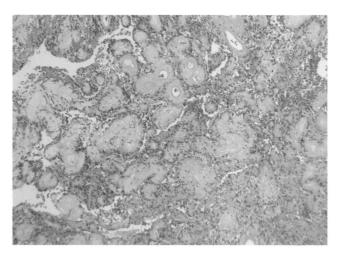

FIGURE 41.1 Lower-magnification appearance of the tumor, showing a vaguely papillary architectural pattern.

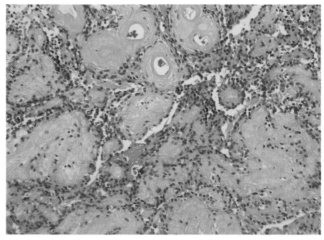

FIGURE 41.2 Higher-magnification view, showing sclerotic vessel changes in the center of papillary structures.

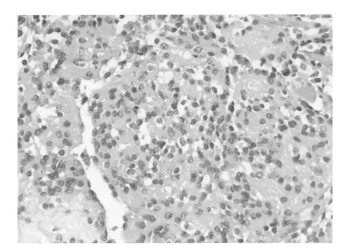

FIGURE 41.3 A more solid-appearing area of the tumor between papillae is marked by a proliferation of rounded cells and hemosiderin-laden macrophages.

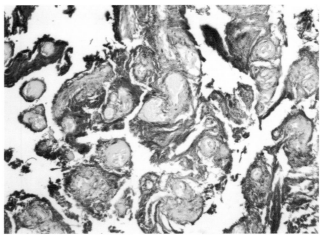

FIGURE 41.4 GFAP immunoreactivity is observed in cells lining the papillae.

arisen in adults—in the cerebral hemispheres, with a predilection for the temporal lobe. On imaging studies, a cystic mass with mural nodule(s) is frequently observable.

As its name suggests, the tumor consists of a papillary architecture, with vascular cores rimmed by GFAP-positive staining glial cells. Vascular sclerotic changes may be prominently evident. Interspersed between the papillary areas is a population

of small, rounded, neuronal cells that demonstrate synaptophysin immunoreactivity. Occasionally, more mature-appearing ganglion cells may be evident. Prominent mitotic activity, vascular proliferative changes, and necrosis are distinctly uncommon in this tumor. The periphery of the lesion may show evidence of gliosis, with Rosenthal fibers and eosinophilic granular bodies. Microcalcifications have been described, as have hemosiderin-laden macrophages, evidence of prior hemorrhage. Cell proliferation markers, such as Ki-67, show very low rates of cell proliferation, typically on the order of less than 2.

Of the tumors that have been reported thus far, all have been associated with long-term survival and have not required adjuvant chemotherapy or radiation therapy.

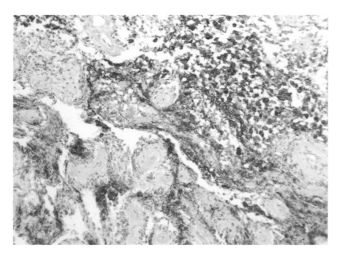

FIGURE 41.5 Synaptophysin immunoreactivity underscores the neural differentiation of the more solid foci of rounded cells situated between the papillae.

References

1. Bouvier-Labit C, Daniel L, Dufour H, et al. Papillary glioneuronal tumour: clinicopathological and biochemical study of one case with 7-year follow up. Acta Neuropathol (Berl) 2000;99:321–6.
2. Kim DH, Suh YL. Pseudopapillary neurocytoma of temporal lobe with glial differentiation. Acta Neuropathol (Berl) 1997;94:187–91.
3. Komori T, Scheithauer BW, Anthony DC, et al. Papillary glioneuronal tumor: a new variant of mixed neuronal-glial neoplasm. Am J Surg Pathol 1998;22:1171–83.

Case 42: Rosette-Forming Glioneuronal Tumor of the Fourth Ventricle

CLINICAL INFORMATION

The patient is a 21-year-old male who presents with headaches and a mildly ataxic gait. On imaging studies, a midline fourth ventricular mass is noted. The lesion appears relatively circumscribed and shows increased signal intensity on T2-weighted images. The lesion is excised, and histologic sections are reviewed.

OPINION

The histologic sections show a well-demarcated tumor, characterized by focal areas marked by rosetted structures. The rosetted structures contain central eosinophilic material, rimmed by a ring of cells with rounded nuclei, indistinct nucleoli, and scant cytoplasm. The majority of the tumor is marked by mildly hypercellular parenchyma, with atypical-appearing astrocytic cells. Mild focal vascular

proliferative changes are observed. In areas, the cells have more rounded nuclei and pericellular clearing. Rosenthal fibers and eosinophilic granular bodies are not noted. Mitotic figures are not observed. There is no evidence of necrosis. On immunostaining, the tumor demonstrates positive staining with antibody to GFAP. The rosetted structures show positive staining, with antibody to synaptophysin, indicating neurocytic differentiation.

We consider the tumor to be a low-grade neoplasm and characterize it as follows: **Fourth Ventricle, Excision—Rosette-Forming Glioneuronal Tumor of the Fourth Ventricle, WHO Grade I.**

COMMENT

The presence of synaptophysin-positive neurocytic rosettes, admixed with a GFAP-positive astrocytoma

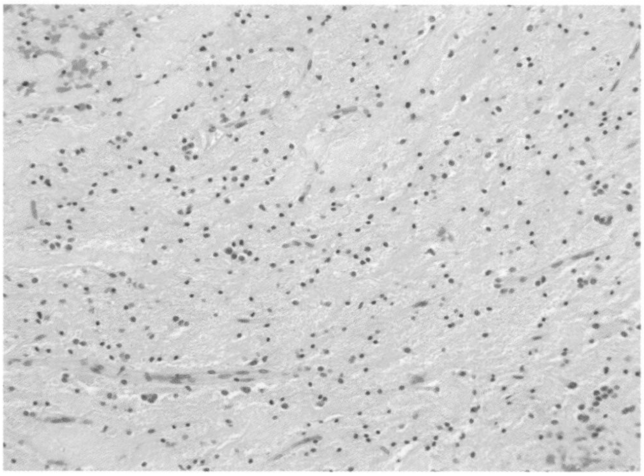

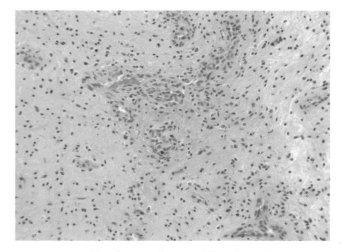

FIGURE 42.1 Intermediate magnification appearance of the tumor, showing a mildly hypercellular neoplasm resembling a low-grade glioma.

FIGURE 42.2 Focal vascular proliferative changes are present. There is no evidence of necrosis and prominent mitotic activity.

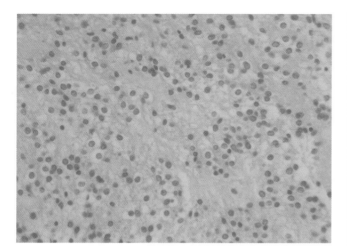

FIGURE 42.3 High-magnification appearance, showing oligodendroglial-like cells, with pericellular clearing in the gliomatous area of the tumor.

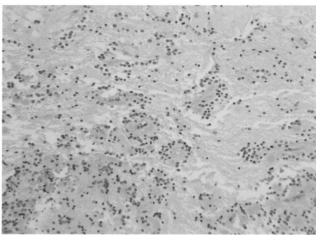

FIGURE 42.4 Characteristic neurocytic rosette-like structures are present in the tumor.

component, supports the diagnosis of a mixed glioneuronal neoplasm.

DISCUSSION

The rosette-forming glioneuronal tumor of the fourth ventricle is a new addition to the WHO classification system. This is a rare tumor, which has been described in both children and adults. As its name suggests, the lesion generally arises in the fourth ventricle

(although anecdotal cases of origin in other locations are reported in the literature). The patients typically present with signs and symptoms related to obstructive hydrocephalus, including headaches, or ataxia. The lesion is generally well circumscribed and microscopically is marked by the presence of synaptophysin-positive neurocytic rosettes or perivascular pseudorosettes, admixed with areas of tumor resembling a low-grade astrocytoma, with elongated tumor

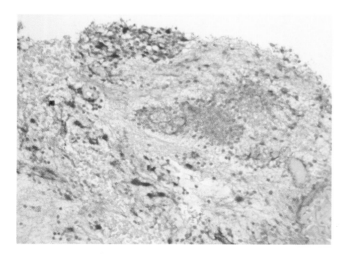

FIGURE 42.5 These rosette-like structures demonstrate positive staining with synaptophysin antibody, indicating neurocytic differentiation.

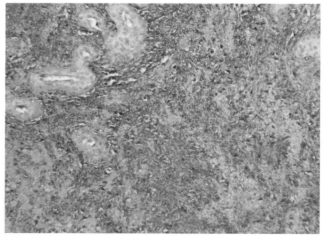

FIGURE 42.6 Much of the remaining tumor demonstrates GFAP immunoreactivity, indicating astrocytic differentiation.

cell nuclei and GFAP-positive cytoplasm. Occasionally, background cells have rounded nuclei, with scant cytoplasm, and resemble oligodendroglial cells. Rosenthal fibers, granular bodies, hemosiderin deposition, and microcalcifications have been variably described in the tumor. Mitotic activity and necrosis are generally absent. Occasional tumors may show hyalinized or sclerosed vessels, vascular thrombosis, and vascular proliferation-type changes. Proliferation markers show low rates of proliferation, in keeping with the general low grade of the tumor. The key to the diagnosis is recognition of the rosette structures and demonstration of both glial and neuronal differentiation in the tumor.

Differential diagnostic considerations include pilocytic astrocytoma, dysembryoplastic neuroepithelial tumor, and neurocytoma. The presence of neurocytic differentiation in this tumor allows distinction from pilocytic astrocytoma. The typical imaging study of a pilocytic astrocytoma (cystic neoplasm with enhancing mural nodule) is not usually observed in the rosette-forming glioneuronal tumor. Dysembryoplastic neuroepithelial tumors usually present as supratentorial lesions in younger patients, often have a multinodular architectural pattern, and generally lack a glial component that resembles pilocytic astrocytoma. Central neurocytomas are usually situated in the lateral third ventricles, demonstrate diffuse neuronal differentiation, and do not contain geographic areas of astrocytic phenotype.

The relatively few cases of this tumor that have been reported in the literature have had a favorable outcome.

References

1. Albanese A, Mangiola A, Pompucci A, et al. Rosette-forming glioneuronal tumor of the fourth ventricle: report of a case with clinical and surgical implications. J Neurooncol 2005;71:195–7.
2. Komori T, Scheithauer BW, Hirose T. A rosette-forming glioneuronal tumor of the fourth ventricle: intratentorial form of dysembryoplastic neuroepithelial tumor? Am J Surg Pathol 2002;25:582–91.
3. Preusser M, Dietrich W, Czech T, et al. Rosette-forming glioneuronal tumor of the fourth ventricle. Acta Neuropathol 2003;106:506–8.
4. Rosenblum MK. The 2007 WHO classification of nervous system tumours: newly recognized members of the mixed glioneuronal group. Brain Pathol 2007;17:308–13.

Case 43: Central Neurocytoma

CLINICAL INFORMATION

The patient is a 32-year-old male who presents with increased headaches. On imaging, a heterogeneous 2.8-cm mass on T1-weighted MRI imaging is noted within the right lateral ventricle. The lesion is subtotally resected, and histologic sections are reviewed.

OPINION

Histologic sections show a proliferation of cells with rounded nuclei and scant eosinophilic cytoplasm. The nuclei have a salt-and-pepper chromatin pattern with an occasional small nucleolus evident. An arcuate capillary pattern is noted in the background of the tumor. Focal dystrophic calcifications are observed. Mitotic activity is not seen. Vascular proliferative changes or necrosis are not present. On immunostaining, the tumor demonstrates diffuse positive staining, with antibody to synaptophysin, and does not stain with antibody to GFAP. A Ki-67 immunostain is performed, and a labeling index of 1.7 noted.

We consider the lesion to be a tumor with neural differentiation and characterize it as follows: **Right Lateral Ventricle, Excision—Central Neurocytoma, WHO Grade II.**

COMMENT

Diffuse synaptophysin immunoreactivity supports a diagnosis of central neurocytoma.

DISCUSSION

Although central neurocytomas are classically tumors that arise in young adults and have a predilection

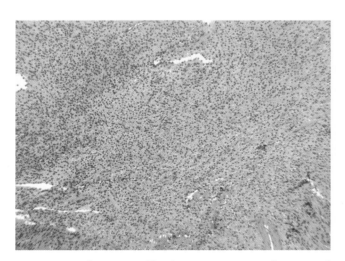

FIGURE 43.1 Low-magnification appearance of a central neurocytoma, highlighting the monotony of the tumor cells.

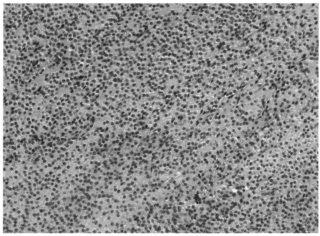

FIGURE 43.2 A prominent arcuate capillary vascular pattern, similar to that seen in oligodendroglioma, may also be observed in central neurocytoma.

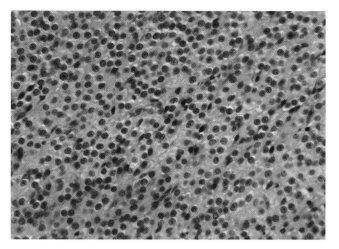

FIGURE 43.3 High-magnification appearance of the cells comprising central neurocytoma. Cells are marked by scant cytoplasm and nuclei with salt-and pepper chromatin pattern.

for the lateral ventricles, the clinical presentation is often related to symptoms associated with increased intracranial pressure. Morphologically, the tumors have a rather monomorphic appearance, consisting of rounded cells, with finely speckled chromatin nuclei and a prominent capillary vascular pattern. Morphologically, these tumors can resemble oligodendrogliomas, as well as rare clear cell ependymomas, particularly given the common intraventricular

location of the central neurocytoma. The key to the diagnosis rests on demonstrating evidence of neural differentiation by immunohistochemistry or ultrastructural examination of the tumor. Cell proliferation indices are generally low, typically less than 2. Central neurocytoma is considered a low-grade lesion; however, the tumor may recur if incompletely resected.

Rare cases of neurocytomas arising outside the ventricular system (extraventricular neurocytomas) have also been described. These tumors are typically well-circumscribed, contrast-enhancing masses that often have a cystic appearance, like their intraventricular counterpart. The presence of a prominent vascular pattern and calcifications raises oligodendroglioma as a differential diagnostic consideration. Again, immunohistochemistry is helpful in arriving at the proper diagnosis.

References

1. Brat DJ, Scheithauer BW, Eberhart CG, et al. Extraventricular neurocytomas: pathologic features and clinical outcome. Am J Surg Pathol 2001;25:1252–60.
2. Giangaspero F, Cenacchi G, Losi L, et al. Extraventricular neoplasms with neurocytoma features. A clinicopathological study of 11 cases. Am J Surg Pathol 1997;21:206–12.

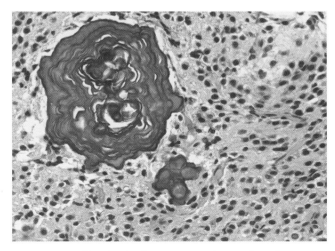

FIGURE 43.4 Focal calcifications are observed in the tumor.

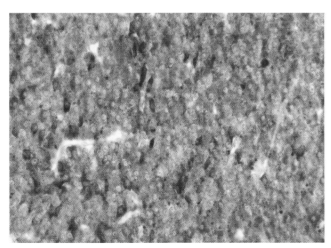

FIGURE 43.5 Diffuse positive immunoreactivity with synaptophysin, indicating neural differentiation, is seen in this tumor.

3. Hassoun J, Soylemezoglu F, Gambarelli D, et al. Central neurocytoma: a synopsis of clinical and histological features. Brain Pathol 1993;3:297–306.

4. MacKenzie IR. Central neurocytoma: histologic atypia, proliferation potential, and clinical outcome. Cancer 1999;85:1606–10.

5. Schild SSE, Scheithauer BW, Haddock MG, et al. Central neurocytomas. Cancer 1997;79:790–5.

6. Yasargil MG, von Ammon K, von Deimling A, et al. Central neurocytoma: histopathological variants and therapeutic approaches. J Neurosurg 1992;76:32–7.

Case 44: Atypical Neurocytoma

The patient is a 39-year-old female who presents with increased confusion. A left lateral ventricular mass, measuring 2.1 cm, is identified and shows marked enhancement after gadolinum injection. The tumor is subtotally resected, and histologic sections are reviewed.

OPINION

Histologic sections show a somewhat monotonous proliferation of generally rounded cells, with scant eosinophilic cytoplasm and salt-and-pepper nuclear chromatin pattern. In focal areas, some degree of nuclear pleomorphism is observable. The background of the tumor has a fibrillary-like appearance, with a prominent arcuate capillary vascular pattern and focal calcifications. Up to 5 mitotic figures per 10 high-power fields are observed. Focal necrosis is also seen. Microvascular proliferation is noted in the tumor. Immunohistochemical staining shows diffuse positive staining with antibody to synaptophysin and paucity of GFAP immunoreactivity. A Ki-67 labeling index of 9.8 is observed.

We consider the lesion to be a tumor with neural differentiation and characterize it as follows: **Left Lateral Ventricle, Excision—Atypical Central Neurocytoma.**

COMMENT

The presence of increased mitotic activity, elevated Ki-67 labeling index, and focal necrosis suggest a more aggressive-behaving tumor.

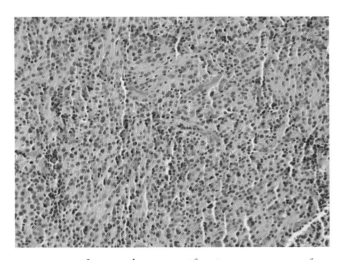

FIGURE 44.1 Intermediate magnification appearance of an atypical neurocytoma, showing a somewhat monotonous proliferation of rounded cells, with fibrillary-like background and a prominent arcuate capillary vascular pattern.

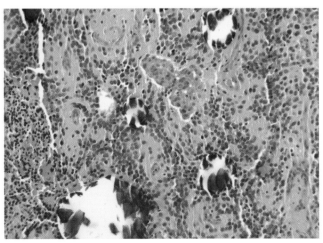

FIGURE 44.2 Focal calcifications and vascular proliferative changes are evident in this tumor.

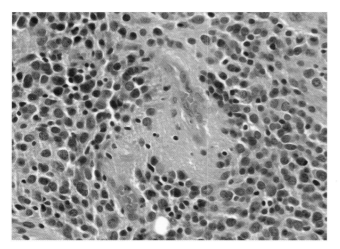

FIGURE 44.3 Focal perivascular pseudorosetting by cells with salt-and-pepper nuclear chromatin pattern is observed.

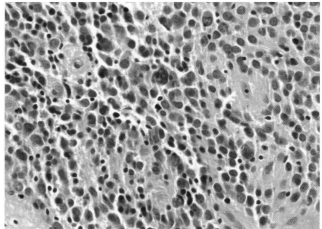

FIGURE 44.4 Focally, nuclear pleomorphism is evident.

DISCUSSION

Although the majority of central neurocytomas, as previously described in Case 43, represent low-grade neoplasms, a subset of tumors may behave in a more aggressive fashion. The morphologic correlates of more aggressive behavior in neurocytomas include increased mitotic activity, vascular proliferative changes, and necrosis. Many of these tumors also have elevated Ki-67 or MIB-1 indices, in excess of 2–3, as in the current tumor. Central neurocytomas, particularly with increased cell proliferation indices, have shown an increased likelihood of recurrence.

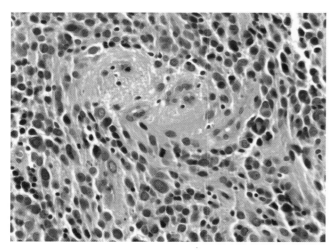

FIGURE 44.5 Readily identifiable mitotic activity is observed in this tumor.

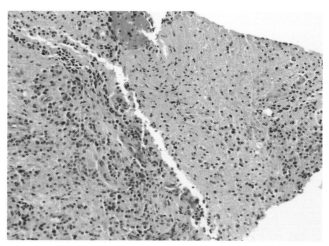

FIGURE 44.6 Focal necrosis is present in the neoplasm.

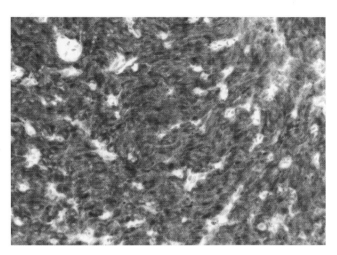

FIGURE 44.7 Diffuse synaptophysin immunoreactivity is present in this tumor.

References

1. MacKenzie IR. Central neurocytoma: histologic atypia, proliferation potential, and clinical outcome. Cancer 1999;85:1606–10.

2. Rades D, Schild SE, Fehlauer F. Prognostic value of the MIB-1 labeling index for central neurocytomas. Neurology 2004;62:987–9.

3. Soylemezoglu F, Scheithauer BW, Esteve J, et al. Atypical central neurocytoma. J Neuropathol Exp Neurol 1997;56:551–6.

Case 45: Extraventricular Neurocytoma

CLINICAL INFORMATION

The patient is a 27-year-old female who is found to have papilledema following work-up for headaches. An MRI scan shows a large left parieto-occipital cyst with an enhancing mural nodule. She undergoes complete gross total excision of the lesion.

OPINION

Sections show a calcified, cytologically bland, moderately hypercellular neoplasm, devoid of necrosis or microvascular proliferation. Numerous hyalinized blood vessels are present throughout the tumor, as is focal hemosiderin pigment. The tumor demonstrates diffuse positive staining, with synaptophysin antibody.

We consider the lesion to be a low-grade neurocytic tumor and characterize it as follows: **Left**

Parieto-Occipital Region, Excision–Extraventricular Neurocytoma, WHO Grade II.

COMMENT

Given the fact that this tumor did not occur within the ventricular system, this neoplasm—which is otherwise histologically identical to central neurocytoma—would be considered an extraventricular neurocytoma. The cystic nature is apparent only on the neuroimaging studies, because the pathologist receives the solid mural nodule portion of the tumor.

DISCUSSION

Extraventricular neurocytoma is a new entity in the 2007 World Health Organization classification system. Although both central neurocytoma and extraventricular neurocytoma are composed of

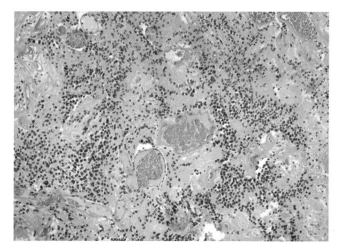

FIGURE 45.1 Lower-magnification appearance of the tumor, demonstrating moderate hypercellularity, hyalinized blood vessels, and vague orientation of tumor cells around blood vessels.

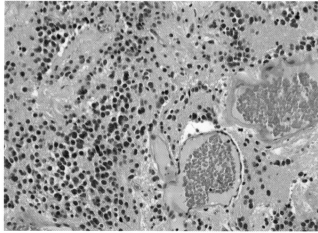

FIGURE 45.2 Intermediate magnification shows the neuropil-like fibrillary background, as well as the slight variability in size of tumor nuclei.

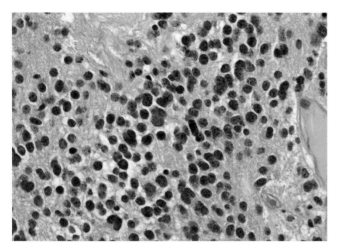

FIGURE 45.3 High-power magnification depicts the salt-and-pepper chromatin pattern of the nuclei and scant cytoplasm.

"uniform round cells that show immunohistochemical and ultrastructural features of neuronal differentiation" (Figarella-Branger et al.), the term "central" neurocytoma is restricted to tumors lying within an intracerebral ventricle, usually the lateral ventricle. Both are WHO grade II neoplasms. Extraventricular neurocytoma may be solid or show a cyst with a mural nodule, as did this case. Tumors are variably contrast-enhancing, and some examples show limited infiltration of tumor cells into adjacent brain.

Making the diagnosis rests on recognizing the monotony of the tumor cells, delicate background fibrillar matrix simulating neuropil, and nuclei with a salt-and-pepper chromatin pattern and scant cytoplasm. The tumor may show intersecting vessels paralleling an endocrine tumor, calcifications, anuclear areas containing delicate fibrillary tumor processes simulating a large rosette, or even perivascular arrangement of tumor cells. Extraventricular neurocytomas are more likely to contain large or intermediate-sized ganglion cells than are central neurocytomas and may be less densely cellular. Suboptimal tissue preservation may even yield perinuclear haloes around the tumor cells. Not surprisingly, oligodendroglioma and ependymoma almost always enter the differential diagnosis.

Application of the immunohistochemical marker synaptophysin clarifies that the tumor is composed of cells with neuronal lineage. Immunostaining is usually strong and diffuse, with maximal immunoreactivity in the anuclear fibrillary zones. The nuclear neuronal marker NeuN is also usually positive. Most cases of extraventricular neurocytoma manifest low mitotic rate and low MIB-1 labeling index.

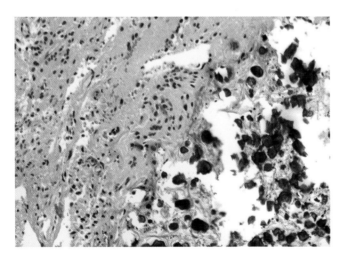

FIGURE 45.4 Calcifications are seen in one-third to one-half of cases of extraventricular neurocytomas.

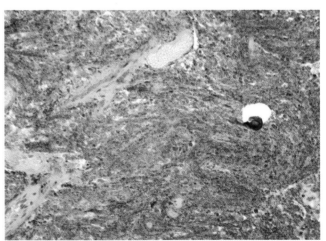

FIGURE 45.5 Strong immunoreactivity for synaptophysin is necessary to distinguish the tumor from an oligodendroglioma or ependymoma.

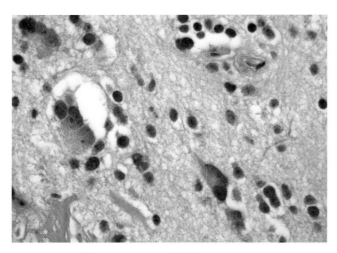

FIGURE 45.6 Many extraventricular neurocytomas contain larger ganglion cells.

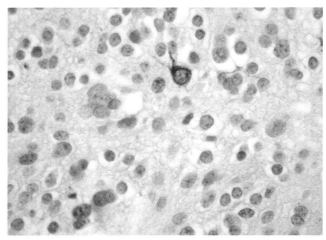

FIGURE 45.7 Anti-neurofilament immunostaining of the scattered individual ganglion cells highlights their neuritic processes.

References

1. Brat DJ, Parisi JE, Kleinschmidt-DeMasters BK, et al. Neuropathology Committee, College of American Pathologists. Surgical neuropathology update: a review of changes introduced by the WHO classification of tumours of the central nervous system, 4th edition. Arch Pathol Lab Med 2008;132:993–1007.
2. Brat DJ, Scheithauer BW, Eberhart CG, et al. Extraventricular neurocytomas. Pathologic features and clinical outcome. Am J Surg Pathol 2001;25:1252–60.
3. Figarella-Branger D, Söylemezoglu, Burger PC. Central neurocytoma and extraventricular neurocytoma. In: Louis DN, Ohgaki H, Wiestler OD, Cavenee WK, Editors. WHO Classification of Tumours of the Central Nervous System. Lyon, FR: IARC Press; 2007. p. 106–9.

Case 46: Paraganglioma

CLINICAL INFORMATION

The patient is a 52-year-old male who presents with a history of progressively increasing lower back pain and sciatica. Imaging of the spinal cord shows a partially cystic, isointense mass in the cauda equina region of the cord on MR imaging. The patient undergoes gross total resection of the mass, and histologic sections are reviewed.

OPINION

Histologic sections of the neoplasm are marked by a proliferation of generally rounded cells. The cells are focally arranged in loose nests, separated by delicate capillaries. Cells have a clear to lightly eosinophilic cytoplasm and nuclei with a salt-and-pepper chromatin pattern. Scattered evidence of nuclear pleomorphism is also noted. The bulk of the tumor cells demonstrate positive staining, with antibodies to chromogranin and neuron-specific enolase. A smaller population of elongated cells at the periphery of the lobules demonstrate S-100 protein immunoreactivity. The tumor does not stain with antibody to GFAP.

We consider the lesion to be a neuroendocrine neoplasm and characterize it as follows: **Cauda Equina Region, Excision—Paraganglioma, WHO Grade I.**

COMMENT

The nested architectural pattern of the tumor and its immunohistochemical profile support a diagnosis of paraganglioma.

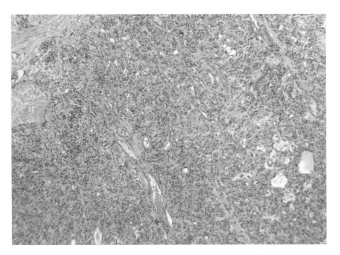

FIGURE 46.1 A solid-appearing architectural pattern is present in this paraganglioma; the zellballen or nested pattern may not be always readily observable on hematoxylin-eosin stained sections.

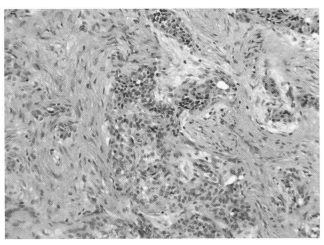

FIGURE 46.2 An area of fibrosis is seen in the tumor, with an entrapped nerve twig.

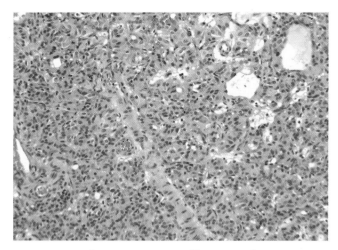

FIGURE 46.3 A prominent capillary vascular pattern is present.

DISCUSSION

Paragangliomas associated with the spinal cord are similar to those that have been described elsewhere in the body. They typically are encapsulated, somewhat well-circumscribed masses that are most commonly encountered in the filum terminale region. Rare cases have been noted to arise in association with nerve roots or in the sellar and suprasellar areas. Most patients are adults at the time of presentation.

Histologically, the tumors are marked by classic nested architectural pattern (zellballen). Occasionally, tumors may have a solid appearance, where nesting is not readily evident, or a trabecular architecture. Scattered pleomorphic nuclei may be observable. Cells generally have a salt-and-pepper chromatin pattern and a variable amount of lightly eosinophilic cytoplasm. Occasional ganglionic cells may be observable in the tumor. By immunohistochemistry, the tumor demonstrates immunoreactivity, with antibodies to chromogranin and synaptophysin. Sustentacular cells, usually located around the perimeter of the cell nests, demonstrate immunoreactivity with antibody to S-100 protein and may demonstrate some positive staining, with antibody to GFAP. Most tumors are quite amenable to surgical resection and have a good prognosis, although recurrence may occur in subtotally resected neoplasms.

Differential diagnostic considerations often involve other tumors commonly arising in the filum terminale region, which include myxopapillary ependymoma, schwannoma, and ependymoma. Schwannomas generally lack a nested architectural pattern, demonstrate diffuse positive staining, with antibody to S-100

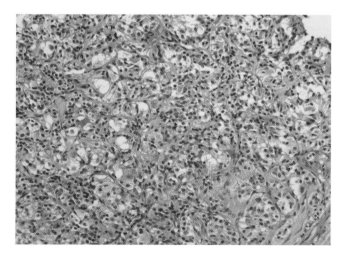

FIGURE 46.4 Intermediate magnification, showing cells with lightly eosinophilic-to-clear cytoplasm.

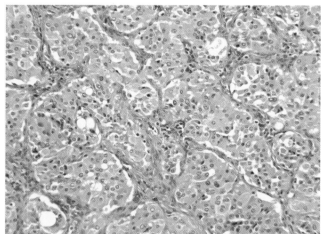

FIGURE 46.5 Eosinophilic cytoplasm is seen in cells arranged in a nested, or zellballen, architectural pattern.

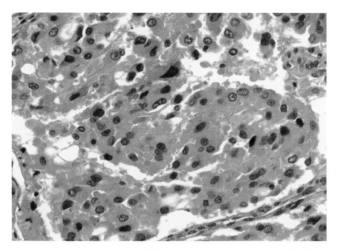

FIGURE 46.6 High magnification, showing scattered pleomorphic nuclei and salt-and-pepper nuclear chromatin pattern.

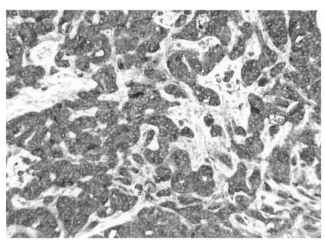

FIGURE 46.7 Neuron-specific enolase positivity is observed in a paraganglioma.

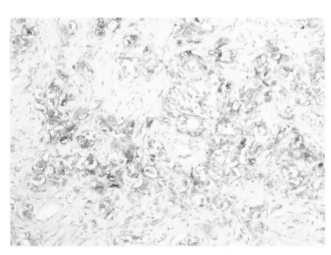

FIGURE 46.8 Positive staining with antibody to chromogranin is characteristic of paraganglioma.

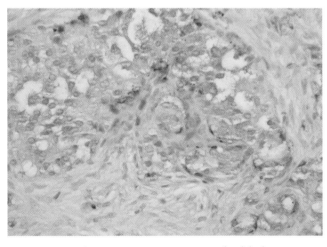

FIGURE 46.9 S-100 immunoreactivity highlights sustentacular cells, primarily situated around the edge of the zellballen nests.

protein, and generally do not stain with antibodies such as chromogranin and neuron-specific enolase. Similarly, diffuse immunoreactivity, with antibody to GFAP, is observable in myxopapillary ependymomas and low-grade ependymomas. Ependymal neoplasms lack immunoreactivity with antibodies such as chromogranin. Rosettes and pseudorosettes that mark ependymomas and the mucin-positive microcystic areas of myxopapillary ependymoma are not features of paraganglioma.

References

1. Aggarwal S, Deck JH, Kucharczyk W. Neuroendocrine tumor (paraganglioma) of the cauda equina: MR and pathologic findings. Am J Neuroradiol 1993;14:1003–7.
2. Moran CA, Rush W, Mena H. Primary spinal paragangliomas: a clinicopathologic and immunohistochemical study of 30 cases. Histopathology 1997;31:167–73.
3. Sonneland PR, Scheithauer BW, LeChago J, et al. Paraganglioma of the cauda equina region. Clinicopathologic study of 31 cases with special reference to immunocytology and ultrastructure. Cancer 1986;58:1720–35.

CLINICAL INFORMATION

The patient is a 57-year-old female with a long history of intermittent headaches who recently develops nausea, vomiting, and paralysis of upward gaze. CT and MRI scanning demonstrates a noninvasive, well-circumscribed, homogeneously enhancing mass in the pineal region, measuring approximately 4 cm in greatest diameter. Histologic sections from the resection specimen are available for review.

OPINION

Sections demonstrate a lobulated mass composed of expanded nests of tumor cells within an anastomosing network of thin-walled blood vessels, with variable adventitial proliferation. Portions of the tumor demonstrate an admixture of moderately pleomorphic tumor cells and relatively abundant fibrillary matrix, with the formation of oversized Homer Wright-type rosettes ("pineocytomatous rosettes"). Other regions of the tumor show oversized nests of unipolar cells generating a delicate fibrillary matrix, demarcated by prominent fibrovascular septae containing chronic inflammatory cells and adventitial proliferation. Mitotic figures are inconspicuous, and coagulative tumor necrosis is not identified.

We consider the lesion to be a pineal tumor and characterize it as follows: **Pineal Region, Removal—Pineocytoma, WHO Grade I.**

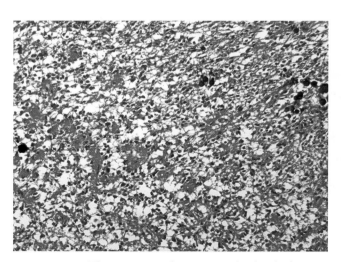

FIGURE 47.1 The non-neoplastic pineal gland demonstrates nests of neuroendocrine cells within a delicate vascular stroma containing microcalcifications.

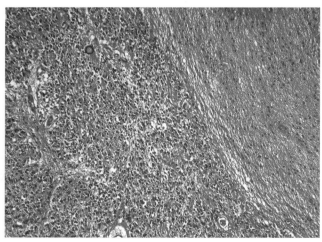

FIGURE 47.2 Glial cyst of the pineal gland with compression of the pineal parenchyma, giving the appearance of hypercellularity, but without the architectural distortion and stromal reaction seen within true pineal parenchymal tumors.

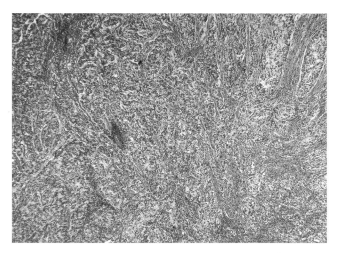

FIGURE 47.3 Low magnification view of expanded lobular architecture comprising pineocytoma. A perivascular lymphocytic infiltrate is present near the center of the photograph.

DISCUSSION

Pineal region tumors in adults are unusual and consist predominately of meningiomas and astrocytic tumors. Pineal parenchymal tumors are rare lesions in adults but consist nearly exclusively of WHO grade I pineocytomas. These tumors consist of expanded nests of cells resembling those of the normal pineal, as well as regions containing diagnostic pineocytomatous

rosettes. The latter resemble Homer Wright rosettes, seen in primitive tumors containing neuroblastic differentiation, except that, in the case of pineocytomatous rosettes, there is a greater amount of fibrillary matrix, and the surrounding tumor nuclei are not mitotically active. The presence of these rosettes, in combination with the absence of primitive neuroectodermal tumor-like differentiation, is highly predictive of benign (WHO grade I) behavior, without risk of leptomeningeal dissemination, and long postoperative survivals, even in patients with subtotal resections. Analogous to "ancient change," described in schwannomas, pineocytomas may contain regions demonstrating marked nuclear enlargement and hyperchromasia. When these changes occupy significant portions of the tumor, some authors refer to them as pleomorphic pineocytomas. Similar to schwannomas, the presence and degree of nuclear pleomorphism do not adversely affect the expected benign behavior of these tumors.

Although current neuroimaging techniques have reduced the number of pineal region biopsies in patients with glial cysts of the pineal (pineal

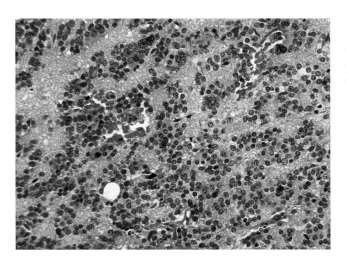

FIGURE 47.4 High magnification view of the upper left region of the previous figure demonstrates pineocytomatous rosettes.

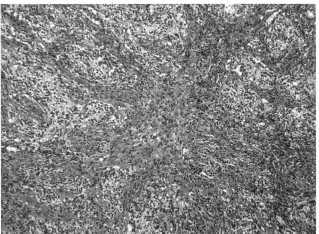

FIGURE 47.5 Expanded nests of neuroendocrine-type cells within a proliferative fibrovascular stroma containing chronic inflammatory cells and adventitial fibroblastic proliferation, are present.

cysts), it is important to be familiar with the appearance of chronically compressed, non-neoplastic pineal parenchyma, in order to avoid the overdiagnosis of tumor in patients who undergo biopsy for an atypical-appearing pineal region cyst. When portions of a pineal cyst are included in biopsy specimens, they are distinguished by the presence of geographic region of fibrillary glial matrix containing Rosenthal fibers, which may be abundant.

References

1. Fakhran S, Escott EJ. Pineocytoma mimicking a pineal cyst on imaging: true diagnostic dilemma or a case of incomplete imaging? AJNR Am J Neuroradiol 2008;29:159–63.

2. Fèvre-Montange M, Szathmari A, Champier J, et al. Pineocytoma and pineal parenchymal tumors of intermediate differentiation presenting cytologic pleomorphism: a multi-center study. Brain Pathol 2008;18:354–9.

3. Lekovic GP, Gonzalez LF, Shetter AG, et al. Role of gamma knife surgery in the management of pineal region tumors. Neurosurg Focus 2007;23:E12.

Case 48: Pineal Parenchymal Tumor of Intermediate Differentiation

CLINICAL INFORMATION

The patient is a 46-year-old male who presents with progressively increasing headaches for several months. An MRI scan is obtained and shows an approximately 2.5-cm midline pineal mass that homogeneously enhances. The differential diagnosis includes meningioma versus pineal tumor. Because of the increasing headaches, the patient is felt to be a candidate for surgical resection. Sections are available for review.

OPINION

Biopsies show a hypercellular, lobulated tumor, composed of aggregates of small blue cells with high nuclear-to-cytoplasmic ratio. Lobules are demarcated by a delicate vasculature devoid of microvascular proliferation; the appearance simulates an endocrine tumor. There are no fibrillar, anuclear zones or large pineocytomatous rosettes. Neither necrosis nor mitotic activity is present. Cytologically, the cells show hyperchromatic nuclei, indistinct nucleoli, and near-absence of cytoplasm.

We consider the pathology to be that of a pineal parenchymal tumor, albeit lacking the features of either a classic pineocytoma or pineoblastoma. We characterize this tumor with intermediate features as follows: **Pineal Gland, Excision—Pineal Parenchymal Tumor of Intermediate Differentiation, WHO Grade II–III.**

COMMENT

Pineal parenchymal tumor of intermediate differentiation (PPTID) occupies a position intermediate between pineocytoma, a WHO grade I tumor usually found in adults, and pineoblastoma, a WHO grade IV

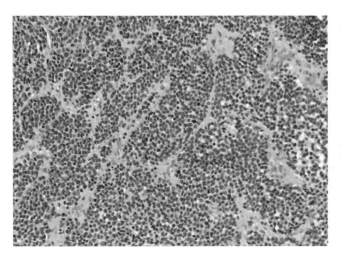

FIGURE 48.1 Low power shows a lobulated tumor devoid of necrosis with lobules defined by delicate vasculature.

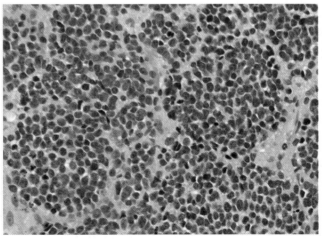

FIGURE 48.2 Higher power shows that the tumor cells possess stippled hyperchromatic nuclei, scant cytoplasm, and rare-to-absent mitoses.

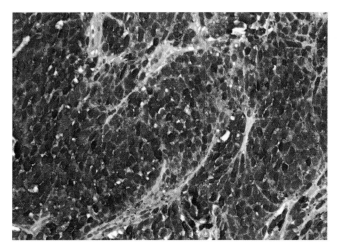

FIGURE 48.3 Strong immunostaining for neuron-specific enolase is present.

tumor usually found in children. Most patients with PPTID are adults. Definite grading criteria to establish whether PPTID should be given a WHO grade II or III designation have not been formally established.

DISCUSSION

Given the rarity of all pineal parenchymal tumors and the often small size of the biopsies obtained from this region, the first goal of the pathologist on a biopsy

from the pineal region is to exclude a metastasis to the pineal/tectal plate region, primary central nervous system germ cell tumor (especially germinoma), and a pineal cyst with adjacent normal pineal gland. Once the diagnosis of pineal parenchymal tumor is established, the next goal is to make a distinction between pineocytoma (WHO grade I), pineal parenchymal tumor of intermediate differentiation (PPTID) (WHO grade II–III), and pineoblastoma (WHO grade IV), because the former is treated by surgical excision alone, and pineoblastoma is treated with radiation and chemotherapy. The PPTID has variable behavior; in general, however, outcome of PPTID is closer to that of pineocytoma than to that of pineoblastoma.

PPTID is the most frequent type of pineal parenchymal tumor, constituting over half of all cases in some series and showing higher frequency than either pineocytoma or pineoblastoma. Several different histological patterns exist. The least frequent is a truly mixed, biphasic tumor, with discrete areas of pineocytoma adjacent to areas of pure pineoblastoma.

More commonly, PPTID has intermediate histologic features. Unlike pineocytoma, PPTID lacks true

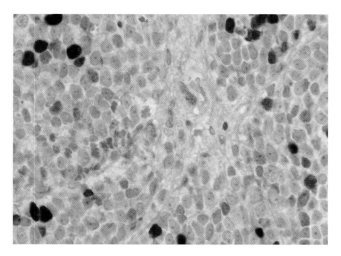

FIGURE 48.4 Strong immunostaining for synaptophysin establishes a neuronal lineage of PPTID and aids in excluding other diagnostic considerations.

FIGURE 48.5 A MIB-1 labeling index is generally 10% or less in PPTID.

rosettes and anuclear fibrillar zones. Unlike pineoblastoma, the tumor lacks brisk mitotic activity or high cell cycle labeling indices. PPTID may either have a diffuse, sheetlike architecture or manifest lobules demarcated by delicate vasculature. Immunostaining for synaptophysin and neuron-specific enolase (NSE) is seen in virtually all pineal parenchymal tumors, albeit with a lower intensity in the higher-grade tumors (pineoblastoma). Chromogranin A and neurofilament staining usually parallel each other and are strongest in pineocytoma (especially in the pineocytomatous rosettes and ganglion cells), variable in PPTID (see the following), and negligible in pineoblastoma. Thus, immunostaining appears to parallel degree of neuronal differentiation in these tumors.

Grading of PPTID has not been established. The largest study to date is that of Jouvet et al., who studied 66 pineal parenchymal tumors accrued over a 23-year time span from 12 centers in France and England. They were able to divide PPTIDs into two subtypes and proposed criteria for grades II versus III, depending on the number of mitoses and whether immunostaining for neurofilaments could be identified (Jouvet et al.). Grade II PPTID had strong immunolabeling for neurofilaments and less than 6 mitoses per 10 HPFs (40X objective), whereas grade III PPTIDs were lobulated or diffuse tumors with either 6 or more mitoses per 10 HPFs or tumors with fewer than 6 mitoses/10 HPFs but no immunostaining for neurofilaments. These criteria have yet to be validated by other studies.

References

1. Jouvet A, Saint-Pierre G, Fauchon F, et al. Pineal parenchymal tumors: a correlation of histological features with prognosis in 66 cases. Brain Pathol 2000;10:49–60.
2. Nakazato Y, Jouvet A, Scheithauer BW. Pineal parenchymal tumour of intermediate differentiation. In: Louis DN, Ohgaki H, Wiestler OD, Cavenee WK, Editors. WHO Classification of Tumours of the Central Nervous System. Lyon, FR: IARC Press; 2007. p. 124–5.
3. Senft C, Raabe A, Hattingen E, et al. Pineal parenchymal tumor of intermediate differentiation: diagnostic pitfalls and discussion of treatment options of a rare tumor entity. Neurosurg Rev 2008;31:231–6.

Case 49: Pineoblastoma

CLINICAL INFORMATION

This 6-year-old male was brought to the emergency room with persistent vomiting. Further questioning elicits a history of intermittent headaches over the past several months. Physical exam reveals Parinaud syndrome (paralysis of upward gaze with light-near dissociation). Neuroimaging shows a 4-cm, heterogeneously enhancing mass within the pineal region, with associated hydrocephalus involving the lateral and third ventricles. The patient undergoes emergency third ventriculostomy, with endoscopic biopsy of the pineal region mass, which is reviewed.

OPINION

Examination of the intraoperative crush preparation discloses a primitive neuroectodermal tumor, composed of cells with moderately pleomorphic and hyperchromatic nuclei, accompanied by indistinct amounts of cytoplasm. Mitotic figures are easily identified. The permanent section slide demonstrates nests of these primitive neuroectodermal cells, separated by anastomosing fibrovascular stromal elements. Neither true rosettes nor perivascular pseudorosettes are identified within the available tissue.

We consider the lesion to represent a primitive neuroectodermal tumor of the pineal gland and characterize it as follows: **Pineal Region, Endoscopic Biopsy—Pineoblastoma, WHO Grade IV.**

DISCUSSION

Although pineoblastomas (or pinealoblastomas) are rare tumors, they comprise approximately 50%

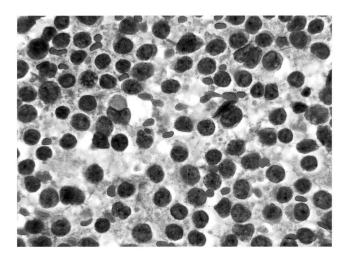

FIGURE 49.1 Intraoperative crush preparation discloses a discohesive sea of hyperchromatic, moderately pleomorphic, mitotically active primitive cells.

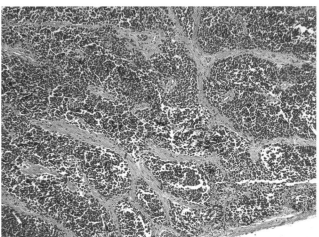

FIGURE 49.2 Low-magnification hematoxylin- and eosin-stained section demonstrates expanded nests of primitive tumor cells, delineated by fibrovascular septae.

147

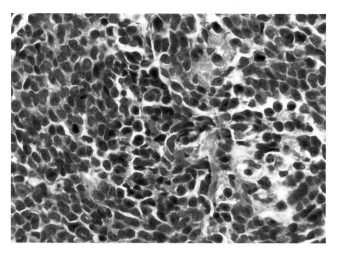

FIGURE 49.3 Densely hypercellular sheets of mitotically active cells, with enlarged hyperchromatic pleomorphic nuclei and indistinct cytoplasm, are seen. Single cell necrosis is readily identified. Neither true nor pseudorosettes are present.

of pineal parenchymal tumors. In addition, they are one of the most common pineal region tumors seen in the first decade of life, second in incidence only to nongerminomatous germ cell tumors, especially immature teratoma. Because of their rarity, they are often included in studies of supratentorial primitive neuroectodermal tumors. However, evidence indicates that pineoblastomas, particularly those seen in children over the age of 3 years, may have a more favorable prognosis and thus should be considered as distinct from a non-pineal region primitive neuroectodermal tumors. Similar to other central nervous system primitive neuroectodermal tumors, pineoblastomas demonstrate a propensity to differentiate long neuronal and glial lineages. However, they may also, on occasion, demonstrate photosensory differentiation (Flexner-Wintersteiner rosettes, fleurettes), similar to retinoblastomas, and often comprise the intracranial component of trilateral retinoblastoma.

Recent studies have demonstrated favorable outcome in children older than 3 years of age at presentation, especially with gross total resection, followed by craniospinal radiation and multiagent chemotherapy.

References

1. Cuccia V, Rodríguez F, Palma F, et al. Pinealoblastomas in children. Childs Nerv Syst 2006;22:577–85.
2. Gilheeney SW, Saad A, Chi S, et al. Outcome of pediatric pineoblastoma after surgery, radiation and chemotherapy. J Neurooncol 2008;89:89–95.
3. Hinkes BG, von Hoff K, Deinlein F, et al. Childhood pineoblastoma: experiences from the prospective multicenter trials HIT-SKK87, HIT-SKK92 and HIT91. J Neurooncol 2007;81:217–23.

Case 50: Yolk Sac Tumor of the Pineal Gland

CLINICAL INFORMATION

The patient is a 17-year-old male who presents with headaches. On imaging, he is noted to have a small mass situated in the pineal gland. A biopsy is performed, and histologic sections reviewed.

OPINION

Histologic sections contain fragments of an epithelioid tumor. The neoplasm is characterized by ribbons and cords of cells and cystic spaces, resembling a vitelline pattern. The cells are somewhat homogeneous in appearance, contain small amounts of eosinophilic cytoplasm, and lack prominent nucleolation. Rare mitotic figures are observed. Eosinophilic droplets are not noted. Focal positive staining with antibody to alpha fetoprotein (AFP) is noted.

We consider the lesion to be a germ cell neoplasm and characterize it as follows: **Pineal Gland, Biopsy— Yolk Sac Tumor (Endodermal Sinus Tumor).**

COMMENT

AFP immunoreactivity supports the diagnosis of yolk sac tumor. Other germ cell tumor components are not identified.

DISCUSSION

Intracranial germ cell tumors are generally midline lesions that arise most commonly in the region of the pineal gland or suprasellar area. There is a male predilection for development of these tumors. Symptomatology may be related to resulting hydrocephalus, Parinaud syndrome (paralysis of upper gaze and conversion related to compression and invasion of the tectal plate), pituitary

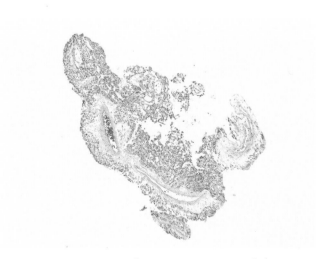

FIGURE 50.1 Low-magnification appearance of the entire biopsy, showing a loose arrangement of cells around blood vessels.

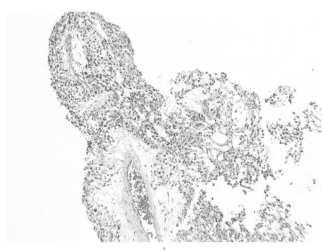

FIGURE 50.2 Higher-magnification, highlighting solid foci, ribbons, and cords of tumor cells adjacent to blood vessels.

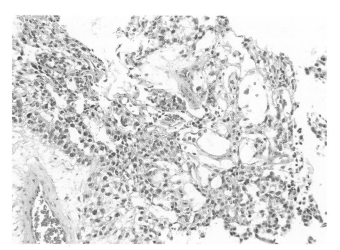

FIGURE 50.3 Intermediate magnification, highlighting the microcystic areas in the tumor.

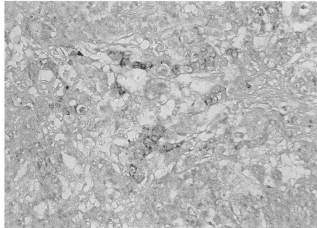

FIGURE 50.4 Focal AFP immunoreactivity confirms the diagnosis of yolk sac tumor.

failure, visual field defects in perioptic chiasmal tumors, and precocious puberty. Imaging appearances can be quite variable and somewhat dependent on the components of the neoplasm. Blood and the cerebrospinal fluid-elevated levels of HCG (beta-human chorionic gonadotrophin), CEA (carcinoembryonic antigen), and AFP may provide clues to the diagnosis and to possible components of the tumor.

The most commonly encountered pattern of intracranial germ cell tumor is germinoma. The tumors may be pure or contain multiple germ cell tumor elements (mixed cell tumors). Yolk sac tumor, or endodermal sinus tumor, is an epithelioid neoplasm in which cells are arranged in sheets, ribbons, cords, or papillae. Areas of the tumor have a loose microcystic appearance, resulting in what is described as a vitelline pattern. Schiller-Duval bodies, if present, are diagnostic; these structures are marked by vessels surrounded by tumor cells projecting into a clear

space also lined by tumor cells. Also, a useful diagnostic clue is the presence of eosinophilic droplets, which stain with Periodic acid-Schiff (PAS). Antibody to AFP can be useful in confirming the diagnosis.

The prognosis is dependent on the components of the germ cells neoplasm, with germinomas being very radiosensitive, and along with teratomas, generally associated with a good prognosis. Yolk sac tumors, along with choriocarcinomas and embryonal carcinomas, tend to behave in a more aggressive fashion.

References

1. Bjornsson J, Scheithauer BW, Okasaki, H, et al. Intracranial germ cell tumors: pathobiological and immunohistochemical aspects of 70 cases. J Neuropathol Exp Neurol 1985;44:32–46.
2. Ho DM, Liutt C. Primary intracranial germ cell tumor. Pathologic study of 51 patients. Cancer 1992;70:1577–1784.
3. Rueda P, Heifetz SA, Sesterhenn IA, et al. Primary intracranial germ cell tumors in the first two decades of life. A clinical, light-microscopic, and immunohistochemical analysis of 54 cases. Perspect Pediatr Pathol 1987;10:160–207.

Case 51: Supratentorial Primitive Neuroectodermal Tumor

CLINICAL INFORMATION

This 3-year-old girl is brought to the hospital because of concerns regarding increased sleepiness and bed-wetting. Physical examination discloses bilateral papilledema, and routine laboratory studies indicate diabetes insipidus. Neuroimaging discloses a large suprasellar mass, with evidence of recent hemorrhage. She is taken to the operating room emergently for surgical resection. The histologic sections are reviewed.

OPINION

The histologic sections confirm the radiographic suspicion of recent hemorrhage, with extravasation of red blood cells showing early autolytic features. The tumor itself is composed of primitive-appearing cells with hyperchromatic nuclei. Structures reminiscent of perivascular pseudorosettes are apparent at low power. However, at higher magnification, the perivascular fibrillary material does not show the radiating pattern expected for perivascular pseudorosettes. Immunohistochemical staining demonstrates immunoreactivity of the tumor cells with both synaptophysin and GFAP. Many of the perivascular regions remain unstained. However, those that demonstrate immunoreactivity are decorated only by synaptophysin antibodies, not antibodies directed against glial filaments.

We consider this lesion to represent a primitive neuroectodermal tumor of the suprasellar region and characterized as follows: **Suprasellar Region, Removal—Primitive Neuroectodermal Tumor, WHO Grade IV.**

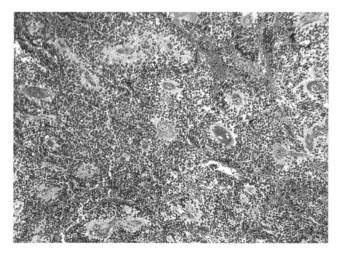

FIGURE 51.1 Low-magnification view shows an embryonal type of tumor with evidence of recent hemorrhage and perivascular rosetting.

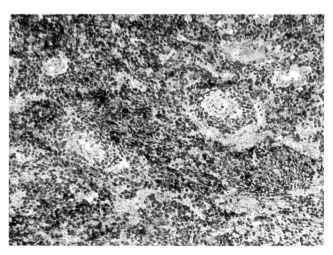

FIGURE 51.2 Synaptophysin immunohistochemical staining labels many of the primitive tumor cells.

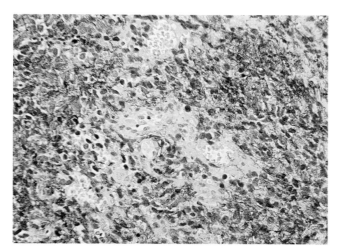

FIGURE 51.3 GFAP immunoreactivity is strongly positive within clusters and sheets of primitive tumor cells. Perivascular regions are unstained.

COMMENT

Immunohistochemical stains with antibodies directed against synaptophysin and GFAP react with primitive tumor cells, consistent with divergent differentiation.

DISCUSSION

As the name implies, supratentorial primitive neuroectodermal tumors are among embryonal central nervous system tumors occurring in the cerebral compartment. Although older studies combined pineoblastomas with other supratentorial primitive neuroectodermal tumors, recently elucidated differences in the behavior of these tumors has led to narrowing of the category of supratentorial primitive neuroectodermal tumors to those occurring within the cerebral hemispheres or suprasellar region. Histologically and immunohistochemically, these tumors resemble the primitive pineal parenchymal tumor, in that they are composed of poorly differentiated neuroepithelial cells that may show divergent differentiation along neuronal and glial cell lineages. Supratentorial primitive neuroectodermal tumors are rare (approximately 2.5% of childhood brain tumors) and occur within early childhood, demonstrating a peak incidence within the first 3 years of life. They most commonly present with symptoms and signs of increased intracranial pressure, as well as focal neurologic deficits dependent on anatomical localization. Disseminated disease at presentation is seen in a minority of patients (approximately 20%), with these patients having an even poorer rate of survival in some

FIGURE 51.4 High-magnification view demonstrates both hyperchromatic pleomorphic primitive tumor cells and perivascular rarefaction, composed of processes resembling those seen with neuroblastic differentiation.

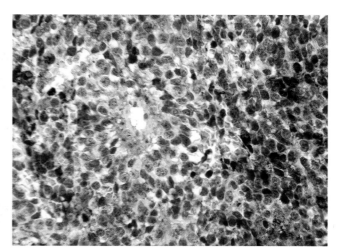

FIGURE 51.5 High-power review of the synaptophysin immunostained section demonstrates strong labeling of tumor cells, accompanied by weak but definite activity within perivascular regions.

studies. The overall 5-year survival for children with supratentorial primitive neuroectodermal tumors is approximately 25%, which is much poorer than that for medulloblastomas. Similar to other primitive tumors of the nervous system, survival is improved by aggressive adjuvant therapy (and, therefore, in children old enough to tolerate such therapy). Supratentorial primitive neuroectodermal tumors demonstrate a second age peak around 30 years, with a similarly dismal prognosis.

In all age groups, neuroimaging tends to demonstrate heterogeneously enhancing masses containing cysts, calcification, necrosis, and hemorrhage. The roles of complete versus partial resection, as well as potential relevance of genetic analyses, are still under investigation in this rare neoplasm.

References

1. Biswas S, Burke A, Cherian S, et al. Non-pineal supratentorial primitive neuroectodermal tumors (sPNET) in teenagers and young adults: Time to reconsider cisplatin-based chemotherapy after cranio-spinal irradiation? Pediatr Blood Cancer 2009;52:796–803.
2. Johnston DL, Keene DL, Lafay-Cousin L, et al. Supratentorial primitive neuroectodermal tumors: a Canadian pediatric brain tumor consortium report. J Neurooncol 2008;86:101–8.
3. Ohba S, Yoshida K, Hirose Y, et al. A supratentorial primitive neuroectodermal tumor in an adult: a case report and review of the literature. J Neurooncol 2008;86:217–24.

Case 52: Classic Medulloblastoma

CLINICAL INFORMATION

The patient is a 6-year-old boy who presents with an approximately 1 year of episodic vomiting, with increased frequency over the past few months. The patient also reports episodic headache, and over the last two months, he has developed ataxia. Physical exam reveals bilateral papilledema and truncal ataxia. Neuroimaging shows a large fourth ventricular tumor with noncommunicating hydrocephalus. Histopathologic sections from the resection specimen are reviewed.

OPINION

Sections demonstrate expansive sheets of primitive tumor cells, typical of the "small round blue cell tumors" of childhood. Careful examination disclosed regions of slightly decreased cellularity, accompanied by increased extracellular matrix reminiscent of intestinal Peyer's patches, as well as areas within the tumor demonstrating classic Homer Wright rosettes. Immunohistochemical stains for synaptophysin and neurofilaments confirm the identity of the Homer Wright rosettes. Immunohistochemical staining for GFAP highlights obviously reactive-appearing astrocytes throughout most of the tumor, with rare foci demonstrating immunoreactivity within less well-developed clusters of somewhat atypical-appearing cells.

We consider the lesion to be an embryonal tumor and characterize it as follows: **Fourth Ventricle, Removal—Medulloblastoma, WHO Grade IV.**

COMMENT

Homer Wright rosettes are identified, consistent with primitive neuroblastic differentiation. GFAP

FIGURE 52.1 Low magnification demonstrates a sea of nuclei without apparent cytoplasm or intervening stroma (the "small round blue cell tumor").

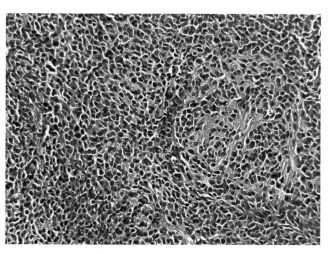

FIGURE 52.2 Nodular foci, demonstrating visible intervening eosinophilic cytoplasm resembling intestinal Peyer's patches.

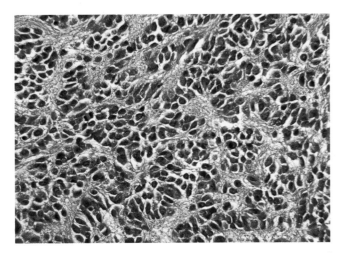

FIGURE 52.3 Classic Homer Wright rosettes, consisting of spherical arrangements of tumor cell nuclei around a fibrillary core, are present.

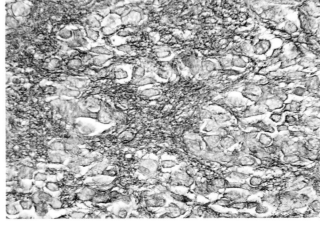

FIGURE 52.4 Immunohistochemical staining for nonphosphorylated neurofilaments establishes the fibrillary cores as primitive neuronal processes.

immunostaining discloses predominately reactive-appearing astrocytes, as well as a small focus of less well-differentiated cells, possibly representing astrocytic differentiation within the tumor.

DISCUSSION

Medulloblastomas are the most frequent malignant pediatric brain tumors and are particularly prevalent during the first decade of life. By definition, medulloblastomas arise within the cerebellum. Patients often remained asymptomatic until the tumor grows to a point where the circulation of cerebrospinal fluid is impaired, leading to hydrocephalus and increased intracranial pressure, with accompanying headaches and (often projectile) vomiting. When it becomes manifest, ataxia is often a late-presenting sign;

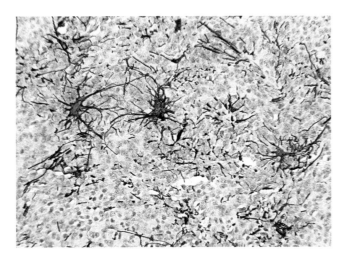

FIGURE 52.5 GFAP immunohistochemical staining demonstrates unmistakable reactive astrocytes throughout much of the primitive tumor.

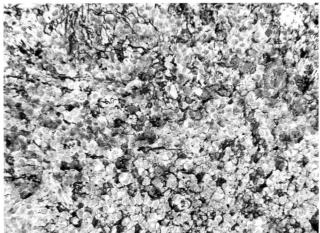

FIGURE 52.6 Rare foci within the tumor demonstrate GFAP labeling within less well-differentiated cells, consistent with true astrocytic differentiation within the tumor.

children with medulloblastomas have often undergone extensive and often repeated evaluation for gastrointestinal disease. Younger children in particular may present with nonlocalizing signs of irritability and failure to thrive. In these patients, early diagnosis may only be possible by careful funduscopic examination and/or neuroimaging.

Despite the status of medulloblastomas as WHO grade IV malignancies and the often protracted periods between symptom onset and surgical resection, current 5-year survivals for patients with classic medulloblastomas range from 70 to 80%. Unfortunately, doses of radiation therapy required for tumor control often result in significant physical and cognitive developmental impairments. Efforts are being made to utilize radiation-sparing protocols in patients with standard risk medulloblastomas, and therefore parallel efforts to define standard and even biologically indolent variants are ongoing. Currently, we recognize classic medulloblastomas as cerebellar primitive neuroectodermal tumors capable of divergent differentiation along neuroblastic and primitive astrocytic lineages. Homer Wright rosettes are indicative of primitive neuroblastic differentiation within medulloblastomas. Although distinctive in their appearance, they are seen in a minority of classic medulloblastomas, and then usually in small widely scattered foci. In the absence of desmoplasia and/or extensive nodularity, the presence of Homer Wright rosettes confers neither improved nor worsened prognosis. Astrocytic differentiation within medulloblastomas can be quite difficult to appreciate, because reactive astrocytes often show some degree of atypia, related to the adverse environment to which they are reacting. True astrocytic differentiation among tumor cells generally is seen in less than 5% of the neoplastic cells. Medulloblastomas demonstrating greater amounts of astrocytic differentiation may demonstrate more aggressive behavior and respond less well to chemotherapeutic regimens tailored toward primitive neuroectodermal tumors, although such tumors are sufficiently rare if they have not been systematically studied. Despite intensive efforts to define histopathologic, immunohistochemical, and molecular signatures related to biologic behavior, tumors not expressing histopathologic features excluding them from the classic medulloblastoma category have so far been resistant to all of our attempts at prognostication.

References

1. Fattet S, Haberler C, Legoix P, et al. Beta-catenin status in paediatric medulloblastomas: correlation of immunohistochemical expression with mutational status, genetic profiles, and clinical characteristics. J Pathol 2009;218:86–94.
2. Rossi A, Caracciolo V, Russo G, et al. Medulloblastoma: from molecular pathology to therapy. Clin Cancer Res 2008 Feb 15;14(4):971–6.
3. Takei H, Nguyen Y, Mehta V, et al. Low-level copy gain versus amplification of myconcogenes in medulloblastoma: utility in predicting prognosis and survival. Laboratory investigation. J Neurosurg Pediatr 2009;3:61–5.

CLINICAL INFORMATION

A 7-year-old healthy boy develops generalized headaches with intermittent vomiting. He then began experiencing difficulties with balance and coordination. A CT scan shows a large enhancing lesion in his posterior fossa, accompanied by hydrocephalus. A MRI discloses a 5-cm mass arising from the floor of the fourth ventricle. A gross total resection is accomplished, and the histologic sections are reviewed.

OPINION

Sections demonstrate a densely cellular tumor, punctuated by pale nodules containing similarly primitive-appearing cells disposed within a delicate fibrillary matrix, vaguely reminiscent of glomeruli within a primitive renal cortex. At higher power, a delicate neuropil-like appearance of the pale islands is appreciated. Tumor cells between the paler islands appear to stream in an Indian file-like pattern. Synaptophysin immunohistochemical staining is strongly reactive within the pale islands, but not within the intervening primitive-appearing tumor cells; whereas, reticulin histochemical staining demonstrates the opposite pattern, a prominent pericellular reticulin, surrounding primitive tumor cells between the synaptophysin positive pale islands. Ki-67 immunostaining labels the majority of the cells between pale islands and a much smaller proportion of those within the islands themselves.

We consider this tumor to be a medulloblastoma variant and characterize it as follows: **Posterior Fossa, Resection—Desmoplastic Medulloblastoma, WHO Grade IV.**

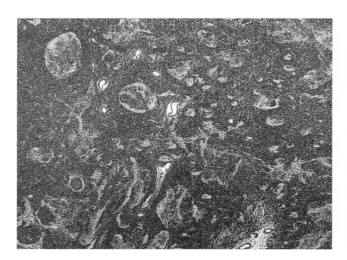

FIGURE 53.1 Low-magnification appearance demonstrates pale islands within a densely hypercellular tumor (vaguely reminiscent of glomeruli within the renal cortex).

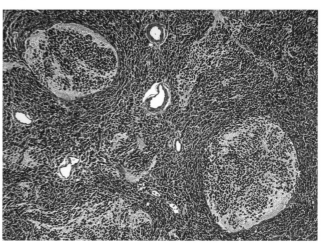

FIGURE 53.2 Pale islands stand out as sharply circumscribed regions of significantly lower cellularity and mitotic activity than the intervening primitive tumor cells.

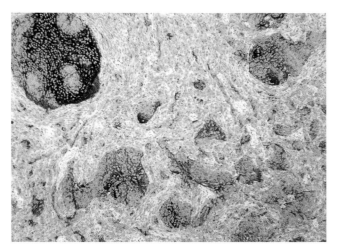

FIGURE 53.3 Synaptophysin immunostaining highlights nodular areas of reactivity corresponding to the pale islands seen on hematoxylin- and eosin-stained slides.

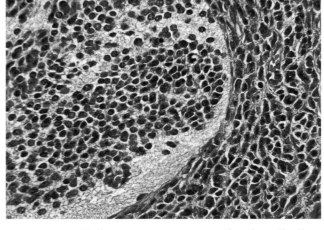

FIGURE 53.4 High power, contrasting the fine fibrillary matrix seen within the better differentiated islands with the subtle yet coarse reticulin network present within the intervening tumor.

DISCUSSION

First recognized as a primitive, yet firm cerebellar tumor that often occurred off the midline in somewhat older children, the desmoplastic medulloblastoma was initially designated as "cerebellar arachnoidal sarcoma." Since then, morphologic continuity with classical medulloblastoma and desmoplasia occurring in the absence of arachnoidal invasion have placed this tumor comfortably within the category of cerebellar medulloblastomas. Desmoplastic medulloblastomas demonstrate a somewhat biphasic age distribution, preferentially occurring both in the adolescent patients (often situated in the lateral lobes of the cerebellum)

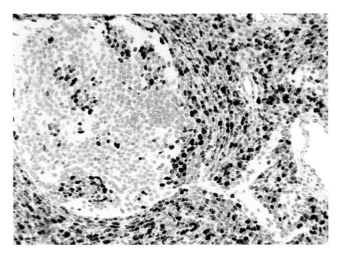

FIGURE 53.5 Ki-67 immunohistochemical staining demonstrates brisk reactivity in the undifferentiated regions of the tumor and sparse clusters of reactivity within the pale islands.

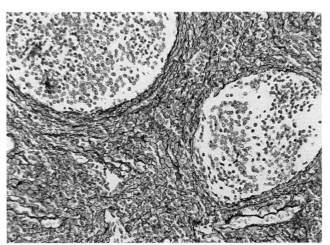

FIGURE 53.6 Reticulin histochemical staining shows a dominant pericellular network of reticulin (accounting for the firm consistency of the tumor) in which are disposed pale, reticulated, free islands of less densely cellular tumor.

and in the first few years of life, they may represent a presenting feature of the nevoid basal cell carcinoma syndrome. The nevoid basal cell carcinoma syndrome, also known as "Gorlin syndrome," is characterized by multiple basal cell carcinomas, odontogenic keratocysts of the jaws, hyperkeratosis of palms and soles, intracranial ectopic calcifications, and rib abnormalities (along with many other infrequently occurring developmental abnormalities and neoplasms). This syndrome results from mutations involving the PTCH1 gene on chromosome 9, which has subsequently also been demonstrated within both syndrome-associated and apparently sporadic desmoplastic medulloblastomas. Although specific therapy based on this molecular defect is not yet available, further investigations into the signaling pathways have provided information that may be useful in future therapeutic endeavors. Currently, desmoplasia within medulloblastomas does not appear to alter significantly the generally favorable prognosis of treated medulloblastomas.

References

1. Crawford JR, Rood BR, Rossi CT, et al. Medulloblastoma associated with novel PTCH mutation as primary manifestation of Gorlin syndrome. Neurology 2009;72:1618.

2. Kool M, Koster J, Bunt J, et al. Integrated genomics identifies five medulloblastoma subtypes with distinct genetic profiles, pathway signatures and clinicopathological features. PLoS ONE 28 2008;3:e3088.

3. McManamy CS, Pears J, Weston CL, et al. Nodule formation and desmoplasia in medulloblastomas-defining the nodular/desmoplastic variant and its biological behavior. Brain Pathol 2007;17:151–64.

Case 54: Medulloblastoma with Extensive Nodularity

CLINICAL INFORMATION

This 2-year-old boy comes to neurosurgical attention after extensive evaluation for delayed walking. A CT study shows a mass within the fourth ventricle. MRI scanning confirms the fourth ventricular mass, which demonstrates a lobulated appearance. Gross total resection is accomplished, and histologic sections are reviewed.

OPINION

Sections demonstrate large, anastomosing nodules of pale, moderately cellular islands, composed of monomorphous cells, with round moderately hyperchromatic nuclei, within a neuropil-like matrix. These nodules comprise the vast majority of cross-sectional areas on the permanent section slides and are separated by strands and islands of more primitive-appearing hyperchromatic neuroectodermal cells. The pale areas react strongly with antibodies to synaptophysin and nonphosphorylated neurofilaments, whereas the intervening primitive cells do not react with either antibody. Ki-67 immunostaining is positive within many of the primitive cells between pale islands, but only labels rare cells within these more differentiated-appearing areas.

We consider this tumor to represent a medulloblastoma variant and characterize it as follows: **Posterior Fossa, Removal—Medulloblastoma with Extensive Nodularity, WHO Grade IV.**

COMMENT

Despite retention of the WHO grade IV designation, a more favorable outcome is recognized for this medulloblastoma variant.

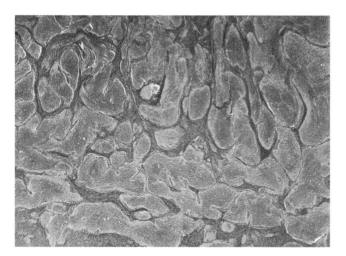

FIGURE 54.1 Low-magnification section demonstrates grossly expanded nodules of tumor, demonstrating advanced neurocytic differentiation separated by intervening islands of less well-differentiated neuroectodermal cells.

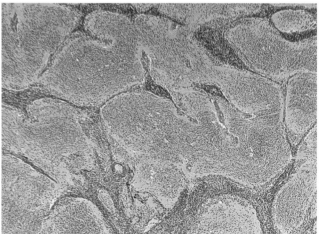

FIGURE 54.2 Higher magnification of the same section demonstrates the monomorphic nuclear appearance of the tumor cells, disposed within the pale islands of neuropil.

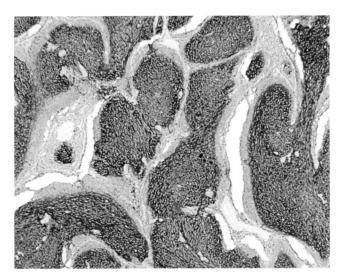

FIGURE 54.3 Synaptophysin immunostaining is strongly and uniformly positive within the anastomosing islands of well-differentiated tumor.

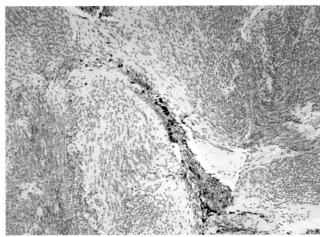

FIGURE 54.4 Immunohistochemical staining for Ki-67 labels a subpopulation of the primitive, intervening, neuroectodermal tumor cells, but not the better differentiated cells, within the pale islands of neuropil.

DISCUSSION

First described by Giangaspero in 1999, the medulloblastoma with extensive nodularity (described previously as "cerebellar neuroblastoma") is a tumor of early childhood, with most children undergoing surgery before the age of 3. This medulloblastoma variant appears similar to the desmoplastic medulloblastoma, but it demonstrates an overwhelming abundance of markedly expanded lobular architecture, with near elimination of intervening primitive neuroectodermal component. In addition, what remains of the less differentiated tumor is often devoid of reticulin. Medulloblastoma with extensive nodularity is significantly more common than either desmoplastic or classic medulloblastoma in patients under the age of 3 years. In addition, approximately 50% of these tumors in this age group are associated with Gorlin (nevoid basal cell carcinoma) syndrome. Because there are some indications that these very young patients with fully developed nodularity may not require aggressive radiotherapy to achieve long-term survival, the diagnosis is

an important one, if somewhat imprecisely defined. At present, the best definition requires radiographic/pathologic correlation: The grossly enlarged nodules should be radiologically visible, described commonly as resembling a "bunch of grapes." In addition to a high association with Gorlin syndrome, association with other familial tumor predisposition syndromes, such as neurofibromatosis, Li-Fraumeni, and fragile X syndrome, have been reported. Therefore, families of patients diagnosed with medulloblastoma with extensive nodularity should be investigated for tumor predisposition syndromes.

References

1. Garrè ML, Cama A, Bagnasco F, et. al. Medulloblastoma variants: age-dependent occurrence and relation to Gorlin syndrome—a new clinical perspective. Clin Cancer Res 2009;15:2463–71.
2. Trembath D, Miller CR, Perry A. Gray zones in brain tumor classification: evolving concepts. Adv Anat Pathol 2008;15:287–97.
3. Verma S, Tavaré CJ, Gilles FH. Histologic features and prognosis in pediatric medulloblastoma. Pediatr Dev Pathol 2008;11:337–43.

Case 55: Anaplastic Medulloblastoma

CLINICAL INFORMATION

This 19-year-old woman presents to the emergency room, complaining of severe headaches and intermittent vomiting that is not accompanied by nausea. Physical exam reveals bilateral papilledema, and neural imaging demonstrates a large enhancing lesion within her fourth ventricle. Histologic sections from the tumor resection are reviewed.

OPINION

Sections show a densely cellular tumor, containing geographic areas of coagulative tumor necrosis. The tumor cells demonstrate an embryonal appearance, consisting nearly entirely of pleomorphic hyperchromatic nuclei, accompanied by barely discernible cytoplasm. At high power, tumor cells show unusual concentric arrangements, in which tumor cells appear to wrap around each other. Occasional microscopic fields contain tumor cells with more abundant cytoplasm and larger nuclei, occasionally containing prominent nucleoli.

We consider this lesion to be a variant of medulloblastoma and characterize it as follows: **Posterior Fossa, Removal—Anaplastic Medulloblastoma, WHO Grade IV.**

COMMENT

Focal large cell differentiation is identified. Because large cell and anaplastic medulloblastomas share many histopathologic features, as well as a dismal

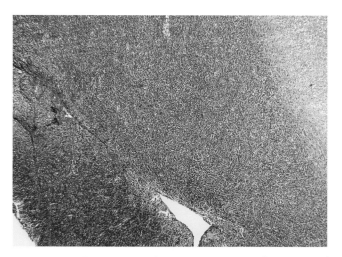

FIGURE 55.1 Low power demonstrates a zonal pattern of differentiation, ranging from a nearly solid blue mass of tumor cells in the lower left corner through a hypercellular, but somewhat less densely packed, region in the center to geographic coagulative necrosis in the upper right.

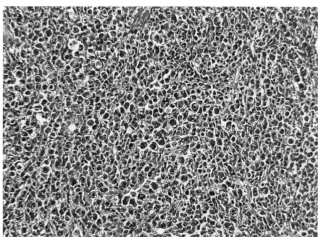

FIGURE 55.2 Medium-power view shows numerous aggregates of concentrically arranged tumor cells, referred to as "cell wrapping."

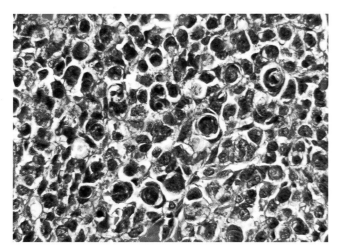

FIGURE 55.3 High power shows prominent cell wrapping, as well as distinct nucleoli, within several of the tumor cells.

prognosis, some authors have suggested that these medulloblastoma subtypes be merged into a single entity that could be referred to as "large cell/anaplastic medulloblastoma."

DISCUSSION

Although all medulloblastomas share a WHO grade IV designation, the vast majority respond favorably to radiation and chemotherapy, resulting in long-term survival for the majority of patients. Unfortunately, this has not been true for the 10 to 15% of patients whose medulloblastomas demonstrate marked anaplasia (characterized by increased nuclear size and pleomorphism, accompanied by "cell wrapping"). Anaplastic medulloblastomas are characteristically encountered in very young patients, often within the first few years of life, but may also be seen in adults, where they comprise approximately 5% of all adult medulloblastomas. Clinical and radiographic features are indistinguishable from those seen in classic medulloblastomas. However, genetic analyses have demonstrated a high frequency of c-Myc overexpression in large cell and anaplastic medulloblastomas. Recent studies have also shown induction of cell cycle progression and increased cell size, by hepatocyte growth factor via activation of the c-Met pathway with consequent c-Myc overexpression. Unfortunately, this has not yet been translated into effective therapy, and the majority of patients with anaplastic and/or large cell medulloblastomas experience recurrence, leptomeningeal and extraneural dissemination, and die within several years of diagnosis despite aggressive therapy.

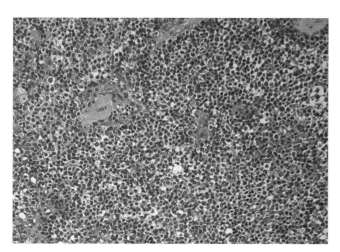

FIGURE 55.4 Several regions of the tumor showed a more amphophilic appearance, secondary to the presence of cells with more abundant cytoplasm.

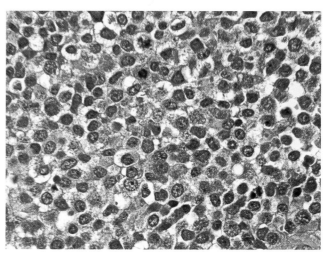

FIGURE 55.5 Areas of large cell differentiation show a brisk mitotic rate, as well as cells with enlarged nuclei containing prominent nucleoli.

References

1. Eberhart CG, Kepner JL, Goldthwaite PT, et al. Histopathologic grading of medulloblastomas: a Pediatric Oncology Group study. Cancer 2002;94:552–60.

2. Pfister S, Remke M, Benner A, et al. Outcome prediction in pediatric medulloblastoma based on DNA copy-number aberrations of chromosomes 6q and 17q and the MYC and MYCN loci. J Clin Oncol 2009;27:1627–36.

3. Rodriguez FJ, Eberhart C, O'Neill BP, et al. Histopathologic grading of adult medulloblastomas. Cancer 2007;109:2557–65.

Case 56: Atypical Teratoid/Rhabdoid Tumor

CLINICAL INFORMATION

The patient is a 16-month-old male who is brought to the Children's Hospital after multiple visits to his pediatrician for unexplained weight loss, failure to thrive, and decreased muscle tone. After extensive work-up, neuroimaging studies are obtained that show a massive posterior fossa tumor, 3.4 × 2.5 × 3.4 cm in dimension, that extends through the foramen of Luschka on the left and Magendie in the midline. The tumor shows heterogeneous contrast enhancement and focal subacute hemorrhage. The decision is made to excise the mass, and histological sections are reviewed.

OPINION

The specimen shows a hypercellular tumor, composed of small cells with vesicular nuclei, variably prominent nucleoli, and eosinophilic cytoplasm. The cytoplasm is more prominent than is seen in most primitive neuroectodermal tumors, including medulloblastomas. The tumor population is usually heterogeneous, but, focally, cells with larger "eye ball" nucleoli and eccentrically placed, globular, eosinophilic cytoplasmic inclusions can be identified, meeting criteria for rhabdoid cells.

After immunohistochemical characterization, we characterize the tumor as follows: **Posterior Fossa, Excision—Atypical Teratoid/Rhabdoid Tumor, WHO Grade IV.**

COMMENT

Atypical teratoid/rhabdoid tumors most often occur in young children under the age of 3 years and may be found in infants.

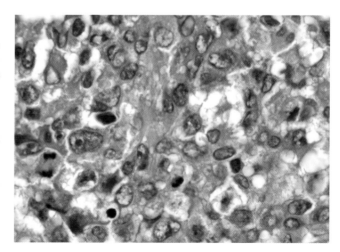

FIGURE 56.1 This AT/RT manifests as a patternless embryonal tumor, composed of cells with spindled or rounded eosinophilic cytoplasm. The cytoplasm is usually more conspicuous than that seen in medulloblastomas or other CNS PNETs.

FIGURE 56.2 High power shows scattered mitoses, but these are few in number in comparison to the exceedingly high cell cycle labeling indices that are recognizable after immunostaining for MIB-1.

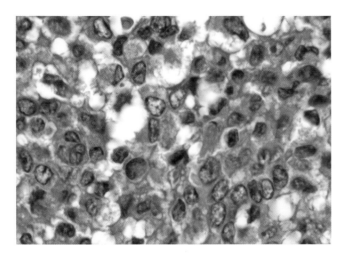

FIGURE 56.3 Nuclei are vesicular, and many, but not all, manifest large nucleoli.

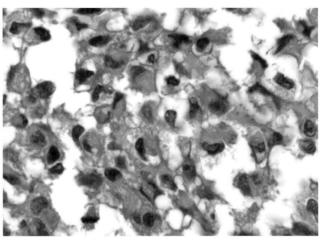

FIGURE 56.4 Rhabdoid cells, with eccentrically placed nuclei and eosinophilic, cytoplasmic ball-like inclusions, can be found in most well-sampled AT/RTs, but these cells can be quite few in number.

DISCUSSION

Atypical teratoid/rhabdoid tumor (AT/RT) is a heterogeneous tumor that usually presents in very young children and only rarely affects either older children (over age 6 years) or adults. Supratentorial sites are slightly more often affected than posterior fossa locations, with cerebral hemispheres and cerebello-

pontine angle being areas of predilection, respectively. AT/RT may seed the cerebrospinal fluid pathways, and in approximately one-quarter of patients, cerebrospinal fluid dissemination is identified at the time of first clinical presentation. Overall, prognosis is poor, and patient response to treatment is worse than is seen for medulloblastomas, even when very aggressive

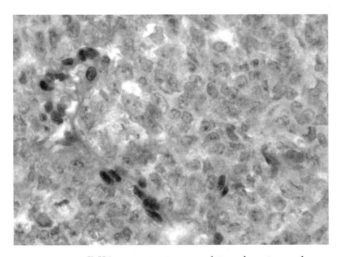

FIGURE 56.5 INI1 protein immunohistochemistry shows loss of immunoreactivity in tumor cell nuclei; positive immunostaining in endothelial cells from blood vessels in the tumor serves as an excellent internal control of staining fidelity.

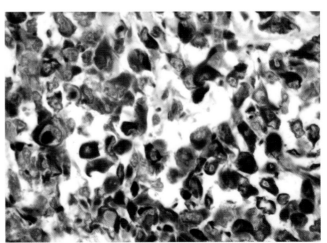

FIGURE 56.6 Vimentin immunostaining usually shows strong cytoplasmic reactivity in the tumor cells and can highlight the ball-like cytoplasmic filaments in the cytoplasm of rhabdoid cells.

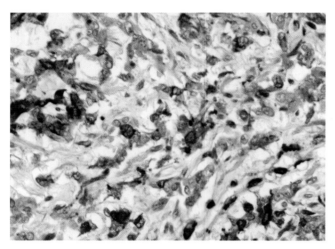

FIGURE 56.7 Although polyphenotypic immunohistochemical expression is almost always detected, staining for some antibodies is more common; immunoreactivity for smooth muscle actin is one of the most frequently detected.

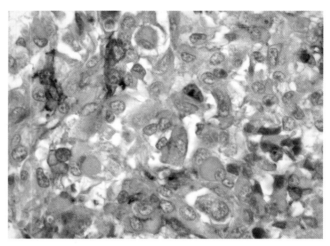

FIGURE 56.8 EMA immunoreactivity is usually also present, in addition to that for vimentin and smooth muscle actin; note that cells with rhabdoid features may not be immunoreactive.

regimens are utilized. Hence, making the pathologic distinction between medulloblastoma and AT/RT is important.

The diagnosis can be difficult because of the rarity of the entity (constitutes 1–2% of all pediatric brain tumors) and the varied histologic appearance. Examples composed solely of classic rhabdoid cells

are rare. More often, AT/RT contains areas with small embryonal appearing cells showing glassy or ball-like eosinophilic cytoplasm, admixed with sheets of cells devoid of cytoplasm and manifesting "small blue cell" primitive neuroectodermal-like features. Mesenchymal areas with spindle cells and myxoid background are also fairly frequent. A purely epithelial appearance, with adenomatous or papillary areas, is uncommon but has been described, making distinction from choroid

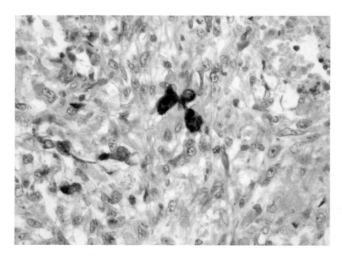

FIGURE 56.9 Patchy immunoreactivity for pancytokeratin (AE1/AE3) can often be seen, but often which cells are positive cannot be predicted based on morphological features at the hematoxylin and eosin level.

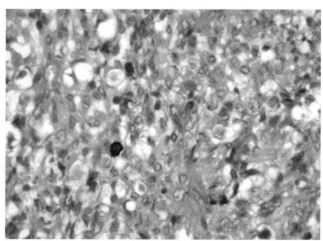

FIGURE 56.10 Focal immunoreactivity for GFAP is present in this case.

plexus carcinoma nearly impossible on hematoxylin- and eosin-stained sections alone.

Fortunately, an immunohistochemical antibody directed against INI1 protein has assisted greatly in making the diagnosis in problematic cases and is considered to be a "sensitive and specific marker" for AT/RT. In most AT/RTs, there is loss of nuclear expression of INI1 protein in the tumor, with retention of nuclear immunostaining in endothelial cells within the blood vessels of tumor. The latter serves as an excellent internal control of staining/technical fidelity. The overwhelming majority of AT/RTs show this nuclear INI1 protein loss, and 75% additionally show deletions or mutations of the INI1 gene on chromosome 22.

An additional helpful feature in making the diagnosis is the polyphenotypic expression of a variety of mesenchymal and epithelial immunohistochemical markers in AT/RT. This polyphenotypic expression pattern differs from the more strictly neuronal and glial lineage markers found in medulloblastomas and in most other primitive neuroectodermal tumors (PNETs).

Vimentin immunostaining is seen in all AT/RTs and can further highlight the cytoplasmic globular filamentous inclusions in the subset of cells with classic rhabdoid features. Epithelial membrane antigen (EMA) and smooth muscle actin are also almost always expressed in AT/RTs, albeit in a patchy pattern. More variable immunoreactivity for cytokeratin, neurofilament protein, GFAP, and synaptophysin is usually found. What is almost never seen is immunoreactivity for germ cell markers, and true germinoma or mixed germ cell histologic features are not present. Hence, AT/RT is "teratoid," or teratoma-reminiscent,

in its ability to show immunohistochemical differentiation along multiple epithelial, mesenchymal, neuronal, and glial lineages, but it does not meet criteria for a true germ cell tumor with teratoma elements.

As is the case with many embryonal tumors, the MIB-1 labeling index is often surprisingly high, in many instances exceeding 50%, even when only scattered mitoses are identifiable. Because a PNET-like small blue cell component is one of the most frequently encountered elements in true AT/RT, some laboratories routinely perform immunostaining for INI1 on all primary small blue neoplasms of the central nervous system (i.e., CNS PNETs) in children, in order not to miss the rare example of a PNET-dominant AT/RT that was perhaps undersampled and devoid of the rhabdoid elements. Haberler et al. have suggested that PNETs without nuclear immunoreactivity for INI1 protein are likely to be undersampled AT/RTs and behave in a more aggressive fashion than conventional PNETs.

References

1. Haberler C, Laggner U, Slavc I, et al. Immunohistochemical analysis of INI1 protein in malignant pediatric CNS tumors: lack of INI1 in atypical teratoid/rhabdoid tumors and in a fraction of primitive neuroectodermal tumors without rhabdoid phenotype. Am J Surg Pathol 2006;30:1462–8.
2. Judkins AR, Burger PC, Hamilton RL, et al. INI1 protein expression distinguishes atypical teratoid/rhabdoid tumor from choroid plexus carcinoma. J Neuropathol Exp Neurol 2005;64:391–7.
3. Judkins AR, Eberhart CG, Wesseling P. Atypical teratoid/rhabdoid tumor. In: Louis DN, Ohgaki H, Wiestler OD, Cavenee WK, Editors. WHO Classification of Tumours of the Central Nervous System. Lyon, FR: IARC Press; 2007. p. 147–9.
4. Takei H, Bhattacharjee MB, Rivera A, et al. New immunohistochemical markers in the evaluation of central nervous system tumors. A review of 7 selected adult and pediatric brain tumors. Arch Pathol Lab Med 2007;131:234–41.

Case 57: Embryonal Tumor with Abundant Neuropil and True Rosettes

CLINICAL INFORMATION

This 3-year-old boy presents with macrocephaly, failure to thrive, and developmental delay. Neuroimaging demonstrates a 9-cm well demarcated, focally enhancing mass within the right frontal and parietal lobes. The intraoperative consultation is read as "malignant glioma—primitive neuroectodermal tumor versus ependymoma." The resection specimen is reviewed.

OPINION

The tumor demonstrates a biphasic appearance and is predominately composed of moderately cellular sheets and nests of primitive-appearing cells, disposed within an abundant fibrillary matrix. Focal, relatively abrupt transitions to dense hypercellularity, with abundant mitotic and apoptotic activity, are present. At the interface between these two regions, primitive rosettes can be identified, many of which contain true lumens. The cells comprising the rosettes demonstrate pleomorphic, hyperchromatic, overlapping nuclei. Immunohistochemical staining for nonphosphorylated neurofilaments is strongly positive within the fibrillary matrix and between rosettes, but not within the cells forming the true rosettes. Scattered GFAP-positive cells and processes are identified within stroma, but not within rosettes. A subpopulation of the rosette-forming cells reacts strongly with antibodies to vimentin.

We consider this lesion to represent a form of cerebral primitive neuroectodermal tumor and characterize it as follows: **Right Frontal and Parietal Lobes, Subtotal Resection—Embryonal Tumor**

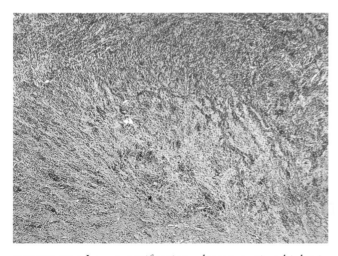

FIGURE 57.1 Low magnification, demonstrating biphasic morphology with an abundant fibrillary matrix present within much of the tumor.

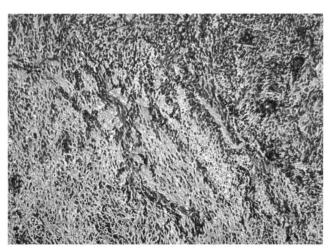

FIGURE 57.2 Relatively abrupt transition into a densely cellular, stromal poor region containing several rosettes is observed.

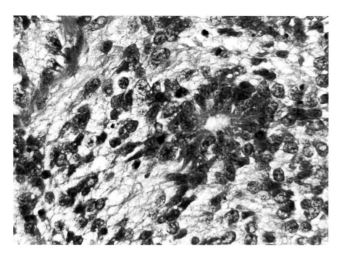

FIGURE 57.3 High-power photomicrograph of a true rosette, surrounded by multiple layers of pleomorphic, hyperchromatic, primitive tumor cells.

with Abundant Neuropil and True Rosettes, WHO Grade IV.

DISCUSSION

Embryonal tumor with abundant neuropil and true rosettes (ETANTR) is a recently distinguished entity still in the process of codification within the classification of primitive central nervous system tumors. First

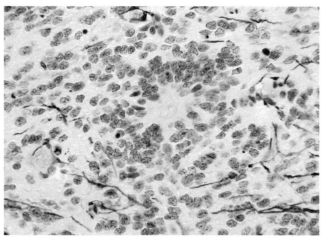

FIGURE 57.4 Immunohistochemical staining for GFAP demonstrates scant glial processes between rosettes.

described in 2000 as "pediatric neuroblastic tumors containing abundant neuropil and true rosettes," less than 40 cases have been described, which are briefly discussed in the current WHO classification of central nervous system tumors as an extremely aggressive type of central nervous system primitive neuroectodermal tumor. The average age at presentation is 24 months, with very few tumors being reported either before 1 year of age or after 4 years of age. There is a predilection

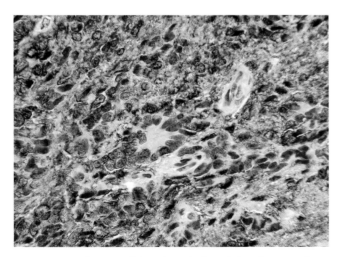

FIGURE 57.5 Immunohistochemical staining for nonphosphorylated neurofilaments demonstrates reactivity within the tumor stroma, but not within the cells composing the rosettes.

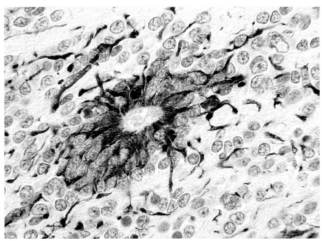

FIGURE 57.6 Vimentin immunohistochemical staining labels a subpopulation of the rosette-forming cells and can also be seen labeling the same stromal glial processes labeled by the GFAP antibodies.

for supratentorial regions, particularly the frontal and parietal lobes, although significant numbers have been described within the brainstem and cerebellum. To date, there appears to be an approximately 2 to 1 female predilection, which distinguishes this tumor from other aggressive central nervous system embryonal tumors of early childhood, in which males appear to be preferentially affected. ETANTRs are also distinctive among central nervous system primitive neuroectodermal tumors in their relative lack of enhancement. Although relatively recent in their description, it is likely that past cases were diagnosed as ependymoblastomas or primitive neuroectodermal tumors with ependymal differentiation.

References

1. Eberhart CG, Brat DJ, Cohen KJ, et al. Pediatric neuroblastic brain tumors containing abundant neuropil and true rosettes. Pediatr Dev Pathol 2000;3:346–52.
2. Gessi M, Giangaspero F, Lauriola L, et al. Embryonal tumors with abundant neuropil and true rosettes: a distinctive CNS primitive neuroectodermal tumor. Am J Surg Pathol 2009;33:211–17.
3. Judkins AR, Ellison DW. Ependymoblastoma: Dear, damned, distracting diagnosis, farewell! Brain Pathol 2008 Dec 17. [Epub ahead of print].

Case 58: Schwannoma with Ancient Change

CLINICAL INFORMATION

The patient is a 72-year-old male who presents with hearing loss. On imaging, a 4-cm right cerebello-pontine angle mass is identified and thought to be either a meningioma or an acoustic neuroma. Surgical resection is undertaken and yields histologic sections, which are reviewed.

OPINION

The resection material shows a spindle-cell neoplasm, with mild hypercellularity and no necrosis. Cells demonstrate elongate nuclei, with pointed tapering ends and wavy eosinophilic cytoplasm. Occasional nuclei show enlargement and hyperchromasia. Hyalinized blood vessels, vascular thrombosis, and hemosiderin are seen. Mitotic figures are not observed.

We consider the findings in this lesion to be consistent with those of a benign schwannoma with degenerative features ("ancient" change) and characterize it as follows: **Right Cerebello-Pontine Angle, Excision—Vestibular Schwannoma, WHO Grade I.**

COMMENT

There is no evidence of malignant features in this vestibular schwannoma (synonymous with acoustic neuroma, neurilemoma). Malignant transformation in schwannomas is rare.

DISCUSSION

One of the more challenging diagnoses in surgical neuropathology at the time of frozen section can be distinguishing a fibroblastic meningioma

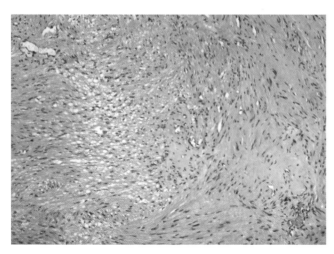

FIGURE 58.1 Low-magnification view of the resection material, showing a mildly hypercellular spindle-cell neoplasm composed of intersecting bands of cells.

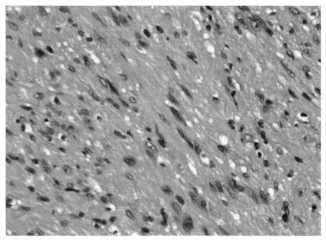

FIGURE 58.2 High-magnification appearance, showing cells with nuclei showing tapering, pointed ends and wavy eosinophilic cytoplasm.

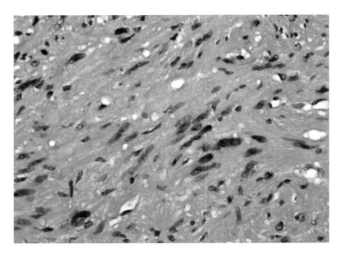

FIGURE 58.3 High magnification, showing other areas containing cells with more hyperchromatic enlarged nuclei, but no mitoses.

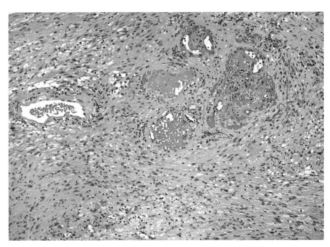

FIGURE 58.4 Prominent vascular hyalinization, vascular thrombosis, and focal hemosiderin pigment deposits are present.

from a schwannoma, especially in the region of the cerebello-pontine angle. The presence of well-developed whorls of cells or psammoma body calcifications makes the diagnosis of meningioma easy, if these features are present. More often, however, one encounters a relatively patternless spindle-cell neoplasm, devoid of even the densely cellular Antoni A tissue alternating with looser, hypocellular, degenerative Antoni B tissue that characterizes schwannomas. Another pitfall can

be in overinterpreting degenerative features, such as nuclear atypia (ancient change), vascular alterations, including thrombosis or clusters of malformation-like vessels, or macrophages in schwannomas. None of these features affect prognosis or grading, although occasionally clinically significant bleeding can occur in benign schwannomas. Microhemorrhages, recent or remote, are more frequent in schwannomas than meningiomas, a feature recently appreciated by neuroradiologists on more sensitive imaging techniques.

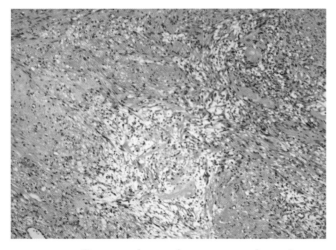

FIGURE 58.5 Occasional areas demonstrate a dense Antoni A area, juxtaposed to looser, degenerative Antoni B tumor tissue.

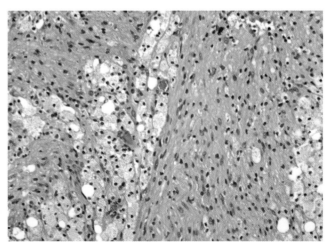

FIGURE 58.6 Clusters of macrophages can be present but are of no prognostic importance.

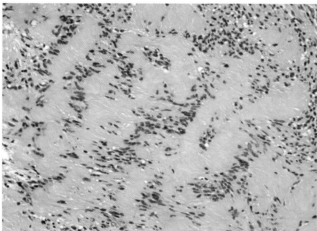

FIGURE 58.7 Antoni A tissue may contain rows of nuclei, aligned parallel to each other, so-called Verocay bodies.

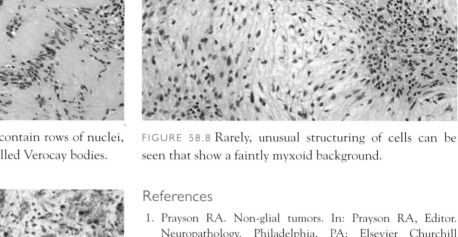

FIGURE 58.8 Rarely, unusual structuring of cells can be seen that show a faintly myxoid background.

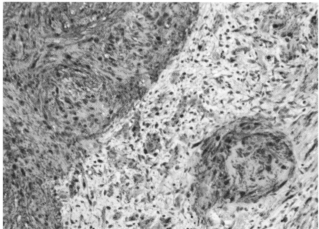

FIGURE 58.9 Strong nuclear and cytoplasmic immunoreactivity for S-100 protein is seen in schwannomas, albeit with less staining in Antoni B degenerative areas; reticulin fibers are also fewer in these areas (red chromagen).

References

1. Prayson RA. Non-glial tumors. In: Prayson RA, Editor. Neuropathology. Philadelphia, PA: Elsevier Churchill Livingstone;2005. p. 489–586.
2. Scheithauer BW, Louis DN, Hunter S, et al. Schwannoma. In: Louis DN, Ohgaki H, Wiestler OD, Cavenee WK, Editors. WHO Classification of Tumours of the Central Nervous System. Lyon, FR; IARC Press;2007. p. 152–5.
3. Thamburaj K. Radhakrishnan VV. Thomas B, et al. Intratumoral microhemorrhages on T2*-weighted gradient-echo imaging helps differentiate vestibular schwannoma from meningioma. AJNR 2008;29:552–7.

Case 59: Neurofibroma

CLINICAL INFORMATION

The patient is a 19-year-old-male with known neurofibromatosis, type I (NF I), who develops recent urinary retention and increasing right leg weakness. Neuroimaging discloses a neurofibroma of proximal nerve root at the level of C2. Intraoperatively, the neurosurgeon thought multiple nerve roots were involved and felt that the patient had a plexiform neurofibroma. Limited resection was undertaken.

OPINION

The resection material shows a bulbous mass, with background mucinous matrix, moderate cell density, clusters of wavy cells with collagen formation

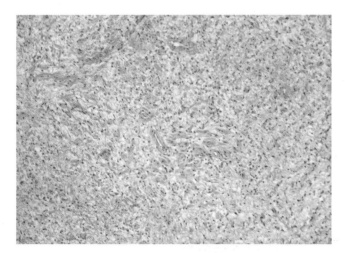

FIGURE 59.1 Lower-magnification appearance of the nerve root mass, showing a relatively hypocellular tumor with spindle cells with wavy cytoplasm associated with bundles of collagen and embedded in a thin, bluish-gray mucoid background matrix; note absence of hyalinization of the small blood vessels in the tumor.

(so-called shredded carrots), and neither necrosis or mitotic activity. Cells posses thin processes and elongate to curved nuclei. Although large neurons are seen within the lesion, these are surrounded by satellite cells, contain cytoplasmic pigment typical of dorsal root ganglion cells, and lack cytological atypia. Thus, they are entrapped ganglion cells in the proximal nerve root plexiform neurofibroma.

We consider the lesion to be a benign peripheral nerve sheath tumor and characterize it as follows: **Proximal Nerve Root, Excision—Neurofibroma, Plexiform, WHO Grade I.**

COMMENT

The assessment of plexiform ("strands of rope," "bag of worms") configuration is best accomplished intraoperatively or on neuroimaging studies, although

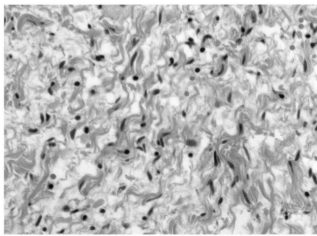

FIGURE 59.2 High magnification shows the curved thin nuclei and wavy cytoplasm of the tumor cells, as well as the absence of mitotic activity.

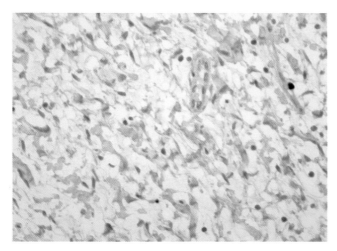

FIGURE 59.3 Only extremely rare nuclear labeling is seen with MIB-1, yielding an index of <1.

often the specimen received by the pathologist shows an involvement of multiple nerve branches or trunks that is necessary to diagnose as a "plexiform" neurofibroma.

DISCUSSION

Neurofibromas present as cutaneous nodules, circumscribed mass in a peripheral nerve (localized intraneural neurofibroma), or plexiform enlargement of a major nerve trunk. They are composed of Schwann cells and fibroblasts, aggregated with wavy collagen and swimming in an Alcian-blue-positive, myxoid background. Extensive collagenization sometimes occurs, forming bundles with the "shredded carrot" appearance. Blood vessels are less hyalinized than they are in schwannomas, and hemorrhage is less frequent. Varying numbers of S-100 positive Schwann cells and neurofilament-positive axons are present within neurofibromas. In proximal nerve root examples such as this one, normal dorsal root ganglion cells can become entrapped. These should not be overinterpreted as being part of a ganglioneuroma. Neoplastic neurons in ganglioneuroma are not surrounded by satellite cells.

Plexiform neurofibromas, especially large ones, are usually associated with patients with NF1. Malignant transformation occurs in a minority of plexiform neurofibromas, estimated to be 5%.

Many nonplexiform neurofibromas are sporadic and unassociated with NF I, and, for the overwhelming majority of cases, the cause is unknown. Rarely, benign neurofibromas and schwannomas can occur as radiation-induced tumors.

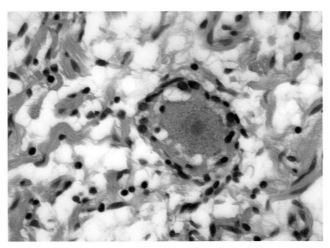

FIGURE 59.5 High-power magnification shows the absence of cytological atypia, the presence of normal satellite cells surrounding the neuron, and the fine brown cytoplasmic pigment typical of normal neuronal cells in this location.

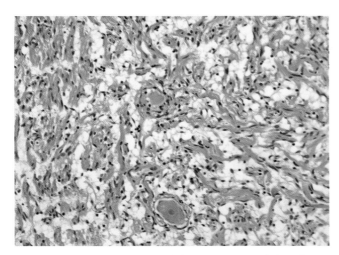

FIGURE 59.4 In some areas of the mass, normal dorsal root ganglion cells are encompassed by the tumor.

References

1. Ferner RE. Neurofibromatosis 1 and neurofibromatosis 2: a twenty-first century perspective. Lancet Neurology 2007;6: 340–51.
2. Scheithauer BW, Louis DN, Hunter S, et al. Schwannoma. In: Louis DN, Ohgaki H, Wiestler OD, Cavenee WK, Editors. WHO Classification of Tumours of the Central Nervous System. Lyon, FR: IARC Press;2007. p. 156–7.
3. Zadeh G, Buckle C, Shannon P, et al. Radiation induced peripheral nerve tumors: case series and review of the literature. J Neurooncol 2007;83:205–12.

CLINICAL INFORMATION

The patient is a 50-year-old female who presents with a 3-cm firm, but painless, nodule in the right calf. She has no past medical history of malignancy. A decision is made to resect the lesion, and histologic sections are reviewed.

OPINION

Biopsies show a well-demarcated, but nonencapsulated, moderately hypercellular, homogeneous solid mass, composed of spindled cells arranged in intersecting fascicles. Whorls of tumor cells are focally prominent. Psammoma body-type calcifications, Verocay bodies, loosened Antoni B tissue, necrosis, and mitotic activity are all absent.

After immunohistochemical studies, we consider the resected lesion as representing a soft tissue perineurioma and characterize it as follows: **Right Calf, Resection—Perineurioma, Soft Tissue Type, WHO Grade I.**

COMMENT

Perineuriomas can be of soft tissue, intraneural, and sclerosing subtypes; this case represents an example of the soft tissue subtype. Most examples are not associated with neurofibromatosis type I or II.

DISCUSSION

Perineurioma of soft tissue type is an uncommon entity that most closely resembles a fibroblastic tumor. Most patients present with a painless mass. In the largest reported series on soft tissue perineuriomas, by Hornick et al., the mean size of the single lesion was 4.1 cm (range 0.3–20 cm), and most occurred in the lower or

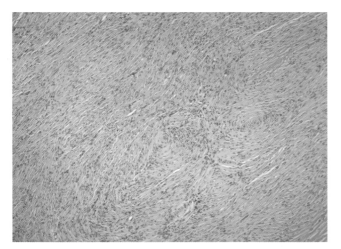

FIGURE 60.1 Low-power view of the lesion shows a homogeneous, solid, spindled cell tumor displaying a fascicled pattern.

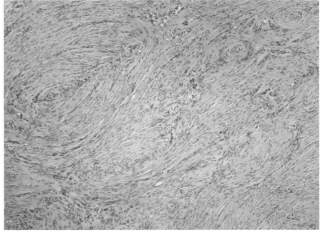

FIGURE 60.2 Medium-power magnification illustrates areas within the same tumor manifesting a slightly more storiform architecture, but no necrosis.

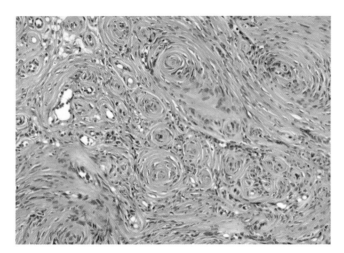

FIGURE 60.3 Medium-power magnification highlights areas with whorls of cells, with resemblance to meningioma.

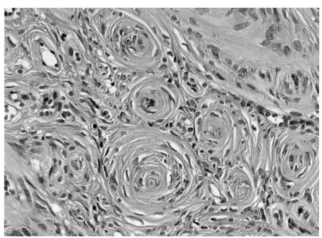

FIGURE 60.4 High-power view shows that blood vessels are delicate and usually devoid of thick hyalinization, as would be typical of schwannoma.

upper limbs or the trunk. Nearly all were grossly well circumscribed. Of the 81 cases, 42 of 81 examples were located in subcutis, 25 of 81 in deep soft tissue, and 9 of 81 in dermis.

Most soft tissue perineuriomas are solid and composed of fascicles of cells, often with a storiform and focally whorled growth pattern. Cells are elongate, wavy, and are surrounded by variable amounts of collagen. Nuclei are thin, elongated, have tapered ends, and devoid of conspicuous

nucleoli, in contrast to the larger, blunt-ended nuclei seen in smooth muscle tumors. Some authors have noted occasional nuclear atypia, but this seems to be degenerative in nature, similar to that seen in "ancient schwannoma," and lacks prognostic significance. Mitoses are usually rare to absent. Paralleling what is seen by electron microscopy, the eosinophilic, bipolar cell cytoplasmic processes are very long and thin. Myxoid background may be found in some cases.

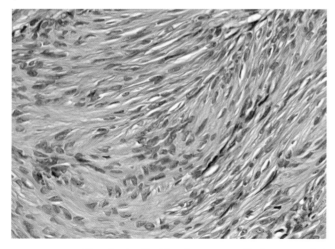

FIGURE 60.5 Cytologically bland tumor cells have nuclei devoid of nucleoli or mitotic activity and resemble fibroblastic cells.

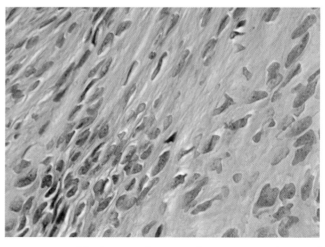

FIGURE 60.6 Nuclei may be very thin is some planes of section, and the cytoplasm is bipolar and very thin as well.

The key feature for making the diagnosis is the strong immunoreactivity for EMA and negative immunoreactivity for S-100 protein and muscle markers. As noted by Giannini et al., however, "EMA reactivity may be difficult to demonstrate without the use of a higher concentration of antisera or of a longer incubation times than are routinely employed in the diagnosis of epithelial neoplasms." Difficult examples require electron microscopic confirmation.

The differential for this benign, WHO grade I, nerve sheath tumor centers around fibroblastic tumors, such as dermatofibrosarcoma protuberans and desmoid tumor (fibromatosis). The first is storiform in pattern and uniformly immunoreactive for CD34, but not for EMA. Desmoid tumors are more infiltrative than most perineuriomas, and again, are EMA-negative. Myxoid soft tissue perineuriomas need to be distinguished from low-grade fibromyxoid sarcoma and low-grade myxofibrosarcoma, both of which lack EMA immunoreactivity. Absence of immunostaining for S-100 protein excludes schwannoma, although both schwannoma and perineurioma have cells that are surrounded by collagen IV- and laminin-immunoreactive basement membrane. Soft tissue perineuriomas also show immunostaining for newer markers, such GLUT-1 and claudin-1.

Intraneural perineuriomas present as enlarged nerve fascicles and used to be called "localized hypertrophic neuropathy." Histologically, they appear quite different than soft tissue perineurioma, in that they manifest tight concentric whorls of EMA-positive cells, yielding "pseudo-onion bulbs" within the affected nerve. Although the soft tissue and intraneural subtypes present very different histologic appearances, both appear to share abnormalities of chromosome 22.

References

1. Boyanton BL Jr, Jones JK, Shenaq SM, et al. Intraneural perineurioma: a systematic review with illustrative cases. Arch Pathol Lab Med 2007;131:1382–92.
2. Giannini C, Scheithauer BW, Jenkins RB, et al. Soft-tissue perineurioma. Evidence for an abnormality of chromosome 22, criteria for diagnosis, and review of the literature. Am J Surg Pathol 1997;21:164–73.
3. Hornick JL, Fletcher CD. Soft tissue perineurioma: clinicopathologic analysis of 81 cases including those with atypical histologic features. Am J Surg Pathol. 2005;29:845–58.
4. Macarenco RS, Ellinger F, Oliveira AM. Perineurioma: a distinctive and underrecognized peripheral nerve sheath neoplasm. Arch Pathol Lab Med 2007;131:625–36.
5. Pina-Oviedo S, Ortiz-Hidalgo C. The normal and neoplastic perineurium: a review. Adv Anat Pathol 2008;15:147–64.

Case 61: Malignant Peripheral Nerve Sheath Tumor

CLINICAL INFORMATION

The patient is a 33-year-old-male with known neurofibromatosis, type I, and a rapidly enlarging right popliteal mass, up to 9 cm in greatest dimension. The decision was made to resect the mass, and histological sections are reviewed.

OPINION

The resection material shows a hypercellular, highly necrotic, focally hemorrhagic spindle neoplasm with brisk mitotic activity. Cells display prominent nucleoli and variable amounts of cytoplasm. Slight palisading of nuclei is seen around some areas of necrosis, a feature not completely exclusive to glioblastomas and recognized in some sarcomas such as malignant peripheral nerve sheath tumor (MPNST). The presence of a benign plexiform neurofibroma nearby ensures that the sarcoma is of peripheral nervous system origin.

We consider the lesion to be a sarcoma and characterize it as follows: **Right Popliteal Nerve, Excision—Malignant Peripheral Nerve Sheath Tumor, WHO Grade IV.**

COMMENT

The grading system for MPNST is similar to that employed for sarcomas in general. This example has very high mitotic activity and extensive necrosis.

DISCUSSION

MPNSTs affect middle-aged adults. Patients with neurofibromatosis, type I, generally are of younger

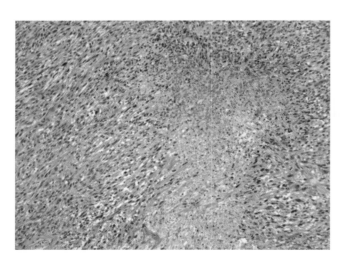

FIGURE 61.1 Lower-magnification appearance of the nerve root mass, showing a hypercellular, spindled tumor with extensive necrosis and embedded in a thin, bluish-gray mucoid background matrix; note absence of hyalinization of the small blood vessels in the tumor.

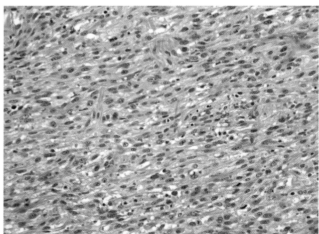

FIGURE 61.2 Intermediate magnification shows spindled cell areas.

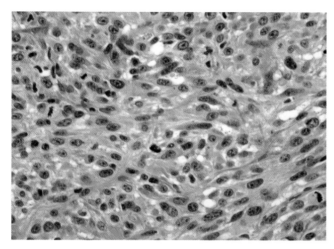

FIGURE 61.3 High-power magnification illustrates areas in the same tumor with more prominent nucleoli and brisk mitotic activity.

age than patients with sporadic cases, explaining the young age of the current case. Larger nerves are more likely affected than smaller nerves, and common sites for MPNST include buttock and thigh, brachial plexus, paraspinal region, and sciatic nerve. Cranial nerve MPNSTs are rare. About one-third to one-half of all MPNSTs arise from neurofibromas, usually plexiform neurofibromas, as in this case. Only rarely do

they arise from other types of benign peripheral nerve sheath tumors, such as schwannomas or ganglioneuromas. It is estimated that 10% of MPNSTs arise years and decades following irradiation.

MPNSTs often begin their growth within the nerve fascicle of origin, but they commonly can break through the epineurium to involve adjacent soft tissues. Many are over 5 cm in diameter when they are removed. Grossly, they vary from being solid tan masses that are deceptively bland-appearing to overtly necrotic and hemorrhagic lesions of massive proportions.

Histologically, tumors exhibit varied patterns, ranging from intersecting fascicles of spindled cells to sheets of relatively patternless cells. Epithelioid cells may be found, with prominent nucleoli. Background mucoid matrix may be identified. The finding of necrosis, often geographic and sometimes surrounded by palisading tumor cells, mandates a grading of WHO grade IV.

Additional neoplastic elements, such as rhabdomyosarcoma, chondrosarcoma, or osteosarcoma, or even intestinal or squamous epithelium, have been documented. These unusual elements tend to be seen

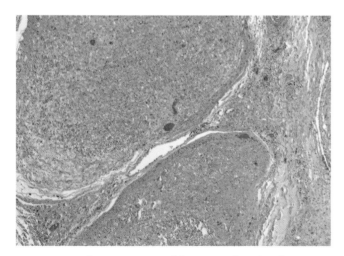

FIGURE 61.4 In some areas of the mass, the plexiform neurofibroma from which this MPNST arose can be identified; note involvement of multiple nerve fascicles by the neurofibroma.

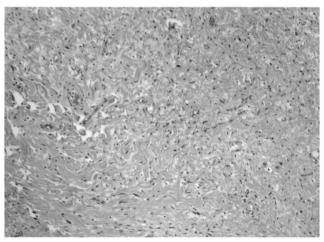

FIGURE 61.5 High-power magnification of the benign plexiform neurofibroma shows dense collagenization and wavy, "shredded carrots" appearance in this area.

in MPNSTs arising in patients with neurofibromatosis, type I.

References

1. Ferner RE. Neurofibromatosis 1 and neurofibromatosis 2: a twenty-first century perspective. Lancet Neurology 2007;16:340–51.

2. Scheithauer BW, Louis DN, Hunter S, et al. Schwannoma. In: Louis DN, Ohgaki H, Wiestler OD, Cavenee WK, Editors. WHO Classification of Tumours of the Central Nervous System. Lyon, FR: IARC Press; 2007. p. 160–2.

Case 62: Cellular Schwannoma

CLINICAL INFORMATION

The patient is a 50-year-old female who is found to have a mass involving the vagus nerve. Resection is undertaken, and histologic sections are examined.

OPINION

The resection material shows an encapsulated, highly cellular, homogeneous solid mass, composed of spindled cells arranged in intersecting fascicles. Whorls of tumor cells are not identified. Psammoma body-type calcifications and Verocay bodies are not seen. The lesion is composed of almost entirely dense Antoni A tissue, with less than 10% of the lesion showing identifiable Antoni B areas.

After immunohistochemical studies, we consider the resected lesion as representing a cellular schwannoma and characterize it as follows: **Vagus Nerve, Resection—Cellular Schwannoma, WHO Grade I.**

COMMENT

Cellular schwannomas are benign and lack metastatic potential. Most examples are solitary and are not associated with neurofibromatosis, types I or II.

DISCUSSION

Cellular schwannoma is, by definition, a schwannoma with high cellularity that is composed almost exclusively of dense Antoni A tissue without well-formed Verocay bodies. An Antoni B pattern may be focally present, but it constitutes no more than

FIGURE 62.1 Low-power view of the lesion shows a homogeneous, solid, spindled cell tumor, devoid of loosened Antoni B areas or Verocay body formation.

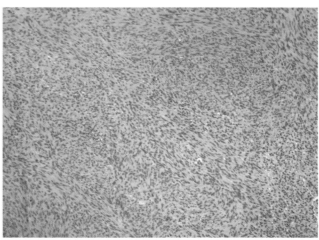

FIGURE 62.2 Cellular schwannoma is more hypercellular than ordinary schwannoma and shows a more uniform pattern at low power. Note the absence of necrosis in this example.

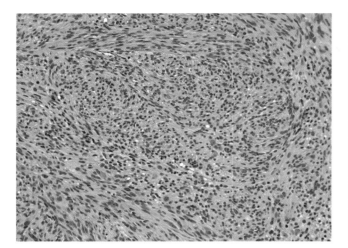

FIGURE 62.3 The tumor is composed of intersecting fascicles of cells, and despite the hypercellularity, there is generally an absence of degenerative nuclear atypia, as is often found in "ancient schwannomas."

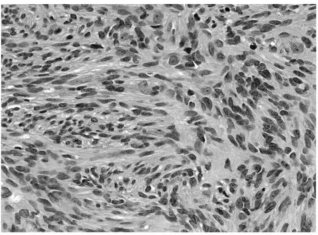

FIGURE 62.4 Cells display elongate nuclei and eosinophilic cytoplasm without distinct cell borders, often identical to that seen in ordinary schwannoma.

10% of the tumor area and is usually confined to subcapsular areas. Cellular schwannomas are similar to ordinary schwannomas in that they are well circumscribed, encapsulated, and microscopically share the presence of hyalinization of tumor vessels and occasional collections of lipid-laden histiocytes. They differ in that they are more hypercellular, have a more uniform architectural pattern, and may show more

conspicuous subcapsular and capsular benign lymphocytic collections than ordinary schwannoma. About one-third of cellular schwannomas arise from a recognizable nerve, as in this case.

Small foci of necrosis can rarely be encountered, but mitoses are found in the majority of cases, usually numbering 1–4 per 10 high-power microscopic fields. The key feature for making the diagnosis is the strong and diffuse immunoreactivity for S-100 protein. The

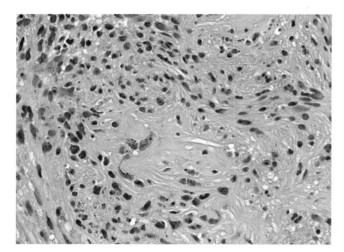

FIGURE 62.5 Cellular schwannomas possess many of the features of ordinary schwannomas, including hyalinization of tumor blood vessels.

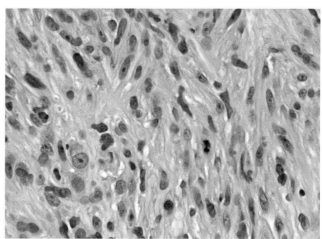

FIGURE 62.6 Mitoses are seen in the majority of cellular schwannomas but generally number from 1–4 per 10 high-power microscopic fields.

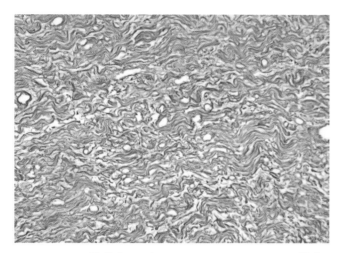

FIGURE 62.7 Cellular schwannomas possess pericellular basement membrane, and cells are individually surrounded by reticulin fibers.

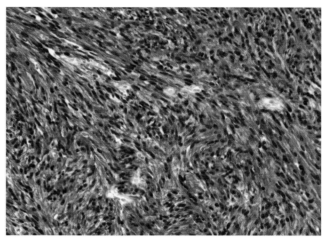

FIGURE 62.8 Similar to ordinary schwannoma and differing from most malignant peripheral nerve sheath tumors, cellular schwannomas show strong diffuse immunoreactivity for S-100 protein.

uniform, abundant, parallel array of wavy, pericellular reticulin in a cellular schwannoma is also a helpful diagnostic feature.

The differential for this benign, WHO grade I, nerve sheath tumor centers around making the distinction from MPNST. The latter is also hypercellular and composed of fascicles of cells, but the nuclei show a higher degree of hyperchromasia and cytologic atypia, and geographic necrosis and higher mitotic accounts are common. S-100 protein is seen in scattered cells in 50–70% of MPNSTs, but they generally lack the diffuse and strong S-100 staining pattern of cellular schwannomas. About 90% of MPNSTs are high-grade lesions, aiding in the distinction from cellular schwannoma.

In one of the original large series, "cellular schwannomas represented 4.6% of benign peripheral nerve tumors operated on at the Mayo Clinic. Median patient age was 47.7 years (range, 15 to 80 years), and the female-to-male ratio was 1.6:1. The principle tumor locations were the para- and intraspinal regions, including the sacrum (64%), extremities (25%), and intracranial space (8%). . . . Surgery was the treatment in all cases. . . . Follow-up revealed recurrences in 11 patients (23.4%): no patient experienced metastasis or died of tumor."

References

1. Casadei GP, Scheithauer BW, Hirose T, et al. Cellular schwannoma. A clinicopathologic, DNA flow cytometric, and proliferation marker study of 70 patients. Cancer 1995;75:1109–19.
2. Scheithauer BW, Woodruff JM, Erlandson RA. Atlas of Tumour Pathology: Tumors of the Peripheral Nervous System. Schwannoma, chapter 7. Washington DC: Armed Forces Institute of Pathology; 1997, p. 138–51.

Case 63: Melanotic Schwannoma

CLINICAL INFORMATION

The patient is a 55-year-old male whose diagnosis is heralded by 2 years of subacute, progressive, left-hand paresthesias, which progressed to involve the entire left upper extremity, with occasional numbness in the left foot and toes. There is associated incoordination of the left hand, significant difficulty typing on a computer keyboard, and problems with dropping objects. Neuroimaging studies show a mass near the cervical spinal cord, at the dorsal root entry zone for C2. The decision is made to resect the lesion, and, intraoperatively, the mass is noted to be jet black.

OPINION

Sections show a heavily pigmented neoplasm, composed of fascicles of cells and devoid of distinct Antoni A and B areas or well-developed Verocay bodies. The spindled and epithelioid cells manifest oval vesicular nuclei with occasional prominent nucleoli. There is no necrosis or mitotic activity. The most striking feature is the presence of dark cytoplasmic pigment, proven to be melanin, within the tumor cells. Unlike a primary or metastatic malignant melanoma in this site, reticulin fibers lie between tumor cells, and minimal mitotic activity and no necrosis are found.

We consider the excised tumor as representing a peripheral nerve sheath tumor and characterize it as follows: **Right Nerve Root, Excision—Melanotic Schwannoma, WHO Grade I.**

COMMENT

There are no psammoma bodies in this example. Over half of patients with psammomatous melanotic

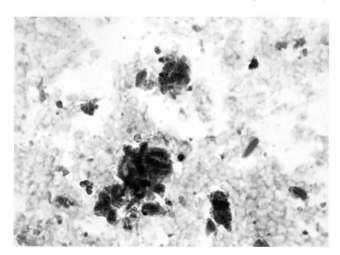

FIGURE 63.1 Intraoperative touch preparation, stained with hematoxylin and eosin, readily shows the heavily pigmented cells in this tumor.

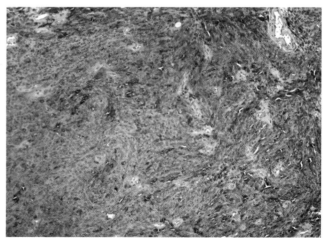

FIGURE 63.2 On low-power magnification, the mass is composed of fascicles of heavily pigmented cells, but no necrosis, Verocay bodies, or distinct Antoni A and B tissue is seen.

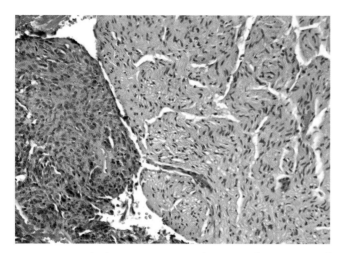

FIGURE 63.3 A close juxtaposition between the pigmented nerve sheath tumor (lower part of photograph) and a non-neoplastic nerve fascicle (upper part) can be seen.

schwannomas have Carney complex, a familial disorder usually transmitted as an autosomal dominant condition. Psammomatous melanotic schwannomas may be multiple. In contrast, non-psammomatous melanotic schwannomas are usually single lesions, not associated with neurofibromatosis, type II, or any other tumor predisposition syndrome.

DISCUSSION

Melanotic schwannomas are rare, circumscribed, but not fully encapsulated tumors that, by immunohistochemistry and electron microscopy, have features of Schwann cell derivation. In addition, they also contain melanosomes and are immunoreactive for melanoma markers. Compared to ordinary schwannomas, these tumors are more highly cellular, show less Antoni A and B distinction, only rare Verocay bodies, a poorly developed reticulin pattern, and more cytologic atypia, including macronucleoli and hyperchromatic nuclei. Epithelioid cells may be present. The amount of melanin pigment is highly variable. Bleaching procedures may be necessary in some cases in order to appreciate fully the cytologic features, mitotic activity, and even degree of necrosis

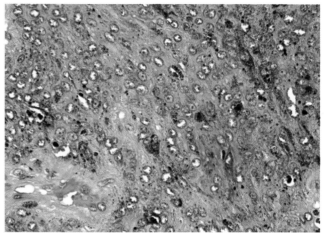

FIGURE 63.4 On high-power magnification, vesicular nuclei and delicate nucleoli are appreciated.

in the tumor, because some examples are extremely heavily pigmented, and the melanin obscures features of the tumor. Melanin pigment can be confirmed by the histochemical Fontana Masson stain. Basement membrane, even if more limited in amount, can be verified by immunostaining for laminin and collagen type IV.

Melanotic schwannoma must be distinguished from metastatic and primary malignant melanoma, mainly on the basis of increased mitotic activity and necrosis. The preoperative imaging

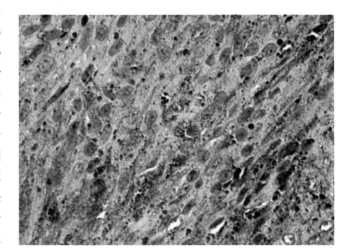

FIGURE 63.5 The absence of mitotic activity can be appreciated in less heavily pigmented areas.

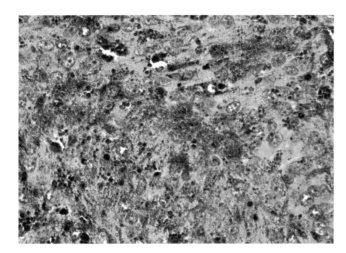

FIGURE 63.6 Melanin totally obscures cytologic detail in some areas and makes the search for mitotic figures more difficult.

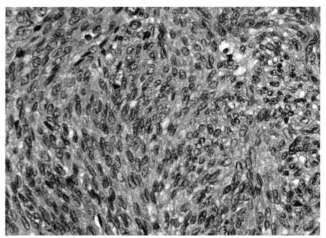

FIGURE 63.7 After bleaching procedures remove the melanin pigment, the fascicled arrangement of tumor cells is more clearly apparent.

findings of a dumbbell-shaped lesion involving a spinal nerve root (especially at cervical or thoracic levels, as in this patient) and the intraoperative and histologic recognition of a melanotic lesion arising from a nerve root are of great assistance in making this diagnosis. These features should sway the pathologist toward a diagnosis of melanotic schwannoma, not a metastasis. The differential diagnosis also includes meningeal melanocytoma

and intermediate-grade melanocytoma, the criteria for which have been published (see reference list). In general, less immunostaining for collagen type IV is seen in melanocytoma than in melanotic schwannoma, but electron microscopy may be necessary to confirm the Schwann cell derivation of melanotic schwannoma.

Melanotic schwannomas are usually benign, but gross total surgical excision with negative margins

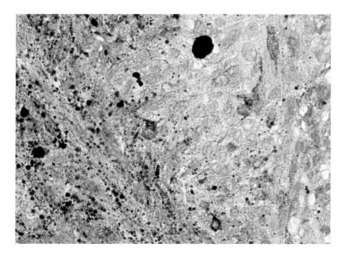

FIGURE 63.8 Fontana Masson histochemical staining confirms that the finely granular, brown pigment was melanin—by the dark, black, positive staining.

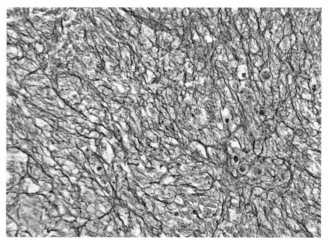

FIGURE 63.9 Reticulin staining in this example shows the classic abundant pericellular reticulin of a Schwann cell tumor, corresponding to abundant basement membrane.

is the optimal treatment. About 10–15% of melanotic schwannomas follow a malignant course, with recurrences and metastases. Bony destruction is more often a feature of malignant than of benign melanotic schwannoma. Unfortunately, it is not possible in individual cases to predict precisely which cases might metastasize, although, in general, tumors with mitotic activity and necrosis are more prone to this behavior. Very prominent macronucleoli are often also present in those cases that metastasize, although some tumors with this feature do not manifest malignant behavior.

References

1. Brat DJ, Giannini C, Scheithauer BW, et al. Primary melanocytic neoplasms of the central nervous systems. Am J Surg Pathol 1999;23:745–54.
2. Brat DJ, Perry A. Melanocytic lesions. In: Louis DN, Ohgaki H, Wiestler OD, Cavenee WK, Editors. WHO Classification of Tumours of the Central Nervous System. Lyon, FR: IARC Press;2007. p. 181–3.
3. Scheithauer BW, Louis DN, Hunter S, et al. Schwannoma. In: Louis DN, Ohgaki H, Wiestler OD, Cavenee WK, Editors. WHO Classification of Tumours of the Central Nervous System. Lyon, FR: IARC Press;2007. p. 154–5.
4. Scheithauer BW, Woodruff JM, Erlandson RA. Atlas of Tumour Pathology: Tumours of the Peripheral Nervous System. Schwannoma, chapter 7. Washington DC: Armed Forces Institute of Pathology; 1997. p. 156–70.

Case 64: Fibrous Meningioma

CLINICAL INFORMATION

The patient is a 62-year-old woman with a prior history of breast carcinoma who presents with headaches and occasional episodes of dizziness. On imaging studies, she is noted to have a contrast-enhancing mass in the left cerebello-pontine angle region on MRI studies. The lesion appears to be separate from the eighth cranial nerve. The mass is excised, and histologic sections are reviewed.

OPINION

Histologic sections show a spindle-cell neoplasm, marked by proliferation of cells with elongated nuclei with rounded nuclear ends and a scant amount of eosinophilic cytoplasm. Cells are arranged in interlacing bundles. Focal whorling of the cells around blood vessels is noted. Only rare mitotic figures are noted. There is no

evidence of calcifications or psammoma bodies. Verocay bodies are not identified. There is no evidence of brain invasion, prominent nucleolation, small cell change, disordered architecture, necrosis, or hypercellularity.

We consider the lesion to be a meningioma and characterize it as follows: **Left Cerebello-Pontine Angle Region, Excision—Fibrous (Fibroblastic) Meningioma, WHO Grade I.**

COMMENT

Morphologic features suggestive of an atypical meningioma are not identified in this tumor.

DISCUSSION

Meningiomas are among the more common nonglial tumors of the central nervous system. Classically,

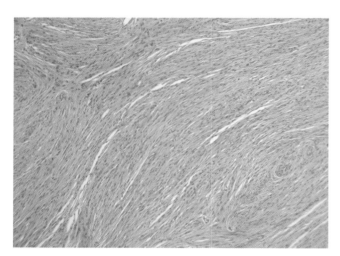

FIGURE 64.1 Low-magnification appearance of the fibrous meningioma, showing spindled cells arranged in large fascicle.

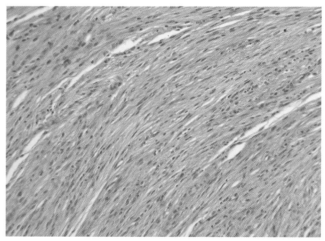

FIGURE 64.2 The cells in fibrous meningioma are rather monotonous in appearance and demonstrate little in the way of nuclear pleomorphism.

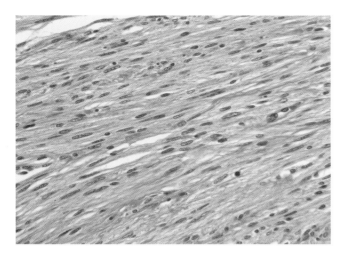

FIGURE 64.3 High-magnification appearance of tumor cells shows elongated nuclei with rounded nuclear ends.

they are dural-based in location and can arise at any age. There is a clear female predominance to cases that are reported in the literature. There is an association of a meningioma with certain malignancies, including breast cancer (as in this patient) and prior radiation.

Histologically, fibrous meningioma is marked by a proliferation of spindled cells, which are often arranged in bundles or fascicles and associated with

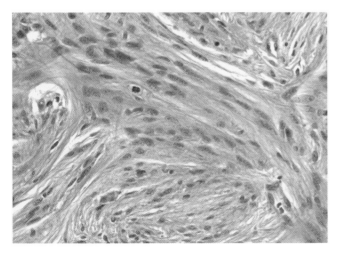

FIGURE 64.4 Rare mitotic figures identified in this fibrous meningioma. The number of mitotic figures was not high enough (4 mitotic figures of 10 high-power fields) to warrant consideration of atypical meningioma.

a collagen-rich matrix. The whorling of cells around blood vessels is a fairly frequent finding. Psammoma bodies, which are not evident in the current tumor, may be present in this lesion. Occasionally, nuclear pleomorphism may be evident and has no impact on grading of the tumor or prognosis.

The main differential diagnostic consideration in this current case includes differentiating this lesion from a schwannoma. The cerebello-pontine angle region is also a frequent site of origin for schwannomas of cranial nerve eight derivation. In contrast to meningioma, schwannomas generally have a biphasic appearance, with Antoni A and Antoni B patterns and Verocay bodies. Schwannomas do not demonstrate much whorling of cells around blood vessels, and they generally lack psammoma bodies. Immunohistochemistry is useful in distinguishing these two tumor types when morphology is not clear. Schwannomas demonstrate diffuse, positive staining with S-100 protein antibody; meningiomas may show weak, focal, positive staining in about 20% of cases. Most meningiomas demonstrate at least focal EMA immunoreactivity, in contrast to schwannomas that do not stain with EMA antibody. Occasionally, the fibrous pattern in meningioma may be admixed

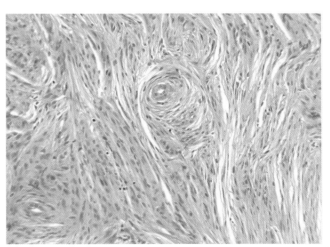

FIGURE 64.5 Focal angiocentric whorling of tumor cells is a characteristic feature of many meningiomas.

with the meningothelial pattern of tumor, in which case the diagnosis of transitional or mixed meningioma can be made. The patient's history of breast carcinoma also raises metastasis in the clinical differential diagnosis. Rare instances of metastatic breast carcinoma to a meningioma have been documented in the literature.

Fibrous meningiomas, along with meningothelial (syncytial) meningiomas, are among the more common patterns of grade I meningiomas. These tumors are quite amenable to surgical excision and have an excellent prognosis. Proliferation markers generally show low rates of cell proliferation in the grade I variants.

References

1. Burger PC, Scheithauer BW. Meningioma. In: Tumors of the Central Nervous System. Washington, DC: AFIP Fascicle 4th Series; 2007. p. 331–62.
2. Perry A, Louis DN, Scheithauer BW, et al. Meningiomas. In: Louis DN, Ohgaki H, Wiestler OD, Cavenee WK, Editors. WHO Classification of Tumours of the Central Nervous System. Lyon, FR: IARC Press;2007. p. 164–72.
3. Prayson RA. Pathology of meningiomas. In: Lee JH, Editor. Meningiomas. Diagnosis, Treatment, and Outcome. London, UK: Springer-Verlag;2008. p. 31–43.

Case 65: Ectopic Meningioma

CLINICAL INFORMATION

The patient is a 46-year-old female who presents with recurrent frontal sinus infections. On imaging studies, a mass lesion is noted, involving a frontal sinus with associated erosion of the adjacent bone. The mass is biopsied, and histologic sections are reviewed.

OPINION

Histologic sections show a normal-appearing respiratory mucosa with a submucosal mass. The mass is comprised of a proliferation of spindled cells with elongated nuclei, scant cytoplasm, and blunt nuclear ends. There is minimal cytologic atypia or nuclear pleomorphism in the tumor cells. An occasional lymphoid aggregate is noted in association with the neoplasm. The adjacent submucosal soft tissue shows focal chronic inflammation and reactive fibroblastic response to the tumor. Mitotic activity, necrosis, prominent nucleolation, small cell change, marked hypercellularity, and disordered architecture are not noted. There is no evidence of psammoma bodies.

We consider the lesion to be an ectopic meningioma and characterize it as follows: **Frontal Sinus, Excision—Fibrous (Fibroblastic) Meningioma, WHO Grade I.**

COMMENT

The tumor morphologically resembles a meningioma arising in an ectopic location.

DISCUSSION

Although the vast majority of meningiomas arise in the brain or spinal cord, most frequently associated

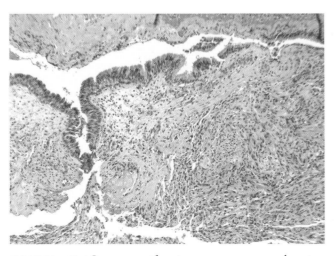

FIGURES 65.1 Low-magnification appearance, showing respiratory mucosa overlying a submucosal tumor.

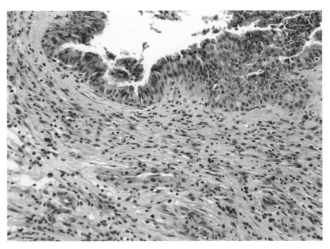

FIGURE 65.2 Adjacent submucosal tissue, uninvolved by tumor, shows chronic inflammation and a fibroblastic reaction.

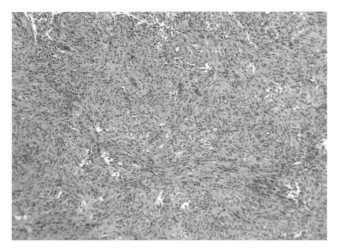

FIGURE 65.3 The tumor is comprised of a proliferation of monomorphic-appearing spindled cells.

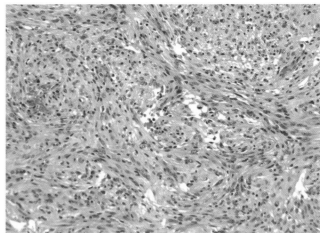

FIGURE 65.4 The tumor cells show minimal nuclear pleomorphism. Nuclear contours are elongated with blunted ends.

with dural tissue, ectopic locations for meningiomas have been described in the head and neck region, including the calvarium, orbit, middle ear, sinuses, and nasopharynx. Less frequently, meningiomas may arise in more distant locations, including skin, lung, and mediastinum; adrenal glands; and retroperitoneum. Because meningiomas in the ectopic locations are a relatively rare occurrence and often an unexpected finding, tumors may present a particular diagnostic challenge, particularly when they demonstrate

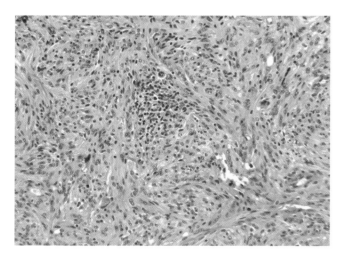

FIGURE 65.5 An occasional lymphoid aggregate is observed in the tumor.

unusual morphologic features. This patient's tumor shows morphology typical of a fibrous meningioma. The presence of psammoma bodies, whorling around vessels, and intranuclear pseudoinclusions may be useful clues that one is dealing with meningioma. The immunohistochemical profile of meningioma tends to be somewhat nondescript. EMA immunoreactivity (observed in approximately 80% of meningiomas) is said to be the most useful in terms of differential diagnosis. Smaller numbers of meningiomas may variably stain with antibodies to S-100 protein and cytokeratin markers. These tumors are generally subtyped and graded according to parameters defined in the central nervous system and spinal cord. Whether this approach is valid in ectopic sites is not known.

References

1. Perzin KH, Pushparaj N. Nonepithelial tumors of the nasal cavity, paranasal sinuses, and nasopharynx: a clinicopathologic study. XIII: meningiomas. Cancer 1984;54:1860–9.
2. Sadar ES, Conomy SP, Benjamin SP, et al. Meningiomas of the paranasal sinuses, benign and malignant. Neurosurgery 1979;4:227–31.
3. Thompson LD, Gyure KA. Extracranial sinonasal tract meningioma: a clinicopathologic study of 30 cases with a review of the literature. Am J Surg Pathol 2000;24:640–50.

Case 66: Clear Cell Meningioma

CLINICAL INFORMATION

The patient is a 42-year-old woman who presents with a mass in the right cerebello-pontine angle region. On imaging, the tumor appears to be a well-demarcated, dural-based mass. The lesion is excised, and histologic sections are reviewed.

OPINION

Histologic sections show a dural-based mass, comprised of a proliferation of cells with abundant clear cytoplasm. The tumor cell's nuclei are frequently eccentrically placed and contain small nucleoli. The overall arrangement of the cells is somewhat disordered (sheeting). Scattered between tumor cells are sclerotic vessels. Bands of collagen are noted, separating groups of cells. The edge of the neoplasm shows focal infiltration of tumor into adjacent soft tissue. Tumor cells in this region resemble the meningothelial pattern of meningioma, marked by cells with eosinophilic cytoplasm arranged in lobules.

We consider the lesion to be a meningioma and characterize it as follows: **Right Cerebello-Pontine Angle Region, Excision—Clear Cell Meningioma, WHO Grade II.**

COMMENT

The predominant pattern of this tumor is that of a clear cell meningioma. The clear cell pattern of meningioma has been associated with increased risk of recurrence.

DISCUSSION

Although the vast majority of meningiomas are grade I lesions, a subset of tumors, because of their increased

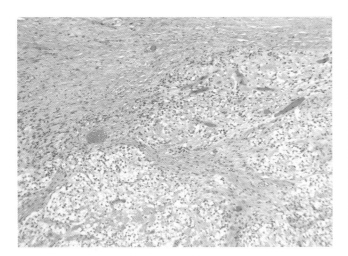

FIGURE 66.1 Low-magnification appearance of the clear meningioma, showing its dural attachment.

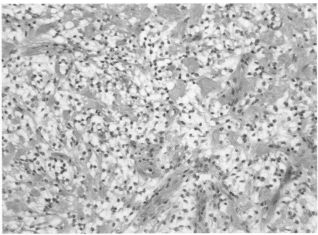

FIGURE 66.2 Intermediate-magnification appearance of the tumor, showing abundant cleared cytoplasm and disordered architectural arrangement of cells.

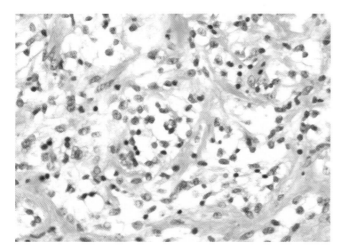

FIGURE 66.3 Cleared cytoplasm and small nucleoli are highlighted in a clear cell meningioma.

risk of a recurrence, are designated as higher-grade lesions. Clear cell meningioma is one such variant that is marked by a proliferation of cells with abundant cleared cytoplasm. The clearing is related to increased cytoplasmic glycogen accumulation, which can be highlighted with PAS staining. The cells in this variant are often arranged in a haphazard fashion, and characteristic meningioma features, such as whorling of cells around vessels and the presence of psammoma bodies, are distinctly uncommon in the vast major-

ity of these tumors. Clear cell meningiomas are more commonly seen in younger patients and seem to have a predilection for arising in the cerebello-pontine angle and cauda equina regions. Again, the importance of making this diagnosis is that these tumors show a propensity for recurrence in a shorter interval of time than grade I variants.

From a differential diagnostic standpoint, distinction of this tumor from other variants of meningioma may be important. This particular lesion, at its periphery, has areas more reminiscent of the grade I meningothelial meningioma pattern. There are no precise guidelines as to what percentage of the tumor must have a clear cell pattern in order to designate the tumor as clear cell meningioma. Because of this, if any appreciable portion of the tumor has clear cell morphology, it is important to indicate this in some way in the pathology report. Occasionally, distinction of clear cell meningioma from metastatic clear cell carcinomas, particularly renal cell carcinomas, may be problematic. Immunomarkers targeted for renal cell carcinomas, such as carbonic anhydrase and RCC antibodies, may be helpful in sorting out this differential diagnosis.

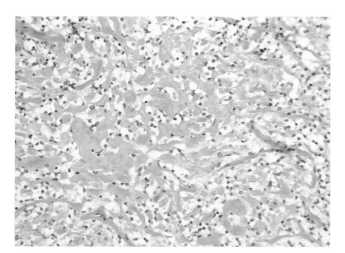

FIGURE 66.4 Focal sclerotic vessel change and bundles of collagen, deposited between groups of cells, are evident in this tumor.

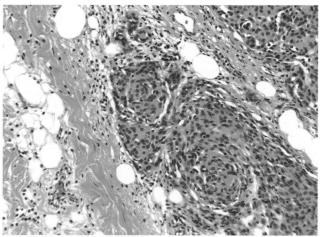

FIGURE 66.5 The periphery of the tumor shows a more conventional-appearing meningothelial (syncytial) pattern of meningioma.

References

1. Carlotti CG Jr, Neder L, Colli BO, et al. Clear cell meningioma of the fourth ventricle. Am J Surg Pathol 2003;27: 131–5.

2. Heth JA, Kirby P, Menezes AH. Intraspinal familial clear cell meningioma in a mother and child. Case report. J Neurosurg 2000;93:317–21.

3. Jallo GI, Kothbauer KF, Silvera VM, et al. Intraspinal clear cell meningioma: diagnosis and management: report of two cases. Neurosurgery 2001;48:218–21; discussion 221–2.

4. Zorludemir S, Scheithauer BW, Hirose T, et al. Clear cell meningioma. A clinicopathologic study of a potentially aggressive variant of meningioma. Am J Surg Pathol 1995;19:493–505.

Case 67: Chordoid Meningioma

CLINICAL INFORMATION

The patient is a 46-year-old female who presents with headaches and a 3.8-cm falcine mass. The mass appears on imaging to be circumscribed. The lesion is excised, and histologic sections are reviewed.

OPINION

Histologically, the mass is marked by a proliferation of generally rounded-to-polygonal cells with eosinophilic cytoplasm and eccentrically placed nucleus. The cells are arranged in cords or trabeculae with intervening mucoid matrix. Focal areas of fibrosis with collagen are observed. Some cells show prominent nucleolation. Occasional mitotic figures (up to 4 MF per 10 HPFs) are observed in this tumor. Focal areas of the neoplasm show a more solid pattern with a less mucoid matrix. The cells in these areas are haphazardly arranged. There is no evidence of necrosis or brain invasion. Prominent small cell change or hypercellularity is not observed.

We consider the lesion to be a variant of meningioma and characterize it as follows: **Falcine Region, Excision–Chordoid Meningioma, WHO Grade II.**

COMMENT

The predominant pattern of the tumor is that of a chordoid meningioma. Chordoid meningiomas are associated with more aggressive behavior and a higher risk of recurrence.

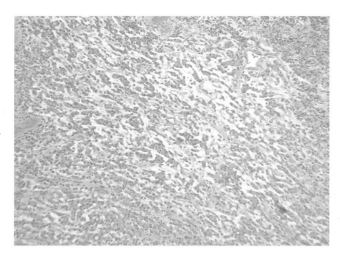

FIGURE 67.1 Low-magnification appearance of a chordoid meningioma, showing cords of cells arranged against a mucoid background.

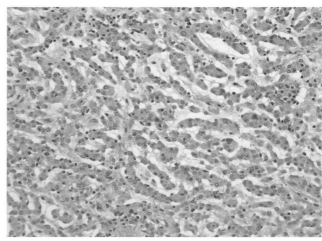

FIGURE 67.2 Higher magnification, showing characteristic architectural features of chordoid meningioma.

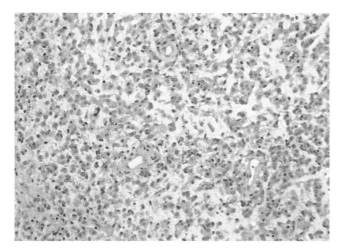

FIGURE 67.3 Focal area, showing more discohesive arrangement of cells against a mucoid background.

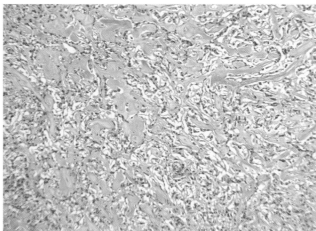

FIGURE 67.4 Focal fibrosis is observed in this tumor.

DISCUSSION

Chordoid meningioma, like clear cell meningioma, represents a morphologic variant of meningioma that has been associated with increased risk of recurrence. Again, like clear cell meningioma, precise criteria are not provided in terms of what percentage of tumor must have a chordoid phenotype to be designated as such. Subsequently, identification of any chordoid pattern in the tumor should be indicated in the pathology report. As the name suggests, the chordoid variant of meningioma resembles chordoma, in that the chordoid-like cells are often arranged in small clusters or trabeculae against a mucoid matrix background. More solid areas often show disordered architecture and, frequently, other features associated with more aggressive behavior in meningioma, such as prominent nucleolation and

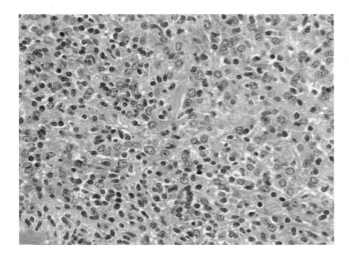

FIGURE 67.5 A more solid focus in a chordoid meningioma is marked by decreased mucoid matrix and cells arranged in a disordered fashion. Many of the cells show prominent nucleolation.

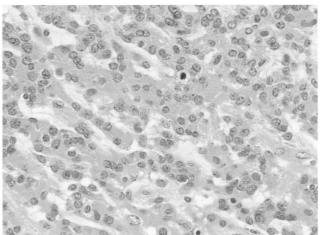

FIGURE 67.6 Mitotic figures, up to 4 MF per 10 HPFs, are observed in this tumor. Using WHO grading criteria, the presence of 4 or more MF per 10 HPFs is also enough to diagnose the tumor as a grade II neoplasm.

prominent mitotic activity (as in the current case), may be observable.

Differential diagnostic considerations typically include a metastatic adenocarcinoma and chordoma. The growth pattern of a chordoid meningioma is somewhat unusual for a metastatic carcinoma. Mucin-positive staining within cells or in glandular lumina is a feature of adenocarcinoma that is not observable in the chordoid meningioma. In contrast to chordoid meningiomas, the vast majority of metastatic muci-nous adenocarcinomas demonstrate diffuse positive staining with a variety of cytokeratin markers; cyto-keratin immunoreactivity in chordoid meningioma is generally focal. The majority of chordomas arise either in the clivus or filum terminale region. A falcine chordoma is extremely unusual. Additionally,

the physaliphorous cell change that is classic for chordoma is usually not observable in chordoid me-ningioma; however, small vacuoles may occasionally be observed in a subset of chordoid meningioma cells. Again, the immunohistochemical profile of chordo-ma also allows for its distinction from the chordoid meningioma, i.e., a more widespread cytokeratin and S-100 protein immunoreactivity in chordoma.

References

1. Couce ME, Aker FV, Scheithauer BW. Chordoid meningi-oma: a clinicopathologic study of 42 cases. Am J Surg Pathol 2000;24:899–905.
2. Kepes JJ, Chen WY, Connors MH, et al. "Chordoid" menin-geal tumors in young individuals with peritumoral lympho-plasmacellular infiltrates causing systemic manifestations of the Castleman syndrome. A report of seven cases. Cancer 1988;62:391–406.

Case 68: Papillary Meningioma

CLINICAL INFORMATION

The patient is an 8-year-old male who presents with confusion and headaches. On imaging studies, he is noted to have a dural-based mass overlying the right frontal-parietal convexity. The lesion is excised, and histologic sections are reviewed.

OPINION

Histologic sections show a cellular, dural-based mass, marked by a disordered arrangement of cells. Tumor cells show a variable amount of eosinophilic cytoplasm and somewhat eccentrically placed nucleus with prominent nucleolus. Prominent mitotic activity (up to 16 mitotic figures per 10 high-power fields) is observed in the tumor. Areas of necrosis are also identified. Focal areas of the tumor have a papillary architectural pattern, marked by fibrovascular cores rimmed by tumor cells. Definite evidence of brain invasion is not identified.

We consider the lesion to be a meningioma variant and characterize it as follows: **Right Frontal-Parietal Convexity, Excision—Papillary Meningioma, WHO Grade III.**

COMMENT

The focal presence of a papillary architectural pattern in meningioma indicates a more aggressive-behaving tumor, with increased risk of tumor recurrence and metastasis.

DISCUSSION

Papillary meningioma is a rare variant that is particularly aggressive in its behavior. The variant

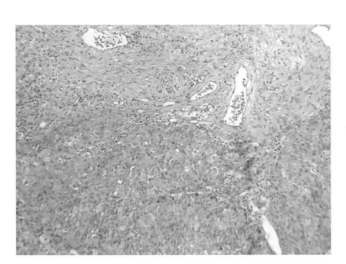

FIGURE 68.1 Low-magnification appearance, showing dural-based attachment of the tumor.

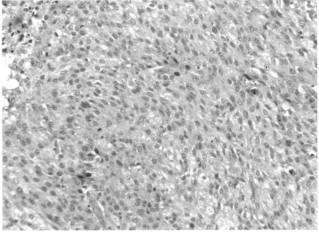

FIGURE 68.2 Intermediate magnification, showing a disordered arrangement of tumor cells and readily identifiable mitotic activity.

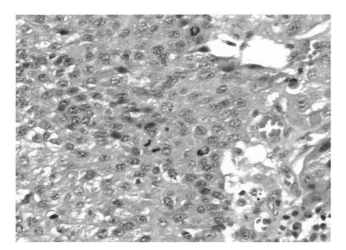

FIGURE 68.3 Mitotic figures are readily identifiable in this tumor.

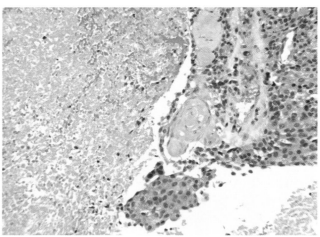

FIGURE 68.4 Focal necrosis is observed in the neoplasm.

shows a predilection for younger patients and is typically marked by a propensity for recurrence and metastasis to distant sites. This variant, as its name suggests, is characterized by a papillary architectural pattern, marked by fibrovascular cores lined by meningothelial cells. More solid areas of the tumor generally show features of high-grade meningioma, including increased mitotic activity, necrosis, brain invasion, hypercellularity, small cell change, prominent nucleolation, and a disordered architecture. In terms of differential diagnosis, care must be taken not to overinterpret discohesive clusters of meningothelial cells as papillary structures. Because of the aggressive behavior of this pattern, these tumors are often surgically excised and treated with adjuvant radiation therapy.

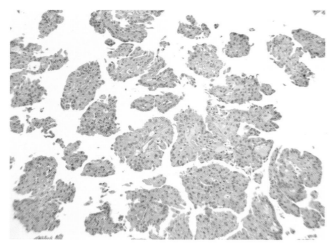

FIGURE 68.5 Low magnification shows areas of tumor with a papillary architecture.

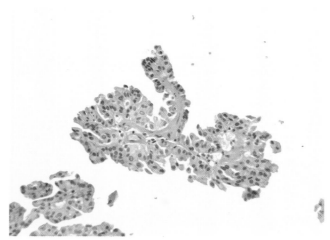

FIGURE 68.6 Intermediate magnification shows papillae, with fibrovascular cores lined by tumor cells.

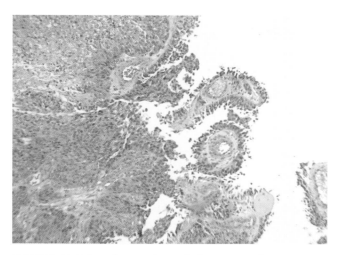

FIGURE 68.7 Another region of the tumor demonstrates the characteristic papillary architecture of papillary meningioma.

References

1. Ludwin SK, Rubinstein LJ, Russell DS. Papillary meningioma: a malignant variant of meningioma. Cancer 1975;36: 1363–73.
2. Pasquier B, Gasnier F, Pasquier D, et al. Papillary meningioma. Clinicopathologic study of seven cases and review of the literature. Cancer 1986;58:299–305.
3. Piatt JH Jr, Campbell, GA, Oakes WJ. Papillary meningioma involving the oculomotor nerve in an infant. Case report. J Neurosurg 1986;64:808–12.

Case 69: Rhabdoid Meningioma

CLINICAL INFORMATION

The patient is a 64-year-old female who presents with headaches of increasing intensity during the last two months. On imaging studies, a right frontal mass, overlying the convexity and attached to the dura, is observed. The lesion is resected, and histologic sections are reviewed.

OPINION

Histologic sections show a dural-based neoplasm, marked by a disordered proliferation of cells with abundant eosinophilic cytoplasm and eccentrically placed nuclei. Prominent nucleoli are observed in many of the cells' nuclei. Occasional cells have an eosinophilic cytoplasmic inclusion. Other areas of the tumor are marked by a proliferation of cells with less cytoplasm and prominent nucleolation.

Mitotic activity is readily observable, up to 22 MF per 10 HPFs. There is no evidence of brain invasion. There is no evidence of necrosis or small cell change. In areas, the tumor cells appear somewhat discohesive, giving the tumor a focal pseudopapillary architectural pattern.

We consider the lesion to be a meningioma and characterize it as follows: **Right Frontal Lobe, Excision—Rhabdoid Meningioma, WHO Grade III.**

COMMENT

The tumor demonstrates focal rhabdoid morphology, which has been associated with more aggressive behavior in meningiomas. Additionally, the mitotic activity is on the order typically observed in anaplastic meningiomas.

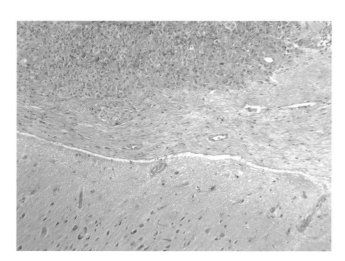

FIGURE 69.1 Low-magnification appearance of the tumor shows its relationship to dura and brain.

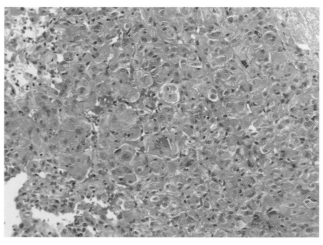

FIGURE 69.2 Intermediate magnification of tumors shows rhabdoid cells with abundant eosinophilic cytoplasm. The cells are arranged in a disordered architectural pattern.

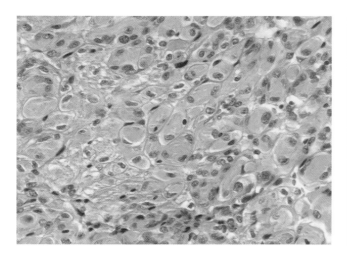

FIGURE 69.3 High-magnification appearance of rhabdoid cell shows cytoplasmic inclusions and prominent nucleolation.

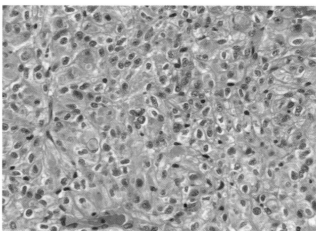

FIGURE 69.4 A disordered architectural pattern is observed in an area of the tumor that does not have a rhabdoid appearance.

DISCUSSION

Rhabdoid meningioma represents a rare variant of aggressive meningioma, marked by the presence of cells with rhabdoid morphology. The rhabdoid morphology is characterized by cells with abundant eosinophilic cytoplasm, containing eosinophilic inclusion-like structures that ultrastructurally consist of aggregates of filaments of intermediate molecular weight. Nuclei in these cells are often eccentrically placed and associated with prominent nucleoli. Similar cells are found in rhabdoid tumors arising elsewhere in the body, as well as the atypical teratoid/rhabdoid tumor of the central nervous system. Many rhabdoid meningiomas also demonstrate features of high-grade meningioma, including markedly increased mitotic activity (as in the current case), disordered architectural pattern arrangement of cells, prominent nucleolation, focal small cell change and hypercellularity,

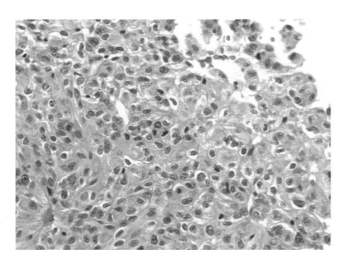

FIGURE 69.5 Prominent mitotic activity is observed in this tumor, in excess of 20 MF per 10 HPFs.

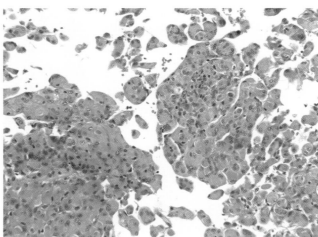

FIGURE 69.6 A discohesive arrangement of cells creates a pseudopapillary appearance.

necrosis, and brain invasion. A subset of these tumors has also been known to metastasize. These tumors notoriously have a poor outcome, with increased risk of focal recurrence and distant metastasis.

References

1. Bannykh SI, Perry A, Powell HC, et al. Malignant rhabdoid meningioma arising in the setting of preexisting ganglioglioma: a diagnosis supported by fluorescence in situ hybridization. Case report. J Neurosurg 2002;97:1450–5.

2. Kepes JJ, Moral LA, Wilkinson SB, et al. Rhabdoid transformation of tumor cells in meningiomas: a histologic indication of increased proliferative activity: report of four cases. Am J Surg Pathol 1998;22:231–8.

3. Perry A, Scheithauer BW, Stafford SL, et al. "Rhabdoid" meningioma: an aggressive variant. Am J Surg Pathol 1998;22:1482–90.

4. Parwani AV, Mikolaenko I, Eberhart CG, et al. Rhabdoid meningioma: cytopathologic findings in cerebrospinal fluid. Diagn Cytopathol 2003;29:297–9.

Case 70: Brain-Invasive Meningioma

CLINICAL INFORMATION

The patient is an 82-year-old female who presents with a seizure. Imaging studies show a 4.2-cm mass, attached to the dura in the right temporal-parietal lobe region. The lesion is resected, and histologic sections are reviewed.

OPINION

Histologic sections show a dural-based neoplasm, marked by a fairly uniform population of cells with oval nuclei and delicate chromatin pattern. Prominent nucleoli are observed focally throughout the tumor. Focal brain invasion is observed in the neoplasm. Rare mitotic figures (up to 2 MF per 10 HPFs) are noted. There is no evidence of necrosis, small cell change, marked hypercellularity, or disordered architectural pattern. Evidence of clear cell, chordoid, rhabdoid, or papillary morphologies is not observed.

We consider the lesion to be a meningioma and characterize it as follows: **Right Temporal-Parietal Lobe Region, Excision—Atypical Meningioma with Brain Invasion, WHO Grade II.**

COMMENT

The presence of brain invasion warrants the diagnosis of a WHO grade II meningioma.

DISCUSSION

Brain-invasive meningiomas are characterized by irregular nests or islands of tumor cells protruding into the subjacent neural parenchyma. This invasion typically

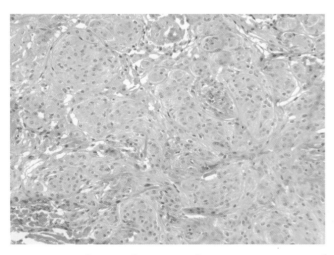

FIGURE 70.1 Intermediate-magnification appearance of the tumor, shows that it has the appearance of a meningothelial (syncytial) meningioma.

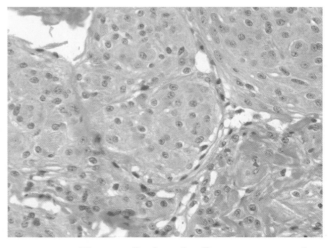

FIGURE 70.2 Tumor cells show focally prominent nucleolation, a feature usually associated with more aggressive behavior in meningiomas.

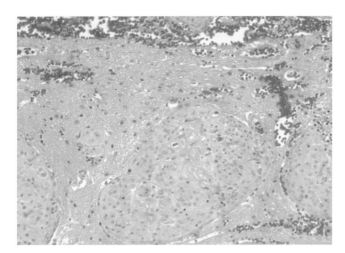

FIGURE 70.3 Intermediate-magnification appearance, shows focal brain invasion by the tumor.

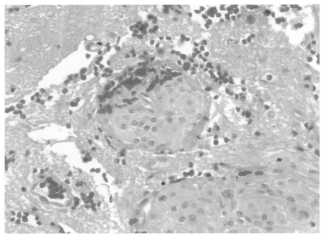

FIGURE 70.4 High-magnification shows an area of brain invasion by tumor is present.

elicits an adjacent reactive astrocytosis. Historically, the presence of brain invasion was equated with a high-grade WHO grade III neoplasm. The most recent updating of the WHO classification in 2007 suggests that brain-invasive meningiomas behave in a fashion more akin to that of WHO grade II neoplasms, in the absence of other criteria that warrant a higher-grade

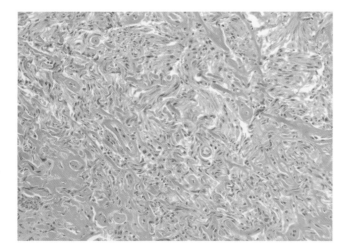

FIGURE 70.5 An area of electrocautery artefact is associated with elongation of cells in the tumor. This artifactual elongation of cells can mimic a fibrous pattern of meningioma.

designation. Many of the invasive tumors demonstrate other histologic features associated with atypical meningiomas, including increased mitotic activity, prominent nucleoli (as in the current case), necrosis, disordered architecture, small cell change, or hypercellularity. The search for the potential presence of an invasive component in meningioma should warrant a careful examination in all meningiomas of the tumor at its deep aspect. In other words, histologic sections should be taken at the interface between the tumor and brain, looking for evidence of invasion. In many of these cases, the surgeon indicates that the lesion is somewhat less circumscribed or is more attached to the brain tissue, warranting removal of brain tissue at the time of surgery.

References

1. Perry A, Louis DN, Scheithauer BW, et al. Meningiomas. In: Louis DN, Ohgaki H, Wiestler OD, Cavenee WK, Editors. WHO Classification of Tumours of the Central Nervous System. Lyon, FR: IARC Press;2007. p. 164–72.
2. Perry A, Stafford SL, Scheithauer BW, et al. Meningioma grading: an analysis of histologic parameters. Am J Surg Pathol 1997;21:1455–65.

Case 71: Atypical Meningioma

CLINICAL INFORMATION

The patient is a 68-year-old female who presents with headaches and a right falcine mass on imaging that measures 3.2 cm in greatest dimension. The lesion is resected, and histologic sections are reviewed.

OPINION

Histologic sections show a neoplasm, characterized by a proliferation of cells arranged in a haphazard, patternless architecture. Prominent vasculature is observed in the tumor. Areas of prominent cellularity and nuclear pleomorphism are present. Individual tumor cells show prominent nucleolation and scattered nuclear cytoplasmic pseudoinclusions. Mitotic figures are readily observable in the tumor, and up to 6 MF per 10 HPFs are present. There is no evidence of small cell change or necrosis. There is no evidence of brain invasion by the tumor.

We consider the lesion to be a meningioma and characterize it as follows: **Right Falcine Region, Excision—Atypical Meningioma, WHO Grade II.**

COMMENT

The increased mitotic activity (in excess of 4 MF per 10 HPFs), disordered architecture, hypercellularity, and prominent nucleolation are consistent with a diagnosis of atypical meningioma.

DISCUSSION

In addition to the histologic subtypes of meningioma (chordoid, clear cell, papillary, and rhabdoid) that are particularly associated with more aggressive behavior,

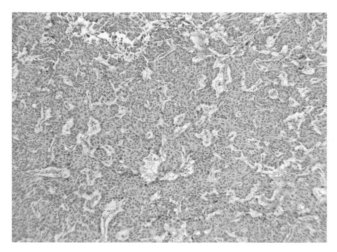

FIGURE 71.1 Low-magnification appearance of a hypercellular meningioma is marked by a haphazard or disordered arrangement of tumor cells and prominent vasculature.

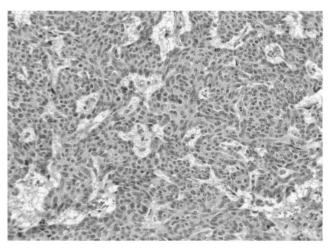

FIGURE 71.2 Intermediate-magnification appearance of the hypercellular, atypical meningioma, shows a disordered architectural pattern.

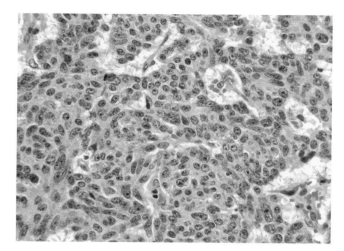

FIGURE 71.3 Prominent nucleoli are observed in tumor cells.

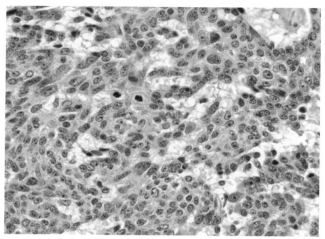

FIGURE 71.4 Mitotic figures are readily identifiable. Up to 6 MF per 10 HPFs are identified in this tumor.

there are a number of other histologic features that portend an increased risk of recurrence and distant spread in meningiomas. The designation of atypical meningioma is used for a tumor that is marked by 4 or more MF per 10 HPFs (a HPF is defined as 0.16 mm²). Alternately, tumors that have three or more other histologic features—including increased cellularity, small cell change with tumor cells marked by high nuclear-to-cytoplasmic ratios, prominent nucleoli,

disordered sheetlike architectural pattern, and necrosis—also warrant a diagnosis of atypical meningioma. As previously discussed in Case 70, tumors that demonstrate evidence of brain invasion are now designated as grade II meningiomas by the WHO. Most of these tumors are well differentiated enough that it is known that they represent meningiomas. Studies that have examined cell proliferation markers, such as Ki-67 or MIB-1, in these tumors have demonstrated an intermediate rate of cell proliferation, compared with the benign or WHO grade I variants of meningioma and the anaplastic or WHO grade III meningioma.

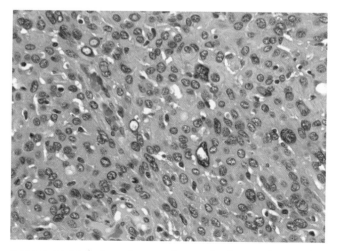

FIGURE 71.5 Nuclear pleomorphism, which is evident in this tumor, is not used in assessing tumor grade in meningiomas. The presence of nuclear pseudoinclusions can be a useful diagnostic clue to the meningothelial derivation of this tumor.

References

1. Abramovich CM, Prayson RA. Histopathologic features and MIB-1 labeling indices in recurrent and nonrecurrent meningiomas. Arch Pathol Lab Med 1999;123:793–800.
2. Perry A. Stafford SL, Scheithauer BW, et al. Meningioma grading: an analysis of histologic parameters. Am J Surg Pathol 1997;21:1455–65.
3. Nakasu S, Li DH, Okabe H, et al. Significance of MIB-1 staining indices in meningiomas: comparison of two counting methods. Am J Surg Pathol 2001;25:472–8.
4. Perry A, Louis DN, Scheithauer BW, et al. Meningiomas. In: Louis DN, Ohgaki H , Wiestler OD, Cavenee WK, Editors. WHO Classification of Tumours of the Central Nervous System. Lyon, FR: IARC Press;2007. p. 164–72.

Case 72: Anaplastic Meningioma

CLINICAL INFORMATION

The patient is a 72-year-old male who presents with weakness in the left arm and generalized fatigue. On imaging studies, he is noted to have a 6.2-cm, focally enhancing tumor, involving the right parietal convexity and attached to the dura. Resection of the tumor is performed, and histologic sections are reviewed.

OPINION

Histologic sections show a markedly cellular tumor, characterized by a haphazard arrangement of tumor cells. Occasional psammoma bodies, suggestive of meningothelial derivation for the tumor, are identified. Focal zones of necrosis are also noted in the tumor. In areas, the tumor cells assume a somewhat spindled appearance, resembling a sarcoma. Prominent numbers of mitotic figures, up to 24 MF per 10 HPFs, are noted in the tumor. Prominent nucleolation is also observed in the neoplasm. The tumor focally shows infiltration of surrounding soft tissue and skull. There is no definite evidence of brain invasion by the tumor. Papillary or rhabdoid features are not noted in the neoplasm.

We consider the lesion to be a high-grade meningioma and characterize it as follows: **Right Parietal Convexity, Excision—Anaplastic (Malignant) Meningioma, WHO Grade III.**

COMMENT

The presence of mitotic activity in excess of 20 MF per 10 HPFs and obviously malignant cytology are consistent with a diagnosis of anaplastic or malignant meningioma.

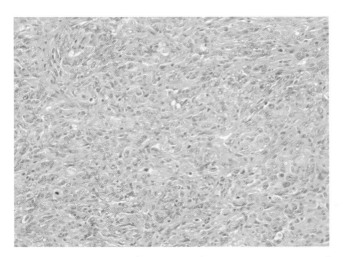

FIGURE 72.1 Intermediate-magnification appearance of the tumor, shows a poorly differentiated neoplasm with disordered architecture.

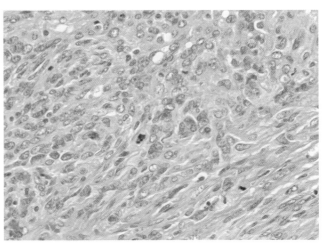

FIGURE 72.2 Increased mitotic activity is present in this tumor. Three mitotic figures in this one high-power field are noted.

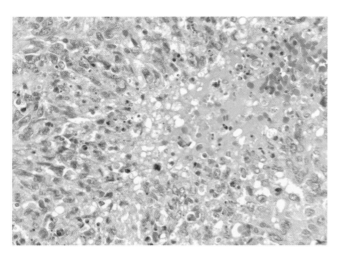

FIGURE 72.3 Necrosis is present.

DISCUSSION

Anaplastic meningiomas often show high-grade cytology, with tumor cells resembling those seen in carcinoma, melanoma, or high-grade sarcoma. These tumors often have exceedingly high mitotic rates, with mitotic indices of 20 or more MF per 10 HPFs. Tumors with either one of these features are generally classified as anaplastic or malignant meningiomas. The significance of the diagnosis is that many of these tumors prove fatal in a relatively short period, with a median survival of less than 2 years in many cases. These lesions, in addition to surgical resection, often warrant adjuvant therapy.

Because these tumors are so poorly differentiated, they often present a diagnostic challenge. Unless there are areas that are more well-differentiated in the tumor, recognition of the lesion as a meningioma can be challenging. The current case demonstrates psammoma body formations, which proves to be useful in delineating the lineage of the neoplasm. Distinction of these tumors from metastatic carcinomas may require the use of keratin immunostains, which generally show diffuse positive staining in carcinomas, and at most, focal weak staining in meningiomas. Differentiation of anaplastic meningioma from metastatic malignant melanoma can also prove to be challenging. Again, immunohistochemistry can be helpful, in that melanomas generally show fairly diffuse S-100 immunoreactivity and immunostaining with antibodies such as Melan-A or HMB 45, two markers that do not stain meningiomas. S-100 immunoreactivity, if present in meningiomas, is often focal and weak. Differentiation of high-grade meningioma from a spindled cell sarcoma can

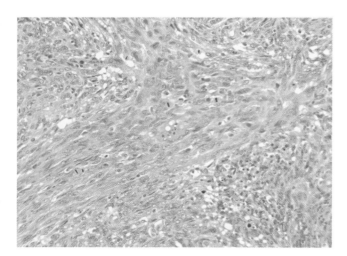

FIGURE 72.4 Areas of the tumor have a spindled, sarcoma-like appearance, with increased mitotic figures.

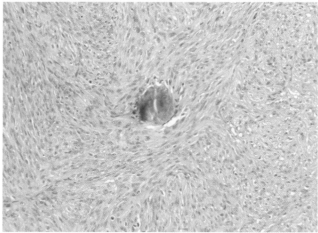

FIGURE 72.5 Rare psammoma bodies in the tumor are helpful in identifying the lesion as a meningioma.

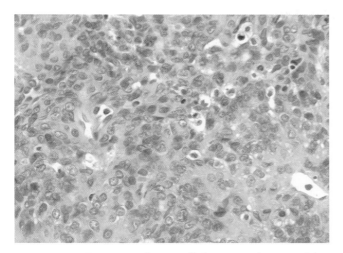

FIGURE 72.6 Prominent hypercellularity is a feature of this tumor.

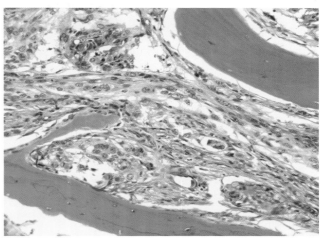

FIGURE 72.7 Infiltration of the skull by tumor is evident.

be difficult. Again, unless there are other clues as to the meningothelial derivation of the tumor or other features suggesting a particular sarcoma type, immunohistochemistry is not helpful in these cases. Rare cases of a sarcomatoid prominent gliosarcoma should also be considered in the differential diagnosis; these tumors generally show some areas of GFAP immunoreactivity, a finding that is not present in meningiomas.

References

1. Jaaskelainen J, Haltia M, Servo A. Atypical and anaplastic meningiomas: radiology, surgery, radiotherapy, and outcome. Surg Neurol 1986;25:233–42.
2. Perry A, Louis DN, Scheithauer BW, et al. Meningiomas. In: Louis DN, Ohgaki H, Wiestler OD, Cavenee WK, Editors. WHO classification of Tumours of the Central Nervous System. Lyon, FR: IARC Press;2007. p. 164–72.
3. Perry A, Scheithauer BW, Stafford SL, et al. "Malignancy" in meningiomas: a clinicopathologic study of 116 patients, with grading implications. Cancer 1999;85:2046–56.

Case 73: Angiomatous Meningioma

CLINICAL INFORMATION

The patient is a 42-year-old female who presents with a right falcine mass, measuring 3.1 cm on imaging studies. The mass is resected, and histologic sections are reviewed.

OPINION

Histologic sections show a dural-based mass, marked by a proliferation of blood vessels. In areas, the blood vessels appear to be almost back to back. Focally, prominent vascular sclerotic changes are noted. In other areas, small collections of atypical-appearing cells with rounded nuclei and eosinophilic cytoplasm are also seen. Intranuclear cytoplasmic pseudoinclusions are noted in some of these cells. Scattered evidence of nuclear pleomorphism in this population of cells is also identified. Mitotic activity, small cell change, necrosis, brain invasion, and prominent nucleolation are not seen. Areas of microcystic degenerative changes are noted. The tumor demonstrates evidence of intravascular embolization.

We consider the lesion to be a meningioma and characterize it as follows: **Right Falcine Region, Resection—Angiomatous Meningioma, WHO Grade I.**

COMMENT

The tumor is marked by a prominent proliferation of benign-appearing blood vessels. Worrisome histologic features indicative of an atypical or anaplastic meningioma are not identified.

DISCUSSION

The angiomatous variant of meningioma is characterized by a prominent proliferation of blood

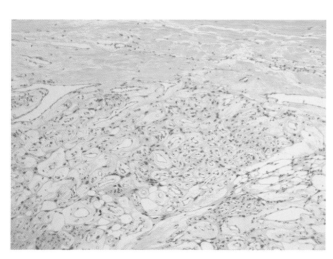

FIGURE 73.1 The tumor is a dural-based mass.

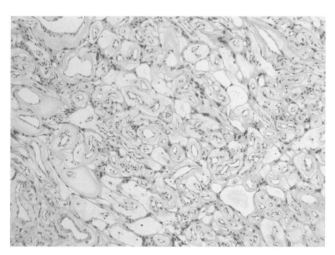

FIGURE 73.2 Back-to-back sclerotic vessels in the tumor can resemble a vascular malformation.

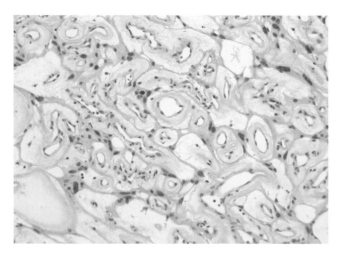

FIGURE 73.3 Intermediate magnification, shows a predominance of blood vessels, with rare atypical meningothelial cells situated between the vessels. The endothelial cells lining the vessels show minimal atypia.

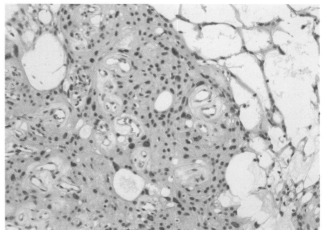

FIGURE 73.4 A more solid-appearing area of the tumor shows microcystic degenerative changes and nuclear pleomorphism of the meningothelial cells.

vessels. In areas of the tumor, the number of blood vessels may be so numerous as to raise vascular malformation as a differential diagnostic consideration. Careful search of these tumors, however, usually yields areas in which meningothelial cells, individually or in clusters or nests, are situated between blood vessels. Vascular sclerotic changes, as in the

current tumor, may be observable in the angiomatous meningioma as well. Hemangioblastomas can rarely arise in the falcine region; the hemangioblastoma is often marked by a stromal cell component that has a vacuolated quality to the cytoplasm. By immunohistochemistry, hemangioblastomas do not demonstrate EMA immunoreactivity, whereas most meningiomas demonstrate at least focal EMA

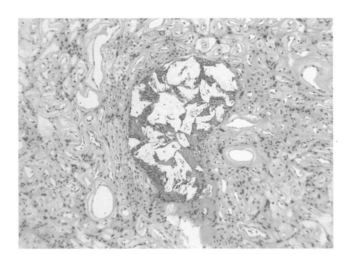

FIGURE 73.5 Focal evidence of embolization is evident in the tumor. Embolization is used preoperatively to reduce intraoperative hemorrhage.

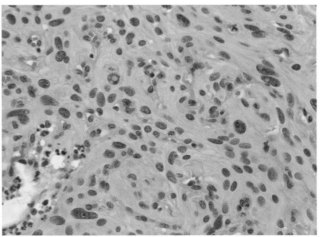

FIGURE 73.6 High-magnification appearance of meningothelial cells, demonstrates cytoplasmic pseudoinvaginations and nuclear pleomorphism.

staining. Hemangiopericytomas may also arise as dural-based masses and can present with a prominent vascular component. The cellular component of hemangiopericytomas is usually more atypical, and mitotic figures are frequently evident. Again, EMA does not usually stain hemangiopericytoma, and many of the cells in the solid areas of hemangiopericytoma frequently demonstrate CD34 immunoreactivity.

As a historical side note, angiomatous meningioma, hemangioblastomas, and hemangiopericytomas used to be collectively referred to as angioblastic meningiomas. These tumors were thought to have a worse prognosis, probably because of inclusion of hemangiopericytomas. With separation of hemangioblastoma and hemangiopericytoma as distinctive entities, the remaining angiomatous meningioma are benign. Use of the term of angioblastic meningioma is no longer advised.

References

1. Burger PC, Scheithauer WB. Meningioma. In: Tumors of the Central Nervous System. Washington, DC: AFIP Fascicle 4th series; 2007. p. 331–62.
2. Hasselblatt M, Nolte K, Paulus W. Angiomatous meningioma. A clinicopathologic study of 38 cases. Am J Surg Pathol 2004;28:390–3.
3. Prayson RA. Pathology of meningiomas. In: Lee JH, Editor. Meningiomas. Diagnosis, treatment, and outcome. London, UK: Springer-Verlag;2008. p. 31–43.

Case 74: Hemangiopericytoma

CLINICAL INFORMATION

The patient is a 62-year-old female who presents with a right parietal mass, growing through the skull and forming a lytic lesion. Because of rich vascularity in the tumor, preoperative embolization is undertaken prior to surgical resection of the lesion. Histologic sections are reviewed.

OPINION

Sections show a highly cellular, relatively pattern-less neoplasm, attached to dura and punctuated by numerous staghorn-shaped blood vessels of varying sizes. Cushions of tumor cells jut into blood vessels. Focal hemorrhage and more extensive necrosis are present, but much of the latter is seen in the same regions where vessels contain intravascular inert

material from preoperative embolization. No whorls of tumor cells or psammoma body calcifications are seen. Cytologically, the tumor is composed of closely juxtaposed atypical cells with elongate to comma-shaped nuclei and ill-defined cytoplasmic borders. Numerous mitotic figures are evident.

We consider the pathology to be that of a hemangiopericytoma with brisk mitotic activity and characterize it as follows: **Dura and Bone From Right Parietal Region, Excision—Anaplastic Hemangiopericytoma, WHO Grade III.**

COMMENT

Hemangiopericytoma is usually attached to dura, and when it extends through bone, as this example did, usually produces a lytic lesion, in contrast to the

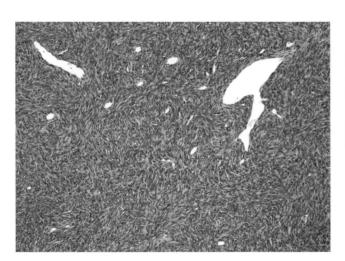

FIGURE 74.1 Low-magnification appearance of hemangiopericytoma shows a patternless tumor, punctuated by staghorn-shaped blood vessels of varying sizes.

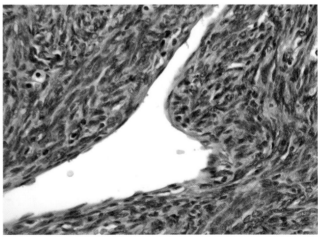

FIGURE 74.2 Medium-power magnification shows cushions of tumor cells to indent blood vessels, although not actually line the blood vessels; this reflects the pericytic lineage of this tumor.

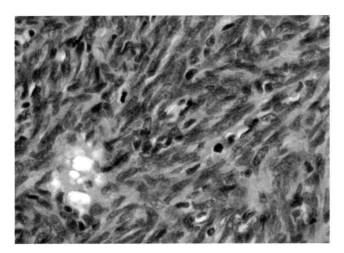

FIGURE 74.3 High magnification illustrates the elongate-to-comma-shaped nuclei of tumor cells, the ill-defined cell borders, and the equidistant spacing of nuclei from each other as a result of the interspersed basement membrane. Note several mitoses in a single field; this tumor had sufficient mitotic activity to classify it as an anaplastic hemangiopericytoma, WHO grade III.

hyperostotic lesion seen with meningiomas involving nearby bone.

DISCUSSION

Hemangiopericytoma is usually a solitary lesion and unassociated with any familial tumor syndrome. It is far less common that meningioma and has a slight predilection for being located in the occipital region, near the confluens of the sinuses. Despite the fact that hemangiopericytoma is usually well demarcated and seemingly able to be totally resected, local recurrence is very frequent, especially if the patient is followed for a sufficiently long period. Tumor may recur more than a decade after the initial resection. Hemangiopericytoma of the central nervous system (CNS) has the distinction of being one of the few primary CNS neoplasms with a propensity to metastasize outside the cranial vault or spinal column. Most patients eventually develop metastatic spread to bone, lung, or liver.

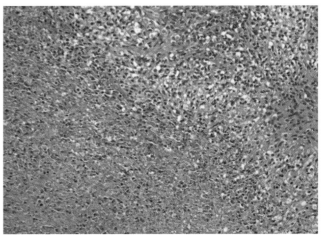

FIGURE 74.4 Several foci of necrosis found in this tumor are likely as a result of the rapidly growing tumor itself, based on the high cellularity and cytologic atypia of the nearby tumor.

Diagnosis is made by identifying a patternless tumor, composed of closely packed cells and punctuated by staghorn-shaped blood vessels. A helpful feature is the presence of each tumor cell being seemingly at equidistant spacing from its neighbor. This corresponds to the extracellular, basement membrane-like material that invests individual

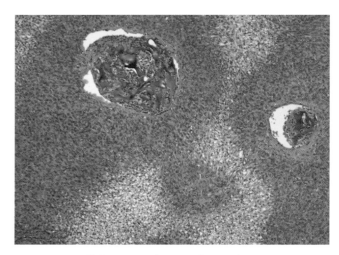

FIGURE 74.5 Other areas show early zonal necrosis, immediately juxtaposed to vessels containing intravascular inert material from the preoperative embolization procedure.

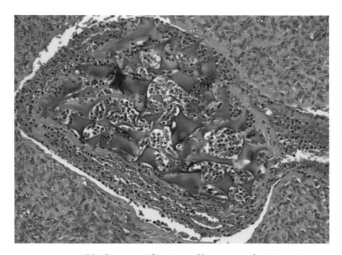

FIGURE 74.6 High magnification illustrates the inert intravascular embolic material.

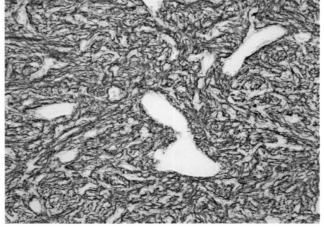

FIGURE 74.7 Abundant reticulin fibers surround individual and small groups of tumor cells.

tumor cells and is highlighted by a rich reticulin network on reticulin stain.

Hemangiopericytoma (HPC) is a low-grade sarcoma of the dura, graded as WHO grade II or III. Anaplastic (WHO grade III) HPCs, according to WHO 2007 classification, are characterized by "brisk mitotic activity (at least 5 mitoses per 10 high power fields) and/or necrosis, plus at least two of the following: hemorrhage, moderate to high nuclear atypia, and cellularity." This example had all of these features,

although, as noted previously, some of the necrosis was best attributed to the preoperative embolization procedure.

Reticulin staining shows abundant reticulin in most cases. HPC is strongly and diffusely immunoreactive for vimentin, shows patchy reactivity for CD34 (in contrast to the diffuse immunoreactivity of solitary fibrous tumor), and usually lacks the strong diffuse

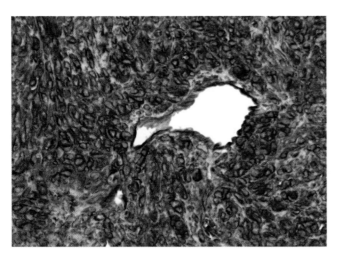

FIGURE 74.8 Hemangiopericytomas always show strong diffuse immunoreactivity for vimentin.

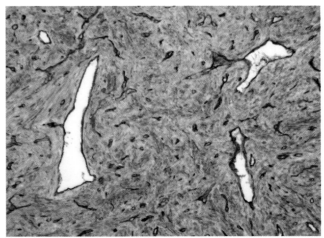

FIGURE 74.9 Patchy CD34 immunoreactivity is usually seen in hemangiopericytoma, in contrast to the diffuse immunoreactivity seen in solitary fibrous tumor; CD34 also highlights the staghorn vasculature.

immunoreactivity for EMA expected in meningioma. However, high-grade (atypical, WHO grade II and anaplastic, WHO grade III) meningiomas also may lose EMA immunoreactivity, and conversely, focal EMA positivity can be seen in HPCs. CD99 and bcl-2 immunoreactivity is seen in the majority of HPCs.

References

1. Giannini C, Rushing EJ, Hainfellner JA. Haemangiopericytoma. In: Louis DN, Ohgaki H, Wiestler OD, Cavenee, WK, Editors. WHO Classification of Tumours of the Central Nervous System. Lyon, FR: IARC Press;2007, p. 178–80.
2. Perry, A, Scheithauer BW, Nascimento AG. The immunophenotypic spectrum of meningeal hemangiopericytoma: a comparison with fibrous meningioma and solitary fibrous tumor of meninges. Am J Surg Pathol 1997;21:1354–60.
3. Prayson, RA. Non-glial tumors. In: Prayson RA, Editor. Neuropathology. Philadelphia, PA: Elsevier Churchill Livingstone;2005. p. 489–536.
4. Rajaram V, Brat DJ, Perry A. Anaplastic meningioma versus meningeal hemangiopericytoma: immunohistochemical and genetic markers. Hum Pathol 2004;35:1413–18.

Case 75: Solitary Fibrous Tumor

CLINICAL INFORMATION

The patient is a 62-year-old female who presents with a right temporal, dural-based mass. On imaging studies, the tumor appears well circumscribed and shows areas of contrast enhancement. The mass measures 2.1 cm. The lesion is excised, and histologic sections are reviewed.

OPINION

Histologic sections show a dural-based mass, marked by a proliferation of spindled cells, arranged in short fascicles. The cellular nuclei have rounded-to-tapered ends and are associated with scant cytoplasm. Between cells is increased collagen deposition. In areas, the cells on cross-section show more rounded nuclei. Intranuclear pseudoinclusions are not noted. Psammoma bodies are not seen. Mitotic figures are

not observed. Immunohistochemical staining shows CD34 immunoreactivity of tumors cells. The tumor does not stain with EMA antibody.

We consider the lesion to be a benign mesenchymal tumor and characterize it as follows: **Right Temporal Convexity, Excision—Solitary Fibrous Tumor.**

COMMENT

The tumor demonstrates CD34 immunoreactivity and does not stain with EMA antibody. This immunohistochemical profile, along with morphologic features of the neoplasm, are consistent with a diagnosis of solitary fibrous tissue.

DISCUSSION

Solitary fibrous tumors are relatively uncommon tumors, usually arising in the meninges in adults. Rare

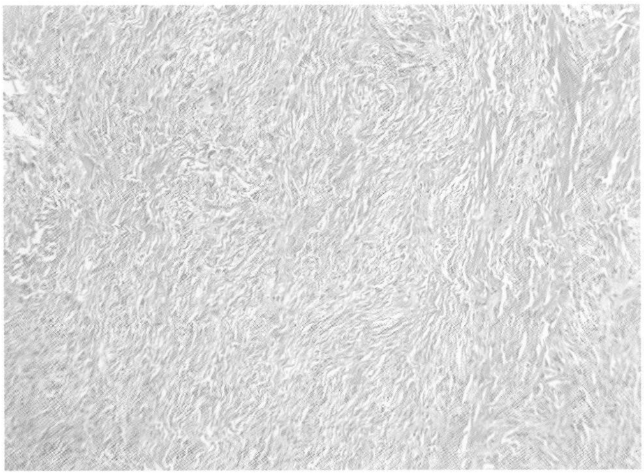

FIGURE 75.1 Low-magnification appearance of a solitary fibrous tumor, showing a proliferation of spindled cells resembling fibrous meningioma.

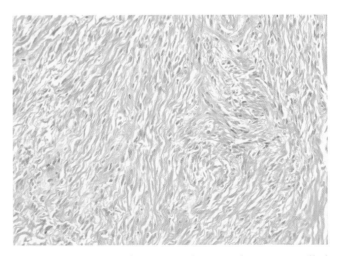

FIGURE 75.2 Intermediate magnification, showing spindled cells with intervening collagen deposition.

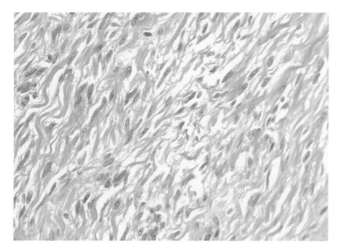

FIGURE 75.3 High-magnification appearance, showing bland nuclei with tapered ends and intervening collagen. Cytoplasmic intranuclear pseudoinclusions, a feature of many meningiomas, are not seen in solitary fibrous tumor.

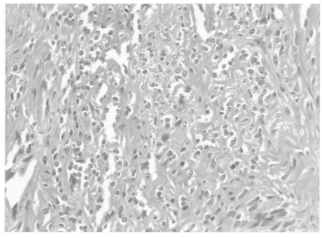

FIGURE 75.4 An area of the tumor where cells are marked by more rounded nuclei.

cases of intraventricular and spinal tumors have been also described. The lesions are generally well circumscribed and marked by a proliferation of spindled-to-rounded cells, with abundant collagen deposition between individual cells and small groups of cells. Spindle-cell tumors can mimic fibrous meningioma, which is usually the major differential diagnostic consideration. In contrast to meningiomas, these tumors

generally lack intranuclear cytoplasmic invaginations or pseudoinclusions and lack psammoma bodies. Immunohistochemistry can be helpful in delineating the lesion from meningioma, in that the majority of these tumors demonstrate fairly extensive immunoreactivity with antibody to CD34 and generally do not stain with antibody to EMA.

Although the majority of these tumors are low-grade lesions with a good prognosis, rare cases of anaplastic tumors with more aggressive histology

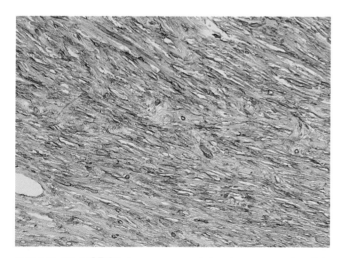

FIGURE 75.5 CD34 immunoreactivity is present in this tumor.

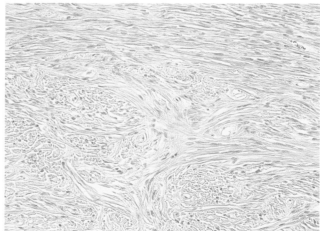

FIGURE 75.6 EMA immunostaining, characteristic of most meningiomas, is not present in this tumor.

have been described. These tumors are marked by increased mitotic activity and necrosis. The anaplastic tumors have a propensity to recur.

References

1. Cummings TJ, Burchette JL, McLendon RE. CD34 and dural fibroblasts: the relationship to solitary fibrous tumor and meningioma. Acta Neuropathol (Berl) 2001;102:349–54.

2. Carneiro SS, Scheithauer BW, Nascimento AG, et al. Solitary fibrous tumor of the meninges: a lesion distinct from fibrous meningioma. A clinicopathologic and immunohistochemical study. Am J Clin Pathol 1996;106:217–24.

3. Tihan T, Viglione M, Rosenblum MK, et al. Solitary fibrous tumors in the central nervous system. A clinicopathologic review of 18 cases and comparison to meningeal hemangiopericytomas. Arch Pathol Lab Med 2003;127:432–9.

Case 76: Primary Sarcoma of the Central Nervous System

CLINICAL INFORMATION

The patient is a 44-year-old male who presents with headaches and is found by neuroimaging studies to have a right frontal lobe mass. The decision is made to excise the lesion surgically, and intraoperatively, no attachment to the dura is detected. Histologic sections are available for review.

OPINION

Sections show a hypercellular, spindled cell neoplasm, with cells arranged in a fascicular pattern. Multifocal zones of necrosis are present, and mitotic rate is very high, exceeding 20 mitoses per 10 high-power microscopic fields. Careful search fails to disclose a coexistent glioblastoma. No smooth muscle, skeletal muscle, or malignant osteoid or cartilaginous elements are present in the sarcoma. The lesion has no continuity with a cranial peripheral nerve.

We consider the lesion to be a high-grade mesenchymal neoplasm and characterize it as follows: **Right Frontal Lobe, Excision—Primary Sarcoma of the Central Nervous System, WHO Grade IV.**

COMMENT

Mixed glioblastoma-sarcomas (gliosarcomas) with a dominant sarcomatous component are also uncommon, but more frequent than pure, nonmeningeal-based primary sarcomas of the brain.

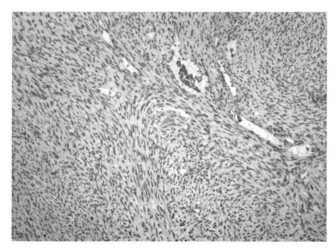

FIGURE 76.1 Low-power magnification appearance of the resected tissue shows a spindled neoplasm with cells arranged in fascicles. No muscle or osteocartilaginous elements are present.

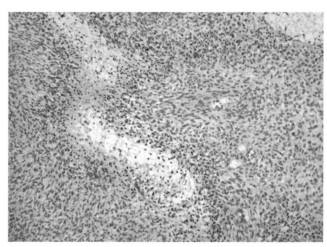

FIGURE 76.2 Low-power magnification allows identification of the extensive zonal, serpinginous necrosis in the high-grade sarcoma.

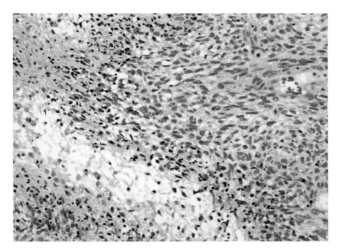

FIGURE 76.3 Intermediate-power magnification shows the karyorrhectic nuclei and slight pseudopalisading around the necrosis that can be seen in some sarcomas.

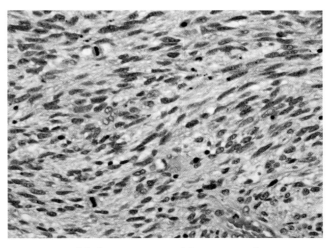

FIGURE 76.4 High-power view of the sarcoma demonstrates the brisk mitotic activity in the high-grade tumor.

DISCUSSION

Primary sarcomas of the central nervous system are very rare. A report in the literature coming from two large institutions was able to generate only 18 examples involving brain or spinal cord over a 30-year period (Oliveira et al.). Gliosarcoma (mixed glioblastoma-sarcoma), postirradiation sarcoma, meningeal sarcoma, and rare examples of sarcoma associated with ependymoma or oligodendroglioma must be excluded. Accurate remote clinical history is necessary in these patients, because decades may elapse between when a patient received cranial irradiation and subsequently developed a radiation-induced sarcoma. No antecedent radiation had been ever given to this patient.

In some instances of mixed glioblastoma-sarcoma (gliosarcoma), the glioblastoma component may be quite small and must be sought diligently by the pathologist. This is particularly true when the

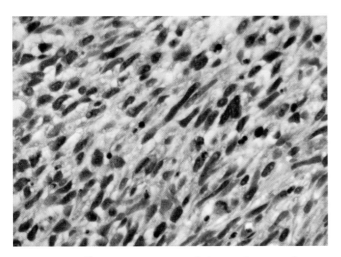

FIGURE 76.5 Sarcoma tumor nuclei are elongate, hyperchromatic, irregular, and without distinct nucleoli.

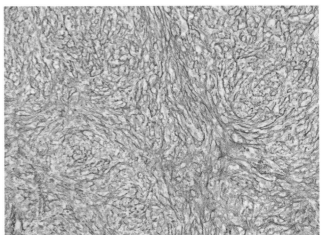

FIGURE 76.6 Reticulin staining demonstrates abundant reticulin fibers within the sarcoma, ruling out a pure, spindled glioblastoma.

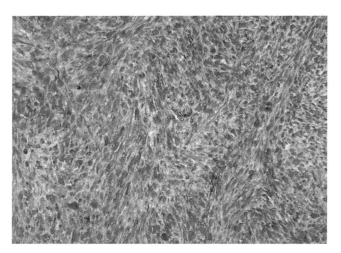

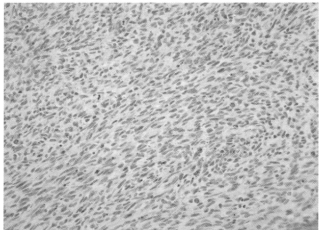

FIGURE 76.7 As is the case with many sarcomas, the only immunoreactivity seen in the tumor is diffuse staining for vimentin.

FIGURE 76.8 S-100 protein immunostaining is negative.

neurosurgeon has selectively removed the more obviously abnormal, cohesive, solid portion of the mixed tumor, leaving the more infiltrative glial portion of the lesion in the patient. No glioblastoma component was identified in this case, and immunostaining for GFAP was negative in several sections.

Another consideration in some cases of primary sarcomas of the brain is a more spindled form of an ordinary glioblastoma, where the glial cells are elongate and mimic a mesenchymal neoplasm. Negative immunostaining for S-100 and GFAP in this case also negated that diagnosis. Very rare intracranial examples of malignant peripheral nerve sheath tumor have been described, but without immunohistochemical evidence of peripheral nerve origin and without location near the skull base location of cranial peripheral nerves, that diagnosis is not possible. Finally, meningeal sarcomas (now synonymous with anaplastic meningioma, WHO grade III) and metastatic sarcomas or intracranial extension of a head and neck sarcoma are considerations. All were excluded in this case.

This example lacked dural attachment and manifests a fibrosarcoma-like pattern, with intersecting fascicles of spindled cells. The lesion is high grade, WHO grade IV, by virtue of its extensive necrosis and brisk mitotic activity. In the series of 18 cases reported by Oliveira et al., 6 of 18 were fibrosarcomas, 5 of 18 were malignant fibrous histiocytomas, and 3 of 16 were undifferentiated sarcomas. Two-thirds were high grade, based on degree of necrosis, mitotic activity, and extent of differentiation. Cerebrum was by far the most common location (83%). An immunohistochemical work-up includes immunostaining for GFAP, S-100, vimentin, desmin, smooth muscle actin, EMA, and CAM 5.2, with additional possible staining for other markers, depending on the light microscopic features.

Prognosis in the largest series of primary sarcomas of the brain and spinal cord was actually slightly better than that for glioblastomas, in that 28% of patients with high-grade sarcomas were alive at 5 years.

References

1. Duffner PK, Krischer JP, Horowitz ME, et al. Second malignancies in young children with primary brain tumors following treatment with prolonged postoperative chemotherapy and delayed irradiation: a Pediatric Oncology Group study. Ann Neurol 1998;44:313–6.

2. Kleinschmidt-Demasters BK, Kang JS, Lillehei KO. The burden of radiation-induced central nervous system tumors: a single institution's experience. J Neuropathol Exp Neurol 2006;65:204–16.

3. Oliveira AM, Scheithauer BW, Salomao DR, et al. Primary sarcomas of the brain and spinal cord: a study of 18 cases. Am J Surg Pathol 2002;26:1056–63.

4. Rodriguez FJ, Scheithauer BW, Perry A, et al. Ependymal tumors with sarcomatous change ("ependymosarcoma"): a clinicopathologic and molecular cytogenetic study. Am J Surg Pathol 2008;32:699–709.

5. Rodriguez FJ, Scheithauer BW, Jenkins R, et al. Gliosarcoma arising in oligodendroglial tumors ("oligosarcoma"): a clinicopathologic study. Am J Surg Pathol 2007;31:351–62.

Case 77: Meningioangiomatosis

CLINICAL INFORMATION

The patient is a 16-year-old male who presents with seizures and a left temporal lobe lesion. On imaging, the lesion appears to be predominantly intracortical in location and has a plaque-like distribution, with low signal intensity on T2-weighted MRI studies. Calcifications are also noted on CT imaging of the lesion. A resection of the lesion is performed, and histologic sections are reviewed.

OPINION

Histologic sections show a proliferation of blood vessels rimmed by spindled cells. Many of the spindled cells have elongated nuclei. The cells are piled up around the blood vessels, predominantly in the cortex, in a stratified fashion. There is minimal cytologic atypia or nuclear pleomorphism to these spindled cells. Occasional psammoma bodies are noted. Some of the vessels show prominent sclerotic changes. Mitotic figures are not identified in the spindled or in the endothelial cells lining vascular lumina. Intervening parenchyma between the blood vessels and the cortex shows gliosis. The overlying meninges shows a tumor, marked by a solid proliferation of spindled cells.

We characterize the lesion as follows: **Left Temporal Lobe, Excision—Meningioangiomatosis with Overlying Fibrous Meningioma, WHO Grade I.**

COMMENT

A subset of meningioangiomatosis cases has been associated with overlying meningioma. There is a

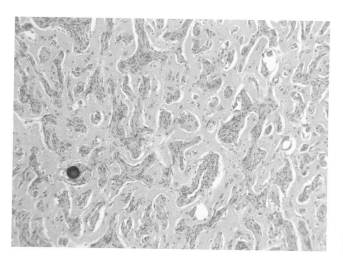

FIGURE 77.1 Low-magnification appearance of the cortex, shows collars of spindled cells arranged around blood vessels. Occasional psammoma bodies are observed.

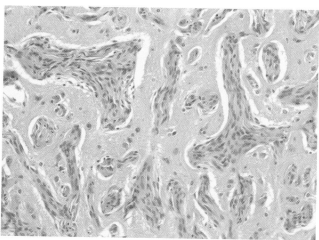

FIGURE 77.2 Intermediate magnification shows a perivascular arrangement of spindled meningothelial cells and fibroblastic cells.

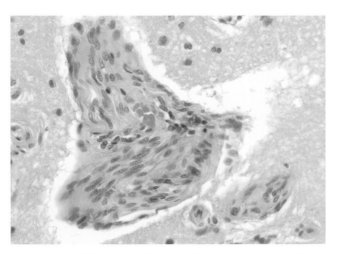

FIGURE 77.3 High magnification, shows minimal cytologic atypia in the cells around blood vessels.

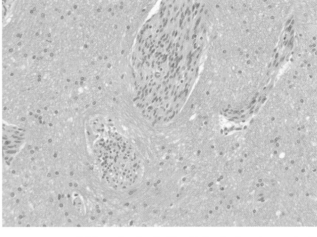

FIGURE 77.4 Although the bulk of the lesion is cortical-based, focal extension of the lesion into the subjacent white matter may be seen.

known association of meningioangiomatosis with neurofibromatosis, type II.

DISCUSSION

Meningioangiomatosis is a rare lesion, which likely has a maldevelopmental basis and is marked by a proliferation of predominantly cortical based vessels, rimmed by collars of spindled meningothelial cells and fibroblasts. Although many of these lesions have a maldevelopmental appearance to them, their

association with overlying meningiomas and certain molecular findings in more recent studies suggest that some of these tumors may represent neoplasms. The entity is known to be associated with neurofibromatosis, type II, and the presence of multifocal lesions is more closely tied to this phacomatosis. Occasional psammoma bodies may be seen in association with the collars of cells around vessels. It is not uncommon for the intervening parenchyma to show gliosis and

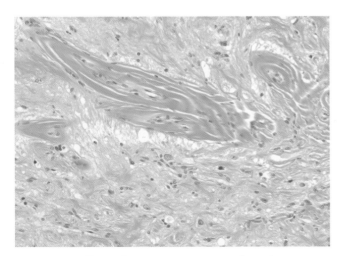

FIGURE 77.5 Foci of prominent perivascular sclerosis may be evident.

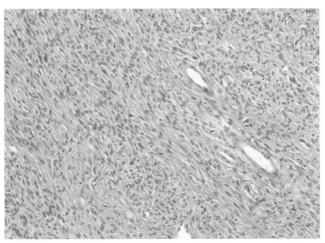

FIGURE 77.6 An overlying WHO grade I fibrous meningioma is observed.

occasionally, neurofibrillary tangles and granulovacuolar degeneration may be observable within cortical neurons in involved areas. Immunohistochemical studies have demonstrated low rates of cell proliferation. EMA immunoreactivity, as seen in meningioma, can be observable in meningioangiomatosis.

The lesion has a distinctive appearance. Differential diagnostic consideration includes a brain-invasive meningioma. The architectural pattern of meningioangiomatosis, however, is unusual for the brain-invasive meningioma, which usually does not invade in a plaque-like fashion. Occasional cases of meningioangiomatosis may show prominent vascular sclerosis; in these cases, the meningothelial and fibroblastic components of the tumor are not as clearly evident. In the lesions with prominent vascular sclerosis, a vascular malformation may enter into the differential diagnosis.

References

1. Halper J, Scheithauer BW, Okazaki H, et al. Meningoangiomatosis: a report of six cases with special reference to the occurrence of neurofibrillary tangles. J Neuropathol Exp Neurol 1986;45:426–46.
2. Perry A, Kurt Kaya-Yapier O, Scheithauer BW, et al. Insights into meningioangiomatosis with and without meningioma: a clinicopathologic and genetic series of 24 cases with review of the literature. Brain Pathol 2005;15:55–65.
3. Prayson RA. Meningioangiomatosis. A clinicopathologic study including MIB1 immunoreactivity. Arch Pathol Lab Med 1995;119:1061–4.
4. Stemmer-Rachamimov AO, Horgan MA, Taratuto AL, et al. Meningioangiomatosis is associated with neurofibromatosis 2 but not with somatic alterations of the NF2 gene. J Neuropathol Exp Neurol 1997;56:485–9.

Case 78: Hemangioblastoma

The patient is a 36-year-old male who presents with an unsteady gait. His past medical history is notable for a father and older brother who both died of renal cell carcinoma. On imaging studies, the lesion is a cyst, with contrast-enhancing mural nodule in the wall of the cyst. The entire lesion measures 2.8 cm. The lesion is resected, and histologic sections are reviewed.

OPINION

Histologic sections show a lesion marked by a proliferation of small caliber capillaries and venous vessels. Between blood vessels are cells with lightly eosinophilic or vacuolated, cleared cytoplasm. Focal microcystic changes are noted. In areas, the lesion shows a moderate degree of nuclear pleomorphism.

Focal dystrophic calcification is observed. The lesion appears to be circumscribed, but not encapsulated. The adjacent parenchyma shows Rosenthal fibers. There is no evidence of mitotic activity or necrosis in the lesion. EMA immunostaining is not observed.

We consider the lesion to be a neoplasm and characterize it as follows: **Left Cerebellum, Excision—Hemangioblastoma, WHO Grade I.**

COMMENT

The tumor does not stain with antibody to EMA. Hemangioblastomas are associated with von Hippel-Lindau disease.

DISCUSSION

Hemangioblastomas are tumors that generally arise in adults and are somewhat more frequently

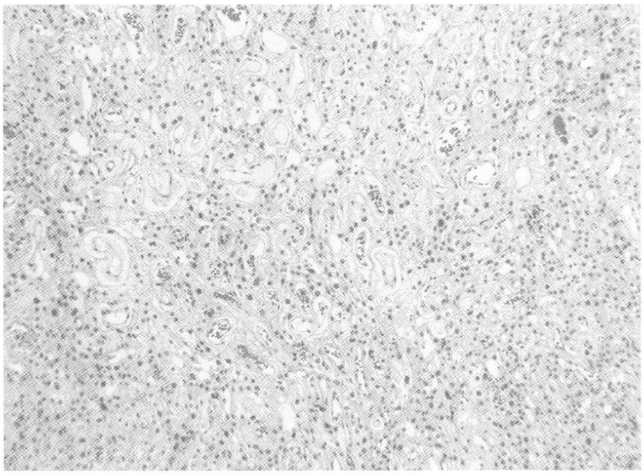

FIGURE 78.1 Low-magnification appearance of hemangioblastoma shows prominent numbers of small vessels with intravenous stromal cells.

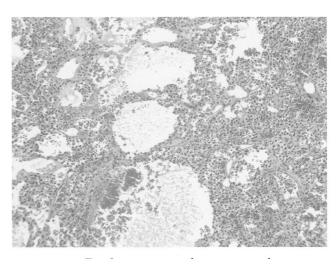

FIGURE 78.2 Focal microcystic degenerative changes are observed in the tumor.

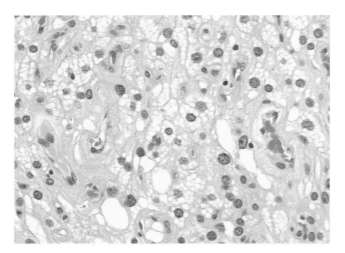

FIGURE 78.3 High-magnification appearance of stromal cells shows vacuolated cytoplasm.

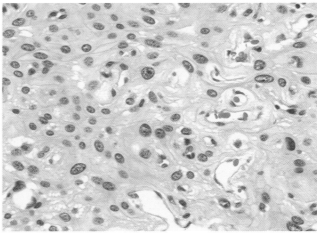

FIGURE 78.4 High-magnification appearance of stromal cells highlights lightly eosinophilic cytoplasm.

encountered in males. The cerebellum is the most common location; however, tumors have been described in the spinal cord or in other dural-based locations in the central nervous system. There is a well-known association of hemangioblastoma with von Hippel-Lindau disease. In the current patient, the family history of a brother and father with renal cell carcinoma raises the possibility of von Hippel-Lindau. There is also a known association of secondary polycythemia vera, with hemangioblastoma, as a

result of the production of erythropoietin in a subset of patients.

Imaging findings demonstrate a characteristic cyst, with enhancing mural nodule configuration. Tumors are often well circumscribed, with gliosis and Rosenthal fiber formations in the adjacent parenchyma. Because pilocytic astrocytomas can also arise in the cerebellum and may have increased Rosenthal fibers and a cyst with enhancing mural

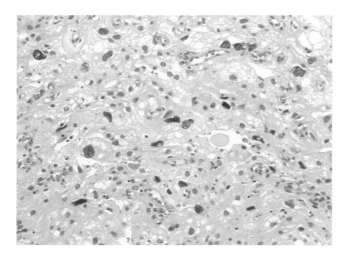

FIGURE 78.5 Pleomorphic cells in a hemangioblastoma do not afford the tumor a worse prognosis.

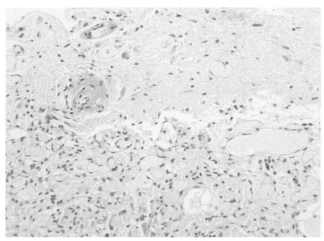

FIGURE 78.6 The hemangioblastomas are well circumscribed, and adjacent parenchyma may show piloid gliosis with Rosenthal fiber formations.

nodule radiographic appearance, tissue taken from the edge of a hemangioblastoma may be misinterpreted as representing a pilocytic astrocytoma. The tumor itself is comprised of a prominent number of small capillaries and venous vessels. Vascular sclerotic changes are often present. The intervening stromal cells may have a light eosinophilic or cleared, vacuolar cytoplasm. Some degree of nuclear pleomorphism may be evident but has no prognostic significance. Mitotic activity is rarely observed, and necrosis is distinctly uncommon in this tumor. These tumors generally demonstrate a low rate of cell proliferation.

The major differential diagnostic consideration is with a metastatic clear cell carcinoma, particularly in patients who have von Hippel-Lindau disease. Antibodies that have been potentially used to distinguish the two tumors include EMA (which stains most renal cell carcinomas positively and hemangioblastomas negatively), inhibin (which stains many hemangioblastomas positively and most renal cell carcinomas negatively), and a variety of renal cell carcinoma-directed antibodies, such as RCC or carbonic anhydrase 9. Metastatic renal cell carcinomas are also more likely to demonstrate areas of necrosis or mitotic activity. The importance of making the distinction lies in the differences in terms of biologic behavior. Hemangioblastomas are considered low-grade lesions, presumably curable with gross total resection.

References

1. Conway JE, Chou D, Clatterbuck RE, et al. Hemangioblastomas of the central nervous system in von Hippel-Lindau syndrome and sporadic disease. Neurosurgery 2001;48:55–62, discussion 62–3.
2. Hoang MP, Amirkhan RH. Inhibin alpha distinguishes hemangioblastoma from clear cell renal cell carcinoma. Am J Surg Pathol 2003;27:1152–6.
3. Neumann H, Eggert H, Weigel K, et al. Hemangioblastomas of the central nervous system. A 10-year study with special reference to von Hippel-Lindau syndrome. J Neurosurg 1989;70:24–30.
4. Wang C, Zhang J, Liu A, et al. Surgical management of medullary hemangioblastoma. Report of 47 cases. Surg Neurol 2001;56:218–26.

Case 79: Meningeal Melanocytoma

CLINICAL INFORMATION

This 39-year-old man with a known right nevus of Ota presents with left homonymous hemianopsia, left hemiparesis, and left hemiapraxia. A CT scan shows a homogeneously enhancing, well-defined mass, involving the right occipital lobe, which is confirmed by MRI. At surgery, the periosteum, bone, and dura mater surrounding the tumor are deeply pigmented, as is the tumor itself. The tumor is densely adherent to the dura mater, but easily dissected away from the brain parenchyma. Sections of the resection specimen are reviewed.

OPINION

The tumor is well demarcated, but not encapsulated. A small amount of neural parenchyma is adherent to the tumor, but not invaded by it. The tumor is composed of fascicles and nests of monomorphous spindle and occasionally, epithelioid cells, with round-to-oval regular nuclei and indistinct nucleoli. Although scattered clusters of tumor cells contain large amounts of melanin pigment, the vast majority of the tumor cells appear nonpigmented. Rare mitotic figures are identified. Coagulative tumor necrosis is absent. Immunohistochemical staining for EMA is negative. Immunostains for vimentin, S-100 protein, and gp100 (HMB 45 antibody) react with the tumor cells.

We consider the lesion to represent a low-grade meningeal melanocytic tumor and characterized as follows: **Right Occipital Lobe of Brain, Excision— Meningeal Melanocytoma.**

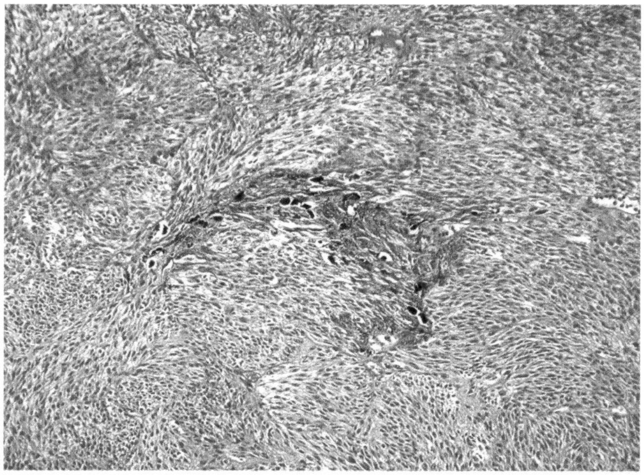

FIGURE 79.1 At low-power magnification, the tumor is composed of fascicles of monomorphous cells without whorl formation. Melanin-containing tumor cells are present in widely scattered clusters.

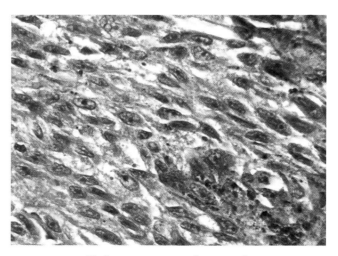

FIGURE 79.2 High-power magnification demonstrates a relatively monomorphous population of spindle shaped cells with small but distinct nucleoli. Although heavily pigmented tumor cells are uncommon, many of the tumor cells contain melanin granules.

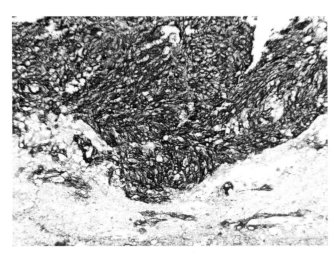

FIGURE 79.3 The tumor cells react strongly with the HMB 45 antibody, which also demonstrates scattered perivascular melanocytes within the adjacent neural parenchyma.

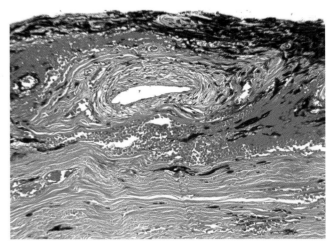

FIGURE 79.4 In this patient, densely pigmented melanocytic cells are identified within accompanying non-neoplastic dura mater, particularly along the epidural surface.

COMMENT

Fascicular growth pattern and low mitotic rate are consistent with "low-grade" meningeal melanocytoma. However, perivascular cortical permeation is considered to indicate "melanocytic tumor of intermediate differentiation." The accumulated literature indicates that all primary melanocytic central nervous system tumors demonstrate a tendency to recur, even after complete surgical resection.

DISCUSSION

Since the establishment of meningeal melanocytoma as a distinct tumor entity in 1972, approximately 100 primary melanocytic tumors of the central nervous system have been reported. Although they may occur throughout the neuraxis, spinal lesions are disproportionately represented—more than half of reported cases have occurred within the spinal canal, usually presenting with radiculopathy secondary to nerve root compression. Primary melanocytic tumors of the central nervous system most commonly present in young adults; fewer than 10 cases have been reported in children. They are believed to be derived from neoplastic transformation of pial melanocytes and, therefore, most commonly present as meningeal masses, although rare intramedullary melanocytomas have been reported. They can be distinguished from meningiomas immunohistochemically—these melanocytic tumors react with S-100 and HMB 45 antibodies, but not with antibody to EMA. Meningeal melanocytomas may be associated with dermal melanocytic lesions, such as oculodermal melanocytosis (nevus of Ota).

In 1999, Dan Brat and colleagues analyzed 33 of these rare tumors (comprising nearly half of the reported tumors at that time) and proposed a three-tiered grading system. Approximately half of their cases consisted of well-differentiated lesions (melanocytomas), characterized by variably pigmented cells arranged in nests and fascicles. This group of tumors demonstrated rare mitotic figures, inconspicuous nucleoli, and absence of parenchymal invasion. With a medium follow-up period of 3 years, none of these tumors recurred. Most of the other half of the tumors in the study were composed of poorly organized, mitotically active cells, with more prominent nucleoli, necrosis, and parenchymal invasion. This group of tumors was classified as primary central nervous system melanoma. Although half of these tumors recurred between 2 and 76 months after surgery, all but one were alive at the time of this publication. In addition, 4 out of 5 totally resected melanomas did not recur. Three of the tumors in the study (10%) could not be easily situated within either category and received the designation of intermediate-grade melanocytic tumor. Therefore, although the grading system proposed for primary central nervous system melanocytic tumors may be helpful in predicting the biologic behavior of these rare tumors, there is very significant overlap. In addition, with longer follow-up intervals, low-grade melanocytomas have shown a tendency toward radiographic recurrence.

References

1. Brat DJ, Giannini C, Scheithauer BW, et al. Primary melanocytic neoplasms of the central nervous systems. Am J Surg Pathol 1999;23:745–6.
2. El-Khashab M, Koral K, Bowers DC, et al. Intermediate grade meningeal melanocytoma of cervical spine. Childs Nerv Syst 2009;25:407–10.
3. Rahimi-Movaghar V, Karimi M. Meningeal melanocytoma of the brain and oculodermal melanocytosis (nevus of Ota): case report and literature review. Surg Neurol 2003;59:200–10.

Case 80: Malignant Melanoma

CLINICAL INFORMATION

The patient is a 15-month-old boy with congenital nevi over 50–60% of his body surface. He had undergone neuroimaging 1 year previously, which had shown a tentorial dural lesion. He presents with recent medial deviation of his right eye, ataxia, vomiting, and loss of consciousness. New imaging studies show a large hemorrhagic lesion of the superior vermis of cerebellum. Resection of his posterior fossa tumor is undertaken, and histologic sections are reviewed.

OPINION

Biopsies show a hemorrhagic, highly necrotic, highly malignant epithelioid tumor. Widespread artifactual pigment is present as a result of the interaction between formalin fixative and fresh blood. The tumor is pleomorphic, amelanotic, and highly mitotically active.

We consider the pathology to be that of a malignant melanoma and characterize it as follows: **Midline Cerebellum, Excision—Malignant Melanoma, Possibly Primary to Central Nervous System, WHO Grade IV.**

COMMENT

There is no obvious systemic or cutaneous primary source for this patient's malignant melanoma; given his previously documented leptomeningeal melanosis, this malignant melanoma may have arisen from leptomeningeal melanocytes.

DISCUSSION

Primary melanocytic neoplasms occur in the central nervous system and can be either benign or malignant. This child displayed neurocutaneous

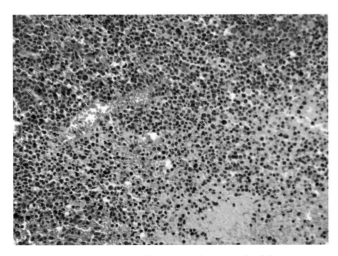

FIGURE 80.1 Low magnification shows a highly necrotic and hemorrhagic epithelioid neoplasm.

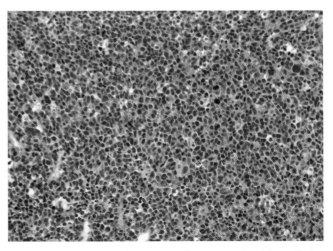

FIGURE 80.2 The malignant melanoma is highly cellular and patternless.

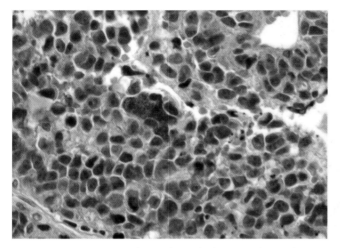

FIGURE 80.3 Large multinucleated pleomorphic cells are present.

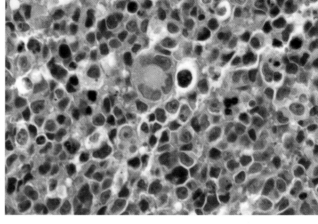

FIGURE 80.4 Nucleoli are prominent, and pleomorphism is evident at higher magnification.

melanosis, a rare phakomatosis typified by large cutaneous nevi, which may cover a significant surface area of the body. This condition is present from birth, but once malignant transformation occurs within the melanocytic population, clinical symptoms develop rapidly. Indeed, this child died within a month after his neurosurgical procedure; permission for autopsy was not obtained, but it is likely that the tentorial lesion seen originally was the primary source of his melanoma.

Histologically, the tumor is composed of epithelioid cells, some of which are large, bizarre, and multinucleated. Cells manifest prominent eosinophilic nucleoli and abundant cytoplasm devoid of melanin pigment, although some central nervous system primary malignant melanomas may be pigmented. Nuclear and cytoplasmic immunoreactivity for S-100 protein and focal cytoplasmic immunoreactivity for Melan-A and HMB 45 corroborate the diagnosis.

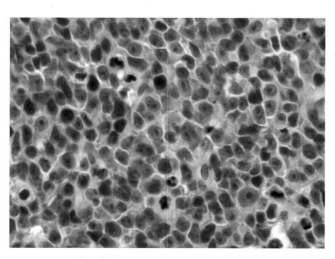

FIGURE 80.5 Brisk mitotic activity is seen.

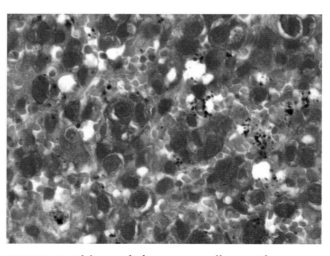

FIGURE 80.6 Many of the tumor cells manifest strong nuclear and cytoplasmic immunoreactivity for S-100 protein (red chromagen).

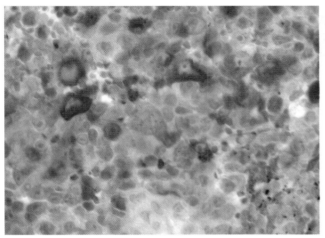

FIGURE 80.7 Significant numbers of tumor cells also show immunoreactivity for Melan-A.

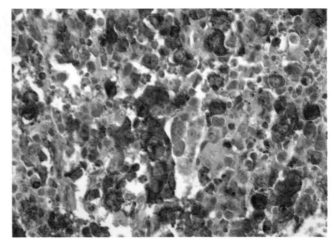

FIGURE 80.8 HMB 45 immunoreactivity is also present.

References

1. Brat DJ, Giannini C, Scheithauer BW, et al. Primary melanocytic neoplasms of the central nervous systems. Am J Surg Path 1999;23(7):745–54.

2. Brat DJ, Perry A. Melanocytic lesions. In: Louis DN, Ohgaki H, Wiestler OD, Cavenee WK, Editors. WHO Classification of Tumours of the Central Nervous System. Lyon, FR: IARC Press;2007. p. 181–3.

Case 81: Lymphoma with First Presentation as Spinal Cord Compression

CLINICAL INFORMATION

The patient is an 18-year-old male who is a very active athlete. He notes worsening leg pain and numbness, as well as spasticity in his lower extremities. A MR scan of the spine demonstrates a large mass, involving thoracic cord levels T3–T6. The mass appears to be located in the epidural space posterior to the spinal cord, with spinal cord compression, and is causing signal changes at T6. Emergent decompression is undertaken, with extensive tumor removal. Histologic sections are reviewed.

OPINION

Sections show sheets of cytologically monotonous, closely packed, hematopoietic tumor cells, occupying the epidural soft tissue space as well as adjacent vertebral bone. Cells manifest very high nuclear-to-cytoplasmic ratios, scant cytoplasm, hyperchromatic nuclei, and moderately distinct nucleoli. Mitotic activity is brisk.

We consider the lesion to be a hematopoietic neoplasm and, after special immunostaining and fluorescence in situ hybridization (FISH) studies, characterize it as follows: **Cerebral Hemispheric Clot, Evacuation—Acute B Lymphoblastic Lymphoma/ Leukemia.**

COMMENT

Acute B lymphoblastic leukemia usually presents with anemia or thrombocytopenia; bone pain or arthralgias are common. Presentation as a mass-like lymphoma is considerably less common.

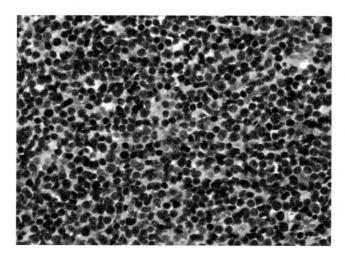

FIGURE 81.1 Intermediate-power magnification appearance shows patternless sheets of monomorphic tumor cells with little necrosis.

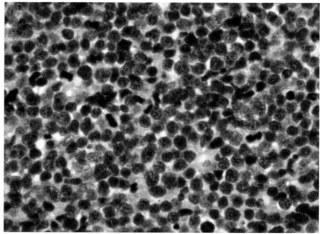

FIGURE 81.2 High-power magnification illustrates the high nuclear-to-cytoplasmic ratio, scant cytoplasm, nuclear hyperchromasia, and mitotic activity of the tumor cells.

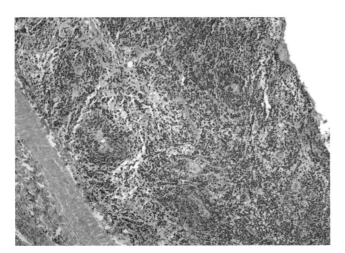

FIGURE 81.3 Low-power magnification illustrates the involvement of fibroadipose tissue by the lymphoma, including a strip of ligament from the epidural space (left lower area).

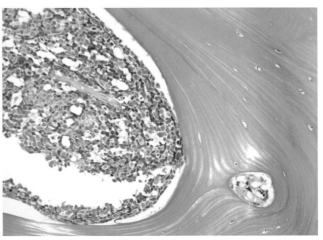

FIGURE 81.4 Low-power magnification also shows that adjacent vertebral bone is involved by the lymphoma.

DISCUSSION

Criteria for diagnosis and classification of leukemias involving the central nervous system are identical to those utilized in other tissues in the body. In this case, the histologic features were those of a lymphoblastic leukemia/lymphoma with very high MIB-1

index of greater than 80%, strong CD10 immunostaining in the lymphoblasts (as is usually the case in acute lymphoblastic leukemia/lymphoma, along with CD24 immunoreactivity), and moderate staining for TdT and CD34. Although another consideration was Burkitt lymphoma, with the high MIB-1 rate and CD10 immunostaining, the additional positive staining for the latter two immunostains negated that consideration. Immunostaining for B cell markers is also seen, with reactivity for CD19 and cytoplasmic CD79a

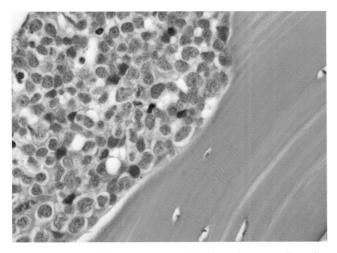

FIGURE 81.5 High-power view of the lymphoma within the bone demonstrates excellent cytologic preservation and the relative, moderate-sized nucleoli in the tumor, contrasting it with several other types of lymphoma, including Burkitt lymphoma.

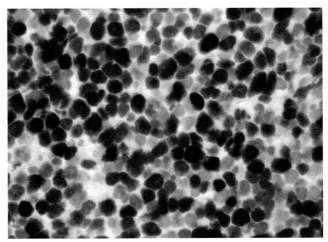

FIGURE 81.6 A very high MIB-1 cell cycle labeling index is present.

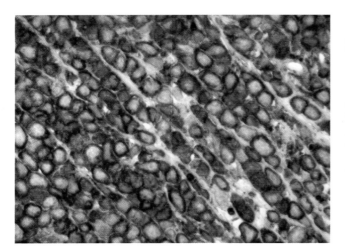

FIGURE 81.7 Strong diffuse immunoreactivity for CD10 is seen in the lymphoblasts in most cases of acute lymphoblastic leukemia/lymphoma.

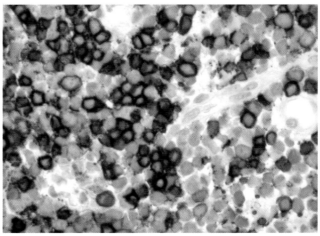

FIGURE 81.8 Patchy immunoreactivity for CD20 is present in this case.

almost always being present, and variable expression of CD22 and CD20. In this example, FISH studies showed no c-MYC translocation, as would have been expected in Burkitt lymphoma, and did show multiple gains of various chromosomes, a feature seen in B lymphoblastic leukemia/lymphoma.

The epidural space is a well-known, albeit uncommon, location for lymphomatous involvement, estimated to occur in less than 3% of all systemic lymphomas. A 10-year retrospective search in one study generated 7 patients who presented initially with back pain, incontinence, and/or lower extremity weakness. By neuroimaging studies, these patients were found to have masses necessitating neurosurgical intervention. Lymphoma types included high-grade non-Hodgkin lymphoma, B cell type (n = 4), indolent B cell lymphoma (n = 1), nodular sclerosing Hodgkin lymphoma (n = 1), and plasmacytoma (n = 1). Advanced disease (stage 4) was subsequently identified in all 7 patients. Despite this, survival varied greatly with therapy, from 3 weeks to almost 6 years, underscoring the need for correct classification of the lymphoma in order to optimize chemotherapeutic choices. The epidural space was

the site of presentation of disease in 4% of all lymphomas diagnosed at our institution.

Epidural lymphomas are systemic lymphomas that present in a critical anatomic location that often requires emergent surgical decompression before a full systemic work-up can be undertaken. The lymphomatous diagnosis may be suspected but is often not proven by tissue biopsy at the time of the neurosurgical procedure. Epidural lymphomas are distinct from both primary central nervous system lymphomas and from primary dural (MALT) lymphomas. Thus, a full work-up for lymphoma classification should be undertaken on tissue received from the epidural space. Usually, adjacent bony involvement is also identified. In some instances, this tissue received from the neurosurgical procedure may be the optimal or only tissue available from the patient on which to perform the work-up for classification of the lymphoma. Therefore, it is important to make the diagnosis of lymphoma/leukemia at the time of intraoperative consultation to allow optimal triaging of tissue for the appropriate studies.

References

1. Brunning RD, Borowitz, M, Matutes E, et al. Precursor B lymphoblastic leukaemia/lymphoblastic lymphoma. In: ES

Jaffe, NL Harris, H Stein, JW Vardiman, Editors. WHO Classification of Tumours of Haematopoietic and Lymphoid Tissues. Lyon, FR: IARC Press;2001. p. 111–14.

2. Chahal S, Lagera JE, Ryder J, et al. Hematological neoplasms with first presentation as spinal cord compression syndromes: a 10-year retrospective series and review of the literature. Clin Neuropathol 2003;22:282–90.

3. Landis DM, Aboulafia DM. Granulocytic sarcoma: an unusual complication of a leukemic myeloid leukemia causing spinal cord compression. A case report and literature review. Leukemia & Lymphoma 2003;44:1753–60.

Case 82: Marginal Zone B-Cell Lymphoma

CLINICAL INFORMATION

The patient is a 44-year-old woman who presents with a dural-based mass, involving the falx and overlying the right frontal convexity. The patient presents with headaches and episodic nausea and vomiting. On imaging, the lesion appears somewhat circumscribed, with contrast enhancement, and a diagnosis of meningioma is entertained. Gross total resection of the lesion is performed, and histologic sections are reviewed.

OPINION

Histologic sections show a cellular lesion, marked by mixed inflammatory infiltrates, involving the dura and underlying leptomeninges. Sheets of predominantly small to medium-sized lymphocytes with a moderate amount of cytoplasm and nuclear irregularities are observed. Some cells show a monocytoid appearance, with cleared cytoplasm and well-defined cell borders. Occasional immunoblastic-like cells, with large vesicular nuclei and prominent nucleoli, are present, as are scattered plasma cells. On low magnification, the inflammatory cells appear to be arranged in a nodular architectural pattern. Prominent numbers of mitotic figures are not evident. Focally, microcalcifications are noted, as are cholesterol clefts with giant cells, the latter indicating previous hemorrhage. Granulomas are not seen. There is no evidence of meningioma. By immunohistochemistry, the tumor cells demonstrate positive staining, with antibodies to CD20 and CD79a, and do not stain with antibodies to CD3, CD10, and CD5. Bcl-2 immunopositivity is also observed in the lesion.

We consider the lesion to be a lymphoproliferative disorder and characterize it as follows: **Falx and**

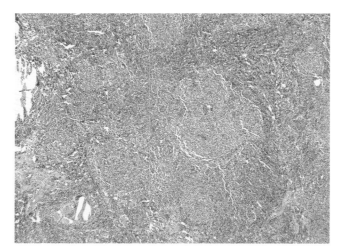

FIGURE 82.1 Low-magnification appearance of the dural mass shows a nodular architectural pattern.

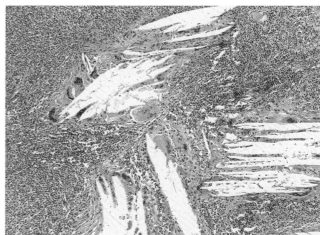

FIGURE 82.2 Focal cholesterol cleft formation, with giant cells indicating previous hemorrhage in the lesion, is observed.

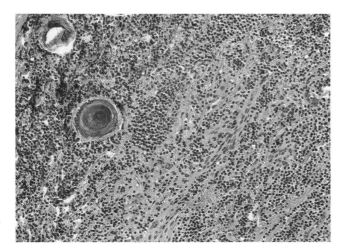

FIGURE 82.3 Focal calcifications, likely representing entrapped psammoma bodies, are present.

Right Frontal Convexity, Excision—Marginal Zone B-Cell Lymphoma.

COMMENT

Marginal zone B-cell lymphomas in the central nervous system are typically indolent tumors that often present as meningioma-like, dural-based masses.

DISCUSSION

Diffuse, large B-cell lymphomas are the most common primary central nervous system lymphomas. Other lymphoma types have been less frequently observed to arise primarily in the central nervous system; among this group is the marginal zone B-cell lymphoma or low-grade B-cell lymphoma of mucosa-associated lymphoid tissue (MALT). The lesion probably represents the most common primary low-grade intracranial lymphoma. Most of these tumors arise in association with the dura and leptomeninges, although rare cases of intracerebral and intraventricular tumor have been reported. Because of their dural location, imaging studies suggest meningioma and prompt surgical resection. In a series reported by Tu et al., 80% of patients were woman with a mean age at diagnosis of 55 years. Presenting symptoms varied and included headaches, nausea, vomiting, visual disturbances, seizures, motor or sensory deficits, ataxia, or gait disturbance.

Histologically, the lesions are marked by proliferation of small lymphocytes, with cleared

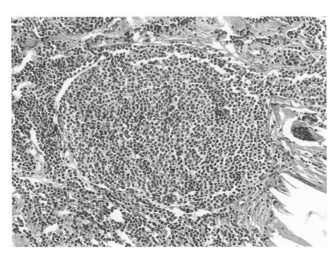

FIGURE 82.4 Intermediate magnification shows a proliferation of small lymphocytic cells, with moderate amount of lightly eosinophilic to cleared cytoplasm, comprise the tumor.

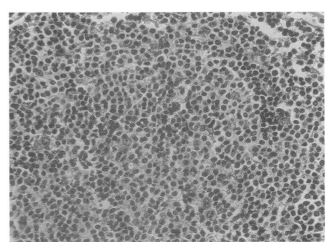

FIGURE 82.5 High-magnification appearance of cells shows irregular nuclear contour with prominent nuclei and cleared cytoplasm.

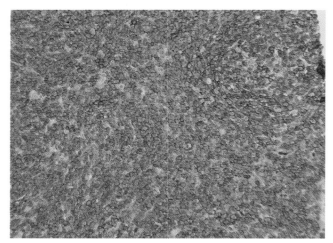

FIGURE 82.6 Diffuse positive staining with antibody to CD20 (B-cell lymphoid marker) is present.

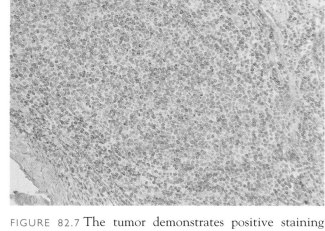

FIGURE 82.7 The tumor demonstrates positive staining with Bcl-2 antibody.

cytoplasm and irregular, centrally located nuclei. Plasmacytic features are variably present. Focal areas of nodular architecture and areas marked by lymphoid follicles may be present. A subset of tumors may demonstrate evidence of amyloid deposition. Similar to marginal zone B-cell lymphomas arising outside the central nervous system, these tumors demonstrate positive staining with B-cell markers (CD20 and CD79a) and do not stain with T-cell markers (CD3).

These tumors tend to have a long-term survival and favorable prognosis.

References

1. Kelley TW, Prayson RA, Barnett GH, et al. Extranodal marginal zone B-cell lymphoma of mucosa-associated lymphoid tissue arising in the lateral ventricle. Leuk Lymphoma 2005;46:1423–7.
2. Tu PH, Giannini C, Judkins AR, et al. Clinicopathologic and genetic profile of intracranial marginal zone lymphoma: a primary low grade CNS lymphoma that mimics meningioma. J Clin Oncol 2005;23:5718–27.

Case 83: Post-Transplant Lymphoproliferative Disorder

CLINICAL INFORMATION

The patient is a 65-year-old male who presents with an approximately 2-month history of progressive short-term memory loss and problems with visual-spatial and executive functions. He has a significant past medical history of having received a kidney transplant 3 years earlier. A medical opinion is sought, and a MRI scan demonstrates multifocal lesions in the brain, the largest of which involve the posterior corpus callosum and right parieto-occipital areas. A stereotactic biopsy of the corpus callosum lesion is undertaken, and sections are available for review.

OPINION

Sections show a cytologically atypical hematopoeitic neoplasm, characterized by large immunoblast-like cells, with vesicular nuclei, prominent nucleoli, and amphophilic cytoplasm surrounding blood vessels. Similar cells are also present in brain parenchyma and associated with even larger numbers of small, non-neoplastic lymphocytes of normal size. Necrosis and brisk astrocytic reaction are also identified. The large cytologically atypical cells mark as B cells with CD20, whereas small non-neoplastic lymphocytes are predominantly CD3-positive T cells. Epstein-Barr virus is detected by in situ hybridization.

We consider the lesion to be a hematopoietic neoplasm and, after immunostaining and polymerase chain reaction (PCR) testing for clonality, characterize it as follows: **Posterior Corpus Callosum, Stereotactic Biopsies—Post-Transplant Lymphoproliferative Disorder, B-Cell Lymphoma, Epstein-Barr Virus-Positive, Monoclonal B-Cell Population Detected by PCR.**

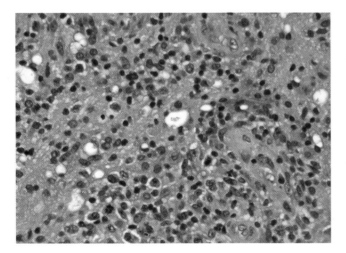

FIGURE 83.1 The hypercellular lesion shows perivascular collections of large, cytologically atypical cells, admixed with variable numbers of small, non-neoplastic lymphocytes and occasional plasma cells.

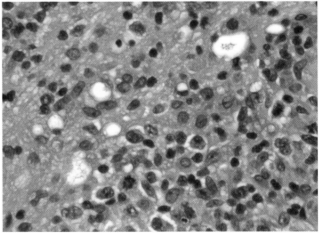

FIGURE 83.2 High-power magnification illustrates the vesicular nuclei and prominent nucleoli in the hematopoeitic tumor, as well as mitoses.

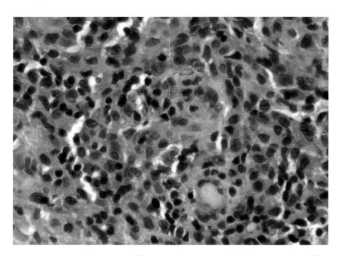

FIGURE 83.3 Tumor cells can be seen within vessel walls, but unlike vasculitis, the hematopoeitic cells manifest severe cytologic atypia.

COMMENT

Most post-transplant lymphoproliferative disorders (PTLDs) are driven by Epstein-Barr virus (EBV), and most are B-cell disorders, existing in a spectrum from polyclonal proliferations to monomorphic B-cell lymphomas. Diffuse, large B-cell lymphomas are usually immunoblastic in type. Far less commonly, anaplastic lymphoma, T-cell lymphoma, plasma cell myeloma, Hodgkin lymphoma, and Hodgkin-like PTLD have been described.

DISCUSSION

PTLD occurs in <2% of solid organ transplant recipients, of which the lowest frequency is in renal allograft recipients, with increasing frequency of PTLD in those who have undergone hepatic, cardiac, or complex heart-lung or liver-bowel allografts. PTLD tends to involve extranodal sites, including the transplanted organ itself and the central nervous system (CNS), especially if the patient was treated with azathioprine-based regimens. The use of tacrolimus-based regimens for immunosuppression has reduced the involvement of the CNS.

Most examples of PTLD in the CNS meet morphologic criteria for a diagnosis of diffuse, large B-cell lymphoma, based on the hypercellularity and cytologic atypia. In brain, tumor cells usually show both perivascular arrangement and sheet-like effacement of the parenchyma, with variable degrees of associated

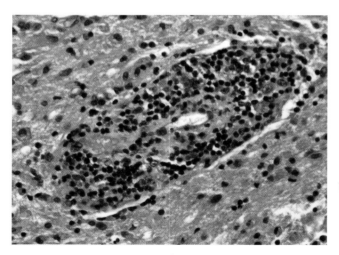

FIGURE 83.4 Some perivascular cuffs of cells consist predominantly of non-neoplastic lymphocytes (which prove to be T cells), with only a few recognizable, larger neoplastic B cells.

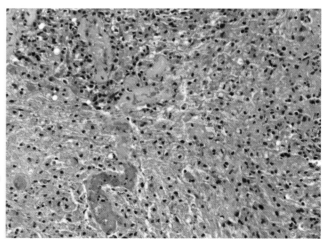

FIGURE 83.5 There may be broad zones of necrosis that prompt consideration of an infectious process, especially infections more frequently seen in immunosuppressed patients, including fungal infection or toxoplasmosis.

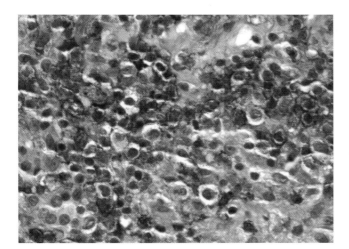

FIGURE 83.6 CD20 identifies the large neoplastic cells as being of B-cell origin.

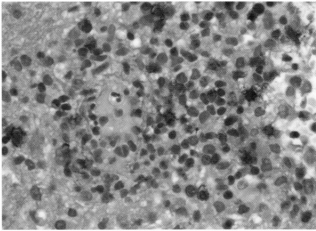

FIGURE 83.7 In some areas of the biopsy, only isolated B cells are seen on CD20 staining, and even some smaller, cytologically normal-appearing B cells can be admixed.

necrosis. Because of the vasocentricity of the lymphoma cells and the accompanying non-neoplastic T cells, vasculitis must be excluded, based on the severity of the cytologic atypia in the hematopoeitic population. The additional finding of a clonal B-cell tumor population on PCR testing supports the diagnosis of B-cell lymphoma in a cytologically atypical process. Heavily necrotic cases of diffuse B-cell lymphoma can also raise consid-

eration of infectious process, especially fungal infection or toxoplasmosis of the CNS. Like most infections, these tend to have a preponderance of T cells rather than B cells, and staining for organisms is positive.

Immunostaining in PTLD-associated, EBV-driven, diffuse, large B-cell lymphomas usually shows positive expression of CD19, CD20, and CD79a. CD43 and CD45RO are also upregulated

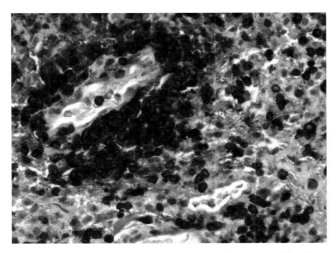

FIGURE 83.8 Large numbers of non-neoplastic T cells often cuff the blood vessels and infiltrate the parenchyma; these CD3-positive cells may overshadow the true, neoplastic, CD20-positive cells.

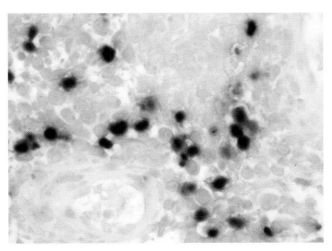

FIGURE 83.9 In situ hybridization for Epstein-Barr virus usually shows large numbers of EBV-positive cells with strong, blue-black, nuclear signal.

in EBV-infected B cells and can be expressed. Many are CD30-positive, even without anaplastic features. Reduction or withdrawal of immunosuppressive medications, with administration of chemotherapy or radiation therapy, can improve prognosis in some cases.

References

1. Harris NL, Swerdlow SH, Frizzera G, et al. Post-transplant lymphoproliferative disorders. In: ES Jaffe, NL Harris, H Stein, JW Vardiman, Editors. WHO Classification of Tumours of Haematopoietic and Lymphoid Tissues. Lyon, FR: IARC Press;2001. p. 264–9.

Case 84: Plasmacytoma

CLINICAL INFORMATION

The patient is a 78-year-old male who presents with fluctuating vision in his right eye. A MRI scan shows a dural-based mass, just superior and lateral to the optic foramen, suggestive of a meningioma. Work-up, however, reveals lytic rib and sacral lesions. The patient is felt to be a candidate for decompression of his right optic nerve, and histologic sections are reviewed from the resected material.

OPINION

Sections show sheets of cytologically monotonous, closely packed, hematopoietic tumor cells, occupying the orbital soft tissue space. Cells manifest only moderate nuclear-to-cytoplasmic ratios, nuclei with clockwork chromatin pattern, moderate amounts of faintly basophilic cytoplasm, and distinct nucleoli. Mitotic activity is brisk.

We consider the lesion to be a hematopoietic neoplasm and, after special immunostaining, characterize it as follows: **Orbital Dura, Biopsy— Plasmacytoma.**

COMMENT

Plasmacytoma is a localized tumoral collection of neoplastic plasma cells. This patient, who had a plasmacytoma on tissue biopsy (a major diagnostic criterion for plasma cell myeloma) and also had lytic bone lesions (a minor diagnostic criterion), met criteria for diffuse disease (plasma cell myeloma). He was subsequently also found to have an M-component in the

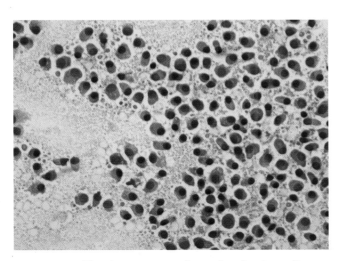

FIGURE 84.1 Touch imprint, performed at the time of intraoperative consultation, shows that the cells in this lesion display cytologic monotony and abundant cytoplasm.

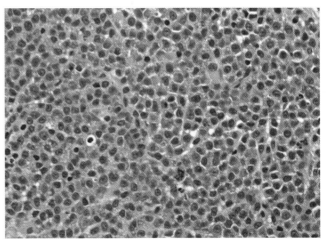

FIGURE 84.2 High-power magnification illustrates the monotonous sheets of tumor cells with moderate nuclear-to-cytoplasmic ratio, basophilic cytoplasm, and clumped nuclear chromatin.

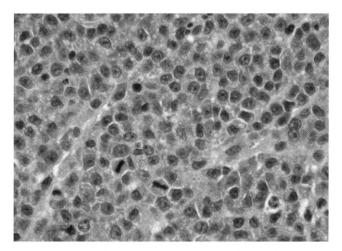

FIGURE 84.3 High-power magnification shows the prominent nucleoli and mitotic activity in this tumor.

urine and serum (free kappa light chains) (another major criterion) and reduced normal serum immunoglobulins (a minor criterion).

DISCUSSION

Making the diagnosis of plasma cell myeloma involves finding systemic body involvement, in addition to the localized tumoral collection of plasma cells seen on this biopsy. Plasmacytoma can be mistaken for a metastatic carcinoma, especially breast carcinoma, thyroid carcinoma, or other relatively monotonous tumor type, such as a neuroendocrine tumor, including pituitary adenoma. Cytokeratin expression in these tumors verifies the diagnosis of metastatic carcinoma and negates the diagnosis of plasmacytoma. Plasmacytoma can also be mistaken for an olfactory neuroblastoma, if the mass occurs in the sinuses or skull base. Both plasmacytoma and olfactory neuroblastoma can be immunoreactive for neuron-specific enolase (NSE) and CD56 (neural cell adhesion molecule, NCAM), but only the former is strongly and diffusely immunoreactive for plasma cell markers such as CD38, CD79a, or CD138.

Benign inflammatory conditions may contain large numbers of plasma cells, especially orbital inflammatory pseudotumor, and thus, they are also diagnostic considerations. However, the cytologic and immunohistochemical monotony of the process argues against a reactive process in this case. Immunostaining or in situ hybridization studies for light chain expression negate a benign reactive process when a monoclonal light chain population is identified. This case expressed kappa light chains exclusively.

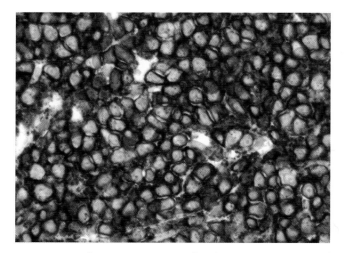

FIGURE 84.4 Immunoreactivity for CD138 is strong and diffuse and negates consideration of a metastatic carcinoma.

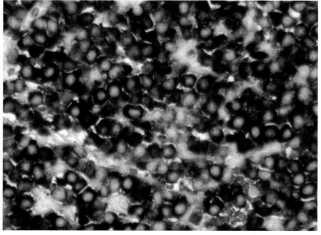

FIGURE 84.5 In situ hybridization signal shows a monoclonal kappa light chain expression in the plasmacytoma.

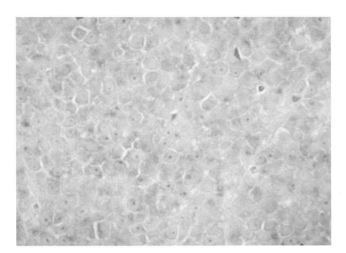

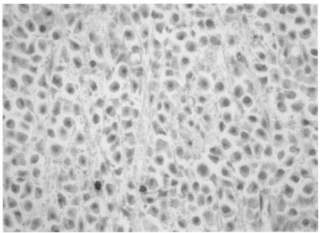

FIGURE 84.6 In situ hybridization signal shows no cells expressing lambda light chain expression in the plasmacytoma.

FIGURE 84.7 As is typically the case in most (but not all) plasma cell neoplasms, this plasmacytoma, as first presentation of plasma cell myeloma, lacks expression for the mature B-cell marker CD20.

The orbital space is a known location for plasma cell myeloma or isolated plasmacytoma. Cranial or spinal dura in other anatomic locations in addition to the orbit is also a known location for plasmacytoma, as well as for various types of low-grade indolent dural lymphoma, including MALT lymphomas.

References

1. Grogan TM, Van Camp B, Kyle RA, et al. Plasma cell neoplasms. In: Jaffe ES, Harris NL, Stein H, Vardiman JW, Editors. WHO Classification of Tumours of Haematopoietic and Lymphoid Tissues. Lyon, FR: IARC Press;2001. p. 142–156.

2. Haegelen C, Riffaud L, Bernard M, et al. Dural plasmacytoma revealing multiple myeloma. Case report. J Neurosurg 2006;104:608–10.
3. Lazaridou MN, Micallef-Eynaud P, Hanna IT. Soft tissue plasmacytoma of the orbit as part of the spectrum of multiple myeloma. Orbit 2007;26:315–18.
4. Sahin F, Saydam G, Ertan Y, et al. Dural plasmacytoma mimicking meningioma in a patient with multiple myeloma. J Clin Neurosci 2006;13:259–61.
5. Thoumazet F, Donnio A, Ayeboua L, et al. Orbital and muscle involvement in multiple myeloma. Can J Ophthalmol 2006;41:733–6.

Case 85: Langerhans Cell Histiocytosis

CLINICAL INFORMATION

The patient is a 9-year-old girl, otherwise healthy, who presents with headaches, occurring over a 2-month period. Neurologic evaluation is normal. MRI reveals a skull-centered mass, extending though the right fronto-parietal skull bone into the epidural space, with focal displacement of the brain in the area of the lesion, but without associated edema. Only a single lytic lesion is identified. The decision is made to excise the skull lesion.

OPINION

Biopsies show a hypercellular tumor, composed of a heterogeneous population of cells, including eosinophils, neutrophils, large multinucleated histiocytes resembling osteoclasts, and a predominant population of medium-sized histiocytes with grooved, folded, or lobulated nuclei. The latter Langerhans cells manifest inconspicuous nucleoli, delicate chromatin, and minimal hyperchromasia. Cytoplasm is devoid of prominent vacuoles, and mitoses are rare.

We consider the pathology to be that of a histiocytic neoplasm without malignant features and, after immunohistochemical studies, characterize it as follows: **Right Fronto-Parietal Skull, Excision— Langerhans Cell Histiocytosis**.

COMMENT

Langerhans cell histiocytosis was referred to in the past as histiocytosis X or Langerhans cell granulomatosis.

DISCUSSION

Langerhans cell histiocytosis (histiocytosis X) is one of three overlapping syndromes, all with similar

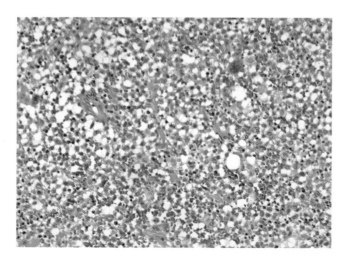

FIGURE 85.1 The section shows a hypercellular tumor, with a heterogeneous population of hematopoeitic elements.

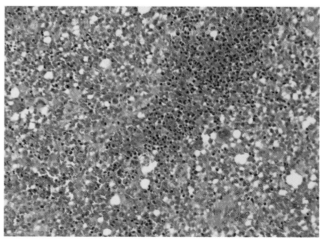

FIGURE 85.2 Small eosinophilic abscesses should not prompt misdiagnosis of a true granulomatous or parasitic infection.

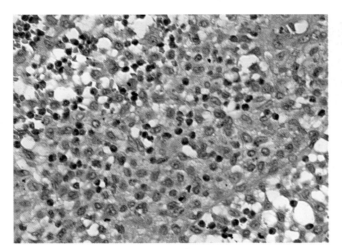

FIGURE 85.3 High magnification illustrates the prominent eosinophils scattered throughout the lesion.

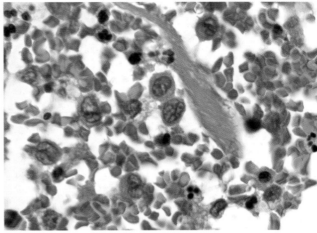

FIGURE 85.4 Langerhans cells manifest folded, indented, and grooved nuclei, delicate chromatin, and small nucleoli.

histologic features, but with the various forms of the disorder defined by the anatomic distribution pattern.

Langerhans cell histiocytosis is the unifocal form of the disease and is usually diagnosed in older children or adults. Bone is the most frequently affected site, particularly the skull (as in this case), but single lesions may also be found in femur, pelvic bones, or ribs.

In Hand-Schüller-Christian disease, there is multifocal involvement, but the multiple lesions are

confined to a single organ system—again, almost always the bone.

Letterer-Siwe disease represents the multifocal, multisystem form of involvement and usually is diagnosed in infants. It may manifest in bones, skin, liver, spleen, and/or lymph nodes.

Prognosis is correlated with the number of organs involved. Although about 10% of patients

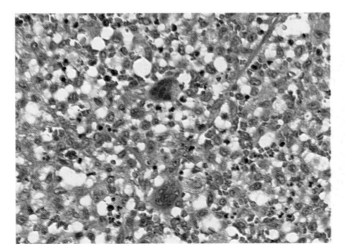

FIGURE 85.5 Multinucleated histiocytes may be prominent and resemble osteoclasts.

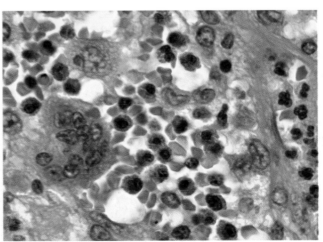

FIGURE 85.6 High-power view illustrates various elements in Langerhans cell histiocytosis: multinucleated cells, eosinophils, Langerhans cells with nuclear grooves, and neutrophils.

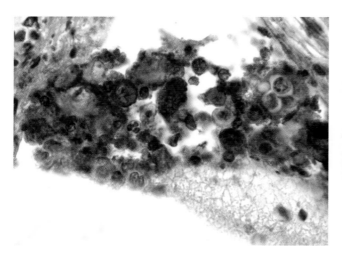

FIGURE 85.7 CD1a immunoreactivity is consistently identified in Langerhans cell histiocytosis within the Langerhans cell population.

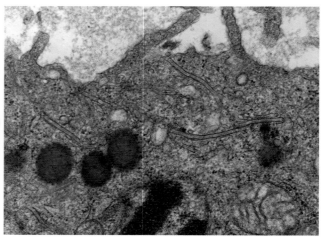

FIGURE 85.8 Electron microscopy shows several intracytoplasmic Birbeck granules, elongate, rodlike structures. The distal distention, forming a "tennis racket," is not always identified and is not present within the granules in this cell, although a median striated line can be seen clearly.

with unifocal disease progress to multisystem disease, even patients with multiple bone lesions have a good prognosis. Overall survival of patients with unifocal disease is 95%.

Histologically, diagnosis rests on identifying the characteristic Langerhans cells, a special type of histiocyte, admixed with variable numbers of eosinophils, neutrophils, and multinucleated histiocytes. Small eosinophilic abscesses can be found in some cases, and such cases should not be mistaken for true infections, such as parasitic and granulomatous abscesses.

Early phases of the condition contain larger numbers of Langerhans cells, whereas older phases show fewer of these cells, with more fibrosis and more foamy macrophages. The identity of the Langerhans cells should be confirmed by immunohistochemical studies. Langerhans cells show "consistent expression of CD1a and S-100 protein. They are usually positive for vimentin, HLA-DR, peanut agglutinin lectin and placental alkaline phosphatase. They are variably

and weakly positive for CD45, CD68, and lysozyme. They are negative for most B-cell and T-cell lineage markers."

Electron microscopy is less often necessary and may be negative because of Birbeck granules being present in a variable percentage of the Langerhans cells. Birbeck granules are rod-, to flask-, to tennis racket-shaped structures that show a median striated line. They are thought to represent a special type of endocytotic structure.

References

1. Weiss LM, Grogan TM, Müller-Hermelink H-K, et al. Langerhans cell histiocytosis. In: Jaffe ES, Harris NL, Stein H, Vardiman JW, Editors. WHO Classification of Tumours: Pathology and Genetics. Tumours of Haematopoietic and Lymphoid Tissues. Lyon, FR: IARC Press;2001. p. 280–2.
2. Ghadially FN. Diagnostic Ultrastructural Pathology: A Self-Evaluation and Self-Teaching Manual. Second Edition. Boston, MA: Butterworth-Heinemann;1998. p. 17.

Case 86: Intravascular Lymphomatosis (Angiotropic Large Cell Lymphoma)

CLINICAL INFORMATION

The patient is a 72-year-old female who presents with right-sided weakness; on imaging, she is noted to have a left-sided infarct. Over the next 2-week period, she develops multiple neural deficits, and on imaging, shows six foci of infarcts in multiple vascular distributions. A vasculitic process is suspected. A biopsy is performed, and histologic sections are reviewed.

OPINION

Histologic sections show an intravascular process, marked by the presence of discohesive, atypical cells with high nuclear-to-cytoplasmic ratios. The adjacent parenchyma shows evidence of an acute infarct, reactive vascular endothelial changes, macrophages, and ischemic-appearing neurons. The atypical cells are confined to vascular lumina. On immunostaining,

the intravascular cells demonstrate positive staining with CD20 antibody. These cells do not stain with antibodies to CD3, muramidase, TdT, cytokeratins AE1/3, or S-100 protein.

We consider the intravascular lesion to be a hematopoietic neoplasm and characterize it as follows: **Left Parietal Lobe Region, Biopsy—Intravascular Lymphomatosis (Angiotropic Large Cell Lymphoma).**

COMMENT

On immunostaining, the tumor cells demonstrates CD20 immunoreactivity, consistent with a B-cell lymphomatous process.

DISCUSSION

Intravascular lymphomatosis is a relatively rare disorder, marked by a proliferation of atypical lymphoid

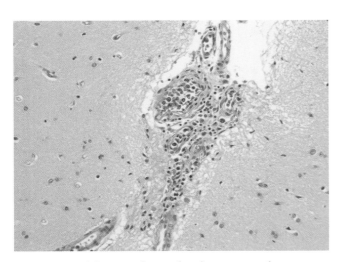

FIGURE 86.1 Meningeal vessels, show atypical-appearing intravascular lymphoid cells.

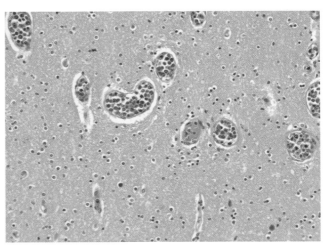

FIGURE 86.2 White matter vessels are also involved by the lymphomatous process.

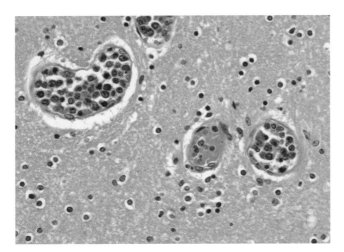

FIGURE 86.3 High-magnification appearance of the atypical-appearing lymphoid cells shows a high nuclear-to-cytoplasmic ratio.

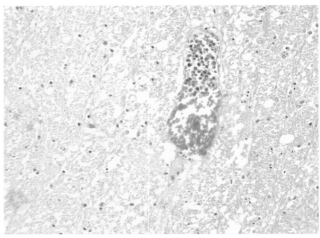

FIGURE 86.4 An area of acute infarct is seen, likely secondary to the intravascular tumor.

cells, confined primarily to vascular lumina. The clinical presentation is often quite variable, depending on the organ involved. Neurologic symptoms include focal neural deficits or dementia in a subset of patients. The characteristic intravascular growth pattern of this tumor has been conjectured to be related to a defect in homing receptors on neoplastic tumor cells. Morphologically, the cells show features

of atypical lymphoid cells, which can be confirmed by immunostaining. The majority of the cases have a B-cell immunophenotype; however, rare cases of intravascular lymphoma of T-cell phenotype have also been reported.

Differential diagnostic considerations include other processes that may have an intravascular location, including leukemia, intravascular spread from a carcinoma, or metastasizing melanoma. The presence of negative immunostains characteristic of

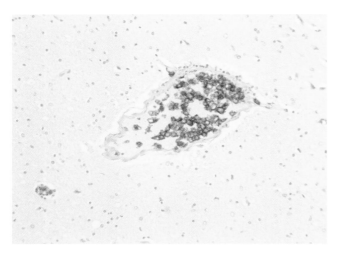

FIGURE 86.5 Most of the tumor cells demonstrate positive staining, with antibody to CD20 (B-cell lymphoid marker).

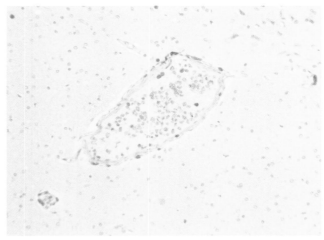

FIGURE 86.6 CD3 immunoreactivity is not present in this tumor.

these various entities helps exclude them from the diagnosis.

The lesion has a particularly aggressive clinical course and does not usually respond well to chemotherapy. In many patients, because of the atypical presentations, the diagnosis is often not made until the time of autopsy.

References

1. Baehring JM, Longtine J, Hochberg FH. A new approach to the diagnosis and treatment of intravascular lymphoma. J Neurooncol 2003;61:237–48.
2. Glass J, Hochberg FH, Miller DC. Intravascular lymphomatosis. A systemic disease with neurologic manifestations. Cancer 1997;71:3156–64.
3. Ponzoni M, Ferreri AJ. Intravascular lymphoma: a neoplasm of 'homeless' lymphocytes? Hematol Oncol 2006;24:105–12.

Case 87: Germinoma

CLINICAL INFORMATION

The patient is a 12-year-old male who presents with respiratory failure of unknown etiology and is found to have aspiration pneumonia. Neurologic evaluation identifies nystagmus, dysmetria, wasting and fasciculations of the tongue, and voice changes suggestive of vocal cord paralysis. MRI shows an enhancing exophytic mass, $5.1 \times 3.2 \times 2.2$ cm, in the medulla, as well as ventriculomegaly. MRI of the spine is negative for cerebrospinal fluid dissemination. Given the site and enhancement characteristics, astrocytoma is favored. The patient subsequently undergoes excisional biopsy of the lesion, and histologic sections are reviewed.

OPINION

Sections demonstrate sheets of large tumor cells, with round vesicular nuclei and prominent nucleoli. Some areas are patternless, whereas, in other areas, a lobular arrangement is formed by delicate fibrovascular septae filled with non-neoplastic lymphocytes. Mitoses are easily appreciated in the large tumor cells. Necrosis is present in this example but is not commonly seen. No other germ cell tumor elements are seen.

We consider the lesion to be a germ cell tumor and characterize it as follows: **Dorsal Brainstem/ Pineal Region, Biopsies—Germinoma.**

COMMENT

Most central nervous system primary germinomas develop in either the suprasellar region or pineal gland. This case is unusual in that it was an exophytic mass in the medulla, a much more common site for astrocytomas than germ cell tumors.

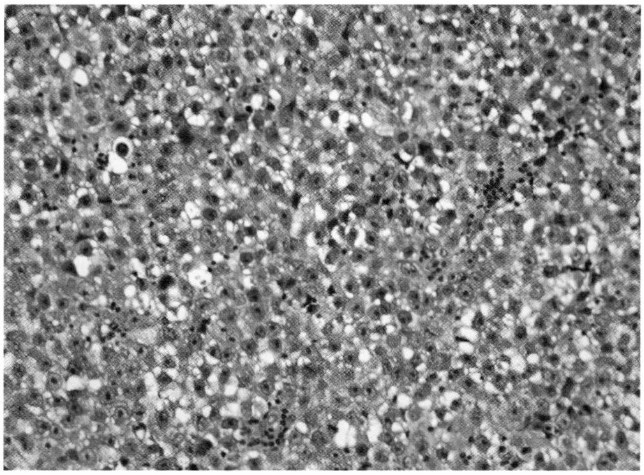

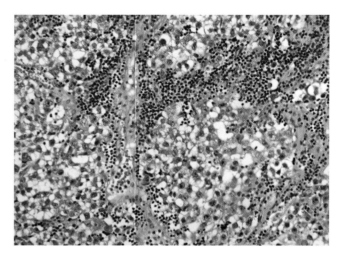

FIGURE 87.1 Low-power magnification appearance of the excision specimen, shows patternless sheets of large cells.

FIGURE 87.2 Other areas in the resected material demonstrate lobules of tumor cells, demarcated by fibrovascular septae containing cytologically benign lymphocytes.

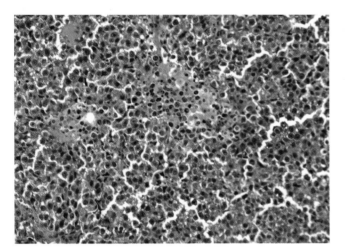

FIGURE 87.3 Small foci of necrosis are evident in this example of central nervous system germinoma.

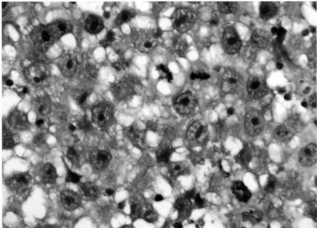

FIGURE 87.4. High-power magnification shows the large vesicular nuclei, prominent nucleoli, and mitoses in the neoplasm.

DISCUSSION

Germinoma is the most common central nervous system germ cell tumor and often occurs in pure form. Large tumor cells can be arranged in patternless sheets or may be punctuated by cords of fibrovascular tissue, yielding a nested or lobular architectural pattern. Variable numbers of non-neoplastic lymphocytes may be present and are usually T cells. Occasional central nervous system germinomas show prominent granulomatous reaction, simulating a tuberculoma or neurosarcoidosis. Granulomatous response may overshadow the tumor cells, making diagnosis difficult.

Although mitoses are easily seen in well-fixed specimens, necrosis is uncommon. Immunohistochemical staining aids in the diagnosis. Cytoplasmic immunoreactivity for c-kit and nuclear immunoreactivity for OCT4 are often seen, with cytoplasmic and cell membrane immunostaining for placental alkaline phosphatase (PLAP) slightly less frequent. NANOG has been shown in some studies to be another useful immunohistochemical marker for central nervous system germinoma.

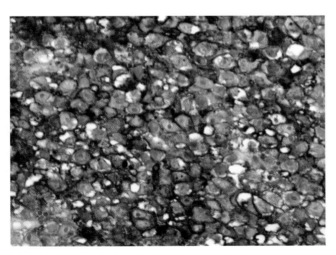

FIGURE 87.5 Cytoplasmic and membranous immunostaining for PLAP is seen in many, but not all, examples of central nervous system germinomas.

References

1. Hattab EM, Pu PH, Wilson JD, et al. OCT4 immunohistochemistry is superior to placental alkaline phosphatase (PLAP) in the diagnosis of central nervous system germinoma. Am J Surg Pathol 2005;29:369–71.

2. Rosenblum MK, Nakazato Y, Matsutani M. CNS germ cell tumours. In: Louis DN, Ohgaki H, Wiestler OD, Cavenee WK, Editors. WHO Classification of Tumours of the Central Nervous System. Lyon, FR: IARC Press;2007. p. 198–204.

3. Santagata S. Hornick JL. Ligon KL. Comparative analysis of germ cell transcription factors in CNS germinoma reveals diagnostic utility of NANOG. J Surg Pathol 2006;30:1613–8.

Case 88: Pineal Teratoma

CLINICAL INFORMATION

The patient is a 19-year-old male who presents with a 1.5-week history of double vision, headaches, nausea, and vomiting. On imaging, a pineal region mass, 4.1 × 2.7 × 3.4 cm, and hydrocephalus are found, and an emergent intraventricular shunt is placed. A decision is made to perform a small endoscopic biopsy, which yields a tumor composed of small blue cells. Pineoblastoma, versus immature nervous system tissue within an immature teratoma, cannot be distinguished on the limited material available. He is treated with radiation and chemotherapy. Subsequently, there is enlargement of his pineal region mass, with a more complex appearance. A larger resection is undertaken, and histologic sections are reviewed.

OPINION

The larger resection shows mature cartilage, loose connective tissue, central and peripheral nervous system tissue, fat and bone. No germ cell tumor or immature nervous system tissue is present on the second surgical procedure.

We consider the lesion to have originally been an immature teratoma, now with maturation after radio- and chemotherapy, and characterize it as follows: **Pineal Gland—Teratoma, Mature.**

COMMENT

Immature teratomas may undergo "maturation" following use of radio- or chemotherapy. In retrospect, the "small blue cell tumor" came from immature, actively proliferating neuroectodermal tissue in the mass. The lesion was never a pineoblastoma. After

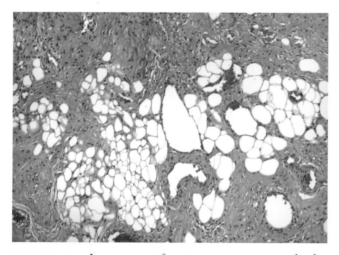

FIGURE 88.1 Lower-magnification appearance of the resected material shows mature fat and connective tissue.

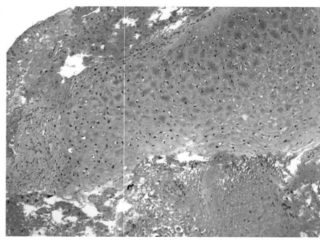

FIGURE 88.2 Cartilage is often abundant in teratomas.

262

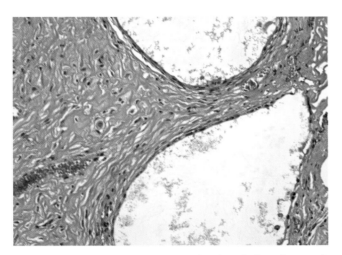

FIGURE 88.3 Cystic areas can be lined by flattened, respiratory-type epithelium and filled with mucous contents.

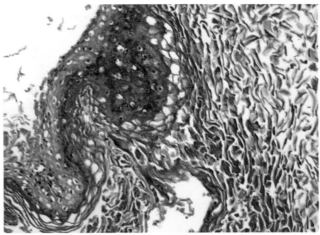

FIGURE 88.4 Cysts with squamous epithelium, keratohyaline layer, and abundant squamous cells simulate epidermoid cyst.

the mitotically active portion of the immature teratoma was ablated by the therapy, the residual, more differentiated portions remained and enlarged over time, with maturation of tissues and accumulation of cystic contents. This phenomenon is known as the "growing teratoma syndrome."

DISCUSSION

Teratomas of the central nervous system may be either mature, immature, or rarely, they may contain a true malignant component. In mature teratomas, skin, brain, and choroid plexus tissues may be seen. Mesodermal tissues include cartilage, bone, fat, and muscle. Cysts may be present and lined by respiratory or enteric type epithelium. Immature teratomas, in contrast, show hypercellular and mitotically active stoma, suggestive of embryonic mesenchymal and/or primitive neuroectodermal elements. The latter may simulate neural

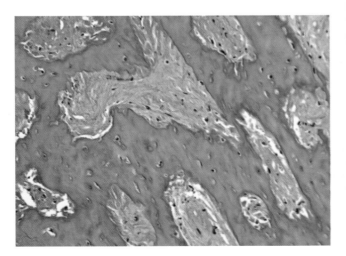

FIGURE 88.5 Bone can be easily identified in many teratomas.

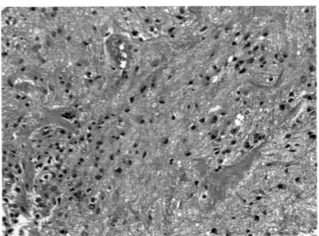

FIGURE 88.6 Mature nervous system tissue shows eosinophilic fibrillar background and easily recognized astrocytes. Note absence of immature neuroepithelium.

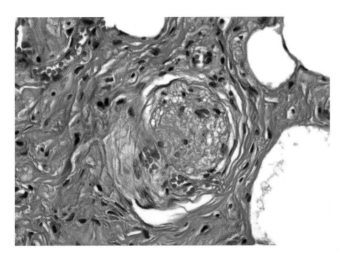

FIGURE 88.7 Well-developed peripheral nerves are scattered throughout the resected tissue.

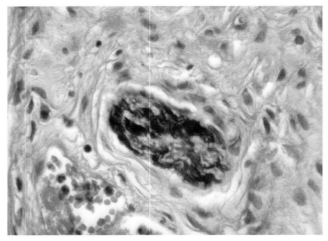

FIGURE 88.8 Some elements within teratomas are more easily verified by immunohistochemistry, such as this peripheral nerve twig with strong reactivity for S-100 protein.

tube. Even clefts containing melanotic neuroepithelium, suggesting retinal differentiation, can be seen.

The "growing teratoma syndrome" can also be seen after treatment for a complex mixed germ cell tumor containing yolk sac, embryonal carcinoma, and/or choriocarcinoma elements and has been well described in germ cell tumors from non-central nervous system sites, including the ovary.

References

1. Bi WL, Bannykh SI, Baehring J. The growing teratoma syndrome after subtotal resection of an intracranial non-germinomatous germ cell tumor in an adult: case report. Neurosurgery 2005;56:188.

2. Rosenblum MK, Nakazato Y, Matsutani M. CNS germ cell tumours. In: Louis DN, Ohgaki H, Wiestler OD, Cavenee WK, Editors. WHO Classification of Tumours of the Central Nervous System. Lyon, FR: IARC Press;2007. p. 198–204.

Case 89: Cystic Craniopharyngioma

CLINICAL INFORMATION

The patient is a 36-year-old male who presents with blurry and double vision, as well as headaches, nausea, fatigue, and decreased libido. Neuroimaging studies show a cystic suprasellar and sellar mass, 2.3 by 1.6 cm. Near-total surgical resection is undertaken.

OPINION

Sections show a collapsed, fibrotic cyst wall and a cyst lining that varies from an attenuated squamous epithelium to a more obvious adamantinomatous appearance. Fibrotic nodules containing cholesterol clefts are evident in some areas. Calcification and islands of ghost cells ("wet keratin") are noted.

We consider the lesion to be a cystic craniopharyngioma and characterize it as follows: **Suprasellar Region, Resection—Cystic Craniopharyngioma, WHO Grade I.**

COMMENT

All symptoms can be attributed to optic chiasm compression and hypopituitarism, with hypogonadism leading to decreased libido and hypoadrenalism with nausea and fatigue.

DISCUSSION

Craniopharyngiomas account for 2–5% of all primary intracranial neoplasms and have a bimodal peak age incidence: in children ages 5–14 years and in adults ages 50–74 years. These tumors arise along the pathway followed during embryological periods by the craniopharyngeal duct before it involutes. Most have a suprasellar component.

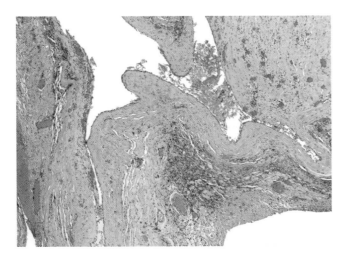

FIGURE 89.1 Low magnification shows collapsed cyst wall; complexity and cyst contents may not be fully apparent on the specimen received by the pathologist.

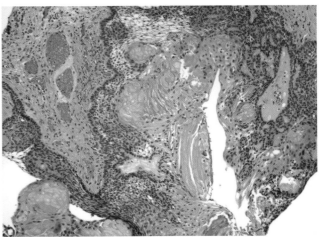

FIGURE 89.2 Adamantinomatous epithelium and squamous epithelium can be seen lining the cyst.

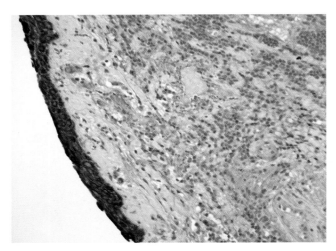

FIGURE 89.3 The attenuated epithelium lining the cyst in some areas is best appreciated by immunostaining for keratins, in this instance CAM 5.2. Note the squamous appearance to the epithelium in this area and the nonimmunoreactive chronic inflammatory cells in the underlying stroma.

Although craniopharyngiomas are WHO grade I neoplasms, their location near the hypothalamus often precludes gross total removal. Many patients require postoperative adjuvant radiation therapy to achieve tumor control. Histologically, almost all

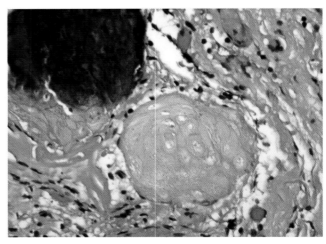

FIGURE 89.4 Calcification and clusters of ghost cells characterize most adamantinomatous and cystic craniopharyngiomas.

pediatric, and most adult, craniopharyngiomas possess calcification and adamantinomatous epithelium. The latter is recognized by intersecting strands and islands of epithelium, with a palisaded basal layer of cells; an intermediate stellate reticulum, which may loosen and degenerate, forming cysts with watery cyst fluid contents; and nodules of "wet keratin." The wet keratin has the appearance of squamous cells, but with loss of

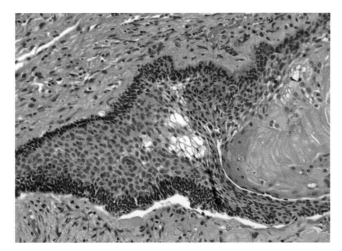

FIGURE 89.5 Adamantinomatous epithelium is characterized by a crowded basal layer of cells; loosening within the epithelium with fluid accumulation may also give rise to cysts in the craniopharyngioma.

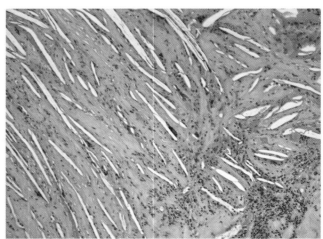

FIGURE 89.6 Nodules of cholesterol clefts, embedded in a fibrotic background, indicate previous, often subclinical bleeding into craniopharyngiomas.

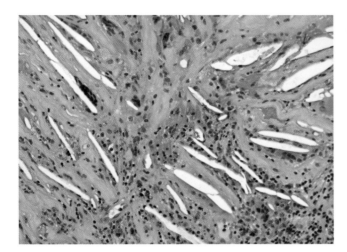

FIGURE 89.7 Higher-power magnification of the cholesterol clefts shows the adjacent hemosiderin pigment deposition, as well as the foreign body giant cell reaction to the material.

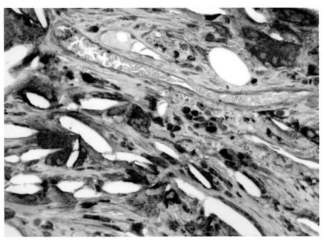

FIGURE 89.8 CD68 immunostaining highlights the foreign body giant cell reaction to the cholesterol debris.

hematoxylin staining, leaving eosinophilic outlines of the nucleus. Dystrophic calcification occurs within these nodules of "ghost cells" (wet keratin). Degeneration of the wet keratin yields the machine oil content in some of the craniopharyngioma cysts. Finding nodules of wet keratin in a small biopsy of a suprasellar mass, even without the viable adamantinomatous epithelium, is diagnostic for craniopharyngioma.

The cholesterol debris and histiocytic reaction, in contrast, are also typical of cystic craniopharyngioma but are only suggestive of the diagnosis of craniopharyngioma if found in isolation without the diagnostic epithelium.

References

1. Burger PC, Scheithauer BW. Tumors of the Central Nervous System. AFIP Atlas of Tumor Pathology. Fourth series, fascicle 7. Washington DC: American Registry of Pathology;2007. p. 461–9.
2. Karavitaki N, Cudlip S, Adams CBT, Wass JAH. Craniopharyngiomas. Endocr Rev 2006;27:371–97.
3. Prayson RA. Non-glial tumors. In: Prayson RA, Editor. Neuropathology. Philadelphia, PA: Elsevier Publishing; 2005. p. 528–30.

Case 90: Papillary Craniopharyngioma

CLINICAL INFORMATION

The patient is a 63-year-old male who notes deterioration in his vision. He sees an ophthalmologist and receives new glasses, but this does not result in improvement. He is then reexamined and found to have bitemporal hemianopsia. Neuroimaging discloses a rim-enhancing lesion, 14 by 6 mm, in the suprasellar cistern with extension to the pituitary gland.

OPINION

Biopsies show fronds of loose, fibrovascular connective tissue, covered by benign squamous epithelium that is devoid of a keratohyaline layer. No dry flaky keratin content is identified. The lesion is devoid of adamantinomatous epithelium or calcifications.

We consider the biopsy as representing a papillary squamous craniopharyngioma and characterize it as follows: **Suprasellar Region Biopsy—Papillary Squamous Craniopharyngioma, WHO Grade I.**

COMMENT

There are no features of an epidermoid cyst, such as dry flaky keratin or a keratohyaline layer. There are no cutaneous adnexae in the cyst wall, as would be seen in a dermoid cyst. Also absent is the typical epithelium of adamantinomatous craniopharyngioma anywhere in the lesion.

DISCUSSION

Papillary craniopharyngioma is considerably less common than adamantinomatous craniopharyngioma

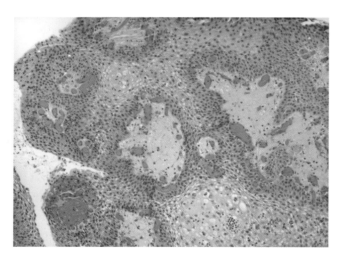

FIGURE 90.1 Pseudopapillary architecture, with fronds of tumor covered by mature squamous epithelium resting on loose fibrovascular tissue, are typical of papillary craniopharyngioma.

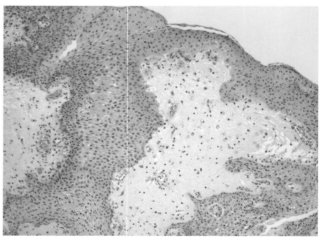

FIGURE 90.2 The surface of the squamous epithelium is not covered by laminate anucleate squamous cells, as would be seen with epidermoid cyst.

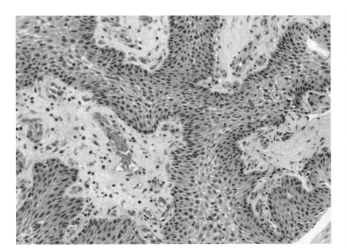

FIGURE 90.3 The squamous epithelium often shows a more hypercellular basal layer, with crowding of nuclei, but this is not as pronounced as in craniopharyngiomas with adamantinomatous epithelium.

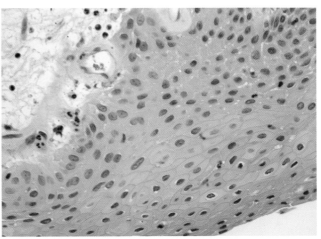

FIGURE 90.4 High-power magnification shows the low nuclear-to-cytoplasmic ratio in the mature squamous cells and absence of mitotic activity.

and occurs almost exclusively in adults. The lesion is usually suprasellar rather than intrasellar, and some examples are located entirely within the third ventricle. The cyst lacks the cholesterol-rich, machine oil-like contents of adamantinomatous cystic craniopharyngiomas. Pseudopapillary architecture may develop somewhat artifactually, when the groups of cell separate one from the other. Nevertheless, the lesions have a relatively distinct MR appearance and are considerably less cystic or calcified than adamantinomatous craniopharyngiomas.

Histologically, papillary craniopharyngiomas are composed of well-differentiated squamous epithelium. No stippled, basophilic, keratohyaline layer is present. Within the squamous epithelium, a basal layer, composed of closely packed cells, is present,

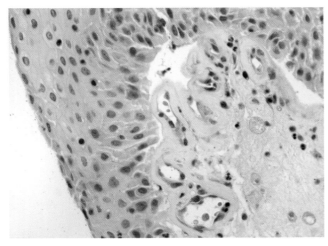

FIGURE 90.5 The fibrovascular stroma in the core of the pseudopapillary tumor may contain macrophages and delicate blood vessels.

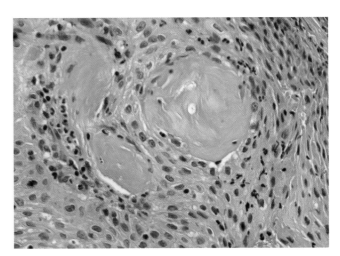

FIGURE 90.6 Scant amounts of wet keratin can occasionally be found in papillary craniopharyngiomas.

but this crowded basal layer is less prominent than that seen in adamantinomatous craniopharyngioma. Nodules of wet keratin, calcifications, and keratin pearls are rare to absent. On very small biopsies, distinction from a Rathke cleft cyst with abundant squamous metaplasia may be impossible without neuroimaging correlation.

References

1. Burger PC, Scheithauer BW. Tumors of the Central Nervous System. AFIP Atlas of Tumor Pathology. Fourth series, fascicle 7. Washington DC: American Registry of Pathology;2007. p. 461–9.
2. Crotty TB. Scheithauer BW. Young WF Jr., et al. Papillary craniopharyngioma: a clinicopathological study of 48 cases. J Neurosurg. 1995;83:206–14.
3. Sartoretti-Schefer S, Wichmann W, Aguzzi A, et al. MR differentiation of adamantinous [sic] and squamous-papillary craniopharyngiomas. AJNR 1997;18:77–87.

Case 91: Granular Cell Tumor of the Pituitary Gland

CLINICAL INFORMATION

The patient is a 62-year-old male who presents with headaches and decreased visual acuity. Imaging studies show a small mass, located in the pituitary gland, that is interpreted as representing a possible adenoma. The lesion is resected, and histologic sections are reviewed.

OPINION

Histologic sections show a circumscribed, nonencapsulated mass, situated in the neurohypophysis. The mass is comprised of a sheetlike proliferation of large rounded cells, with granular eosinophilic cytoplasm. Nuclei are eccentrically placed, with a delicate chromatin pattern. Mitotic figures are not observed. There is no evidence of necrosis. On immunohistochemical staining, the tumor demonstrates diffuse positive staining, with antibody to S-100 protein. The tumor does not stain with antibodies to GFAP or to anterior pituitary hormones.

We consider the lesion to be a low-grade neoplasm and characterize it as follows: **Pituitary Neurohypophysis, Excision—Granular Cell Tumor, WHO Grade I.**

COMMENT

Granular cell tumors represent low-grade neoplasms, which are potentially curable with gross total resection.

DISCUSSION

Granular cell tumor represents the most common neoplasm arising in the neurohypophysis and infundibulum of the pituitary gland. Many of these tumors are

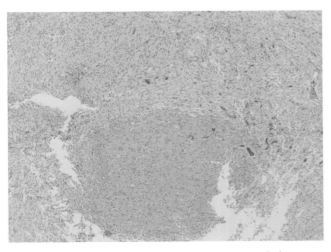

FIGURE 91.1 Low-magnification appearance of the neurohypophysis shows a circumscribed, eosinophilic nodule representing the tumor.

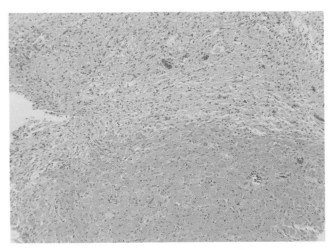

FIGURE 91.2 Intermediate magnification shows a circumscribed interface between the tumor and adjacent neurohypophysis.

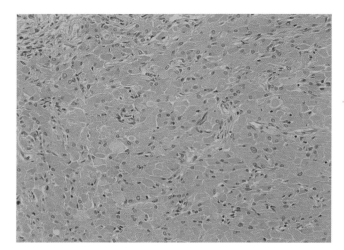

FIGURE 91.3 High-magnification appearance of the tumor cells shows abundant granular eosinophilic cytoplasm and eccentrically placed nucleus.

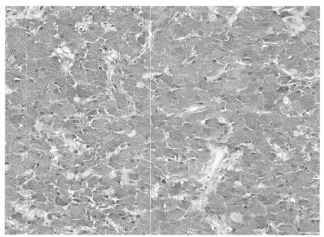

FIGURE 91.4 The tumor demonstrates diffuse positive staining with antibody to S-100 protein.

small and represent incidental findings at autopsy. Occasionally, the tumors may be large enough to present clinically with decreased visual acuity or endocrine deficiency. On imaging, they appear as contrast-enhancing, circumscribed lesions. Microscopically, they resemble their counterparts elsewhere in the body and are marked by a proliferation of large cells with distinctive granular cytoplasm. Nuclei are often eccentrically placed, with delicate chromatin. The granules may be highlighted with PAS staining. Occasional tumors may demonstrate a focal spindled cell pattern. Perivascular chronic inflammation may also be evident. On immunohistochemistry, the tumors demonstrate diffuse positive staining with antibodies to S-100 and vimentin, but do not stain with antibody to GFAP or to antibodies targeting hormones produced in the adenohypophysis. Ultrastructurally, the granular quality of the tumor cells cytoplasm is related to increased number of large lysosomes.

Differential diagnostic considerations most commonly include pituitary adenoma, particularly when the exact location of the lesion is not evident. The granular quality of the cytoplasm is a distinctive characteristic of this tumor, which is not present in the adenomas. In spindled cell areas of granular cell tumor, the neoplasm may resemble pituicytoma or pilocytic astrocytoma. Both of these entities demonstrate GFAP immunoreactivity and are also marked by other findings, including Rosenthal fibers and granular bodies. Rare cases of granular cell differentiation in astrocytomas has been described, particularly in a small number of glioblastoma. Granular cell differentiation in glioblastoma may resemble the cells seen in a granular cell tumor, and key to recognition is identifying the more recognizable glioblastomatous portion of the tumor.

Granular cell tumors of the pituitary gland represent low-grade neoplasms and are curable with gross total resection.

References

1. Cohen-Gadol AA, Pichelmann MA, Link MJ, et al. Granular cell tumor of the sellar and suprasellar region: Clinicopathologic study of 11 cases and literature review. Mayo Clin Proc 2003;78:567–73.
2. Nishioka H, Ii k, Llena JF, et al. Immunohistochemical study of granular cell tumors of the neurohypophysis. Virchows Arch B Cell Pathol Incl Mol Pathol 1991;60:413–17.
3. Schaller B, Kirsch E, Tolnay M, et al. Symptomatic granular cell tumor of the pituitary gland: case report and review of the literature. Neurosurgery 1998;42:166–70; discussion 170–1.

CLINICAL INFORMATION

The patient is a 55-year-old male who presents with adrenal insufficiency and a serum sodium of 111 ng/dl. He is begun on cortisol, and neuroimaging is obtained. MRI shows an enhancing lesion in the sella, which extends upward and measures 1.8 cm in diameter. He has visual problems, and visual field test shows bitemporal hemianopsia. A decision is made to resect the lesion, and histologic sections are reviewed.

OPINION

Sections show a mildly hypercellular neoplasm, comprised of aggregates of plump, eosinophilic cells with abundant cytoplasm. Nuclei manifest an open chromatin pattern, are oval, and contain small nucleoli.

No tight whorls of cells, psammoma body calcifications, mitoses, or necrosis are found.

We consider this lesion to be a low-grade tumor and characterize it as follows: **Suprasellar Region, Excision—Pituicytoma, WHO Grade I.**

COMMENT

This neoplasm is a rare, low-grade tumor that is distinct from other pituitary region masses, such as pituitary adenoma, craniopharyngioma, Rathke cleft cysts, or pilocytic astrocytoma.

DISCUSSION

Pituicytoma is a newly described entity in the 2007 World Health Organization (WHO) classification system. Most patients are adults (mean age 48 years),

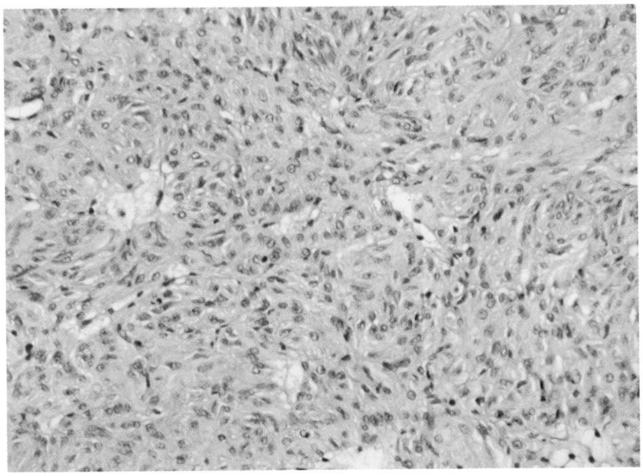

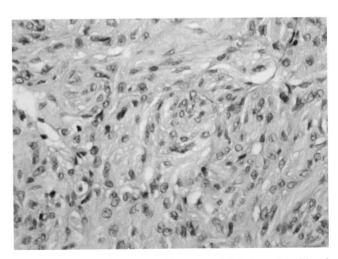

FIGURE 92.1 Low-magnification appearance of the neoplasm shows the absence of necrosis, tight whorls of cells, or calcification. Note the small aggregates and nests of tumor cells.

FIGURE 92.2 Higher magnification highlights the bland open nuclei and delicate small nucleoli in the tumor cells of pituictytoma.

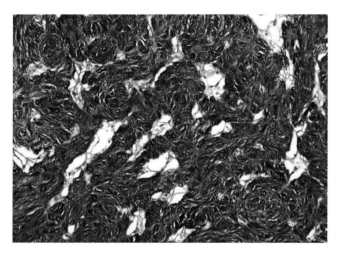

FIGURE 92.3 Strong immunoreactivity for S-100 protein is seen in all cases.

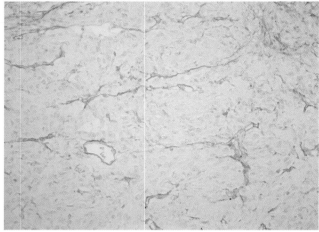

FIGURE 92.4 Absence of abundant reticulin fibers between individual tumor cells negates consideration of schwannoma.

and MR shows solid, discrete, enhancing lesions, either in the sella or suprasellar space, often mistaken for pituitary adenoma. Histologically, the tumor is composed of sheets and nests of plump spindle cells with oval nuclei and small nucleoli. Unlike pilocytic astrocytomas that can also occur in this area, pituicytoma lacks Rosenthal fibers, eosinophilic granular bodies, or a biphasic architectural pattern. Mitoses are rare to absent, and MIB-1 cell cycle labeling is low.

On immunohistochemistry, tumor cells are always strongly immunoreactive for vimentin and S-100 protein, but only variably positive for GFAP. No immunostaining for neuronal markers, such as synaptophysin or neurofilament protein, is ever found. Thus, unlike normal posterior pituitary gland, no axons are seen in the tissue on neurofilament immunostaining. Immunostaining for EMA is focal and weak, in rare instances, and usually not present at all.

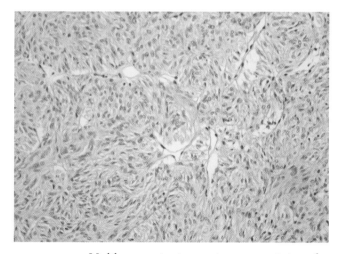

FIGURE 92.5 Unlike meningioma, immunostaining for EMA is almost always negative.

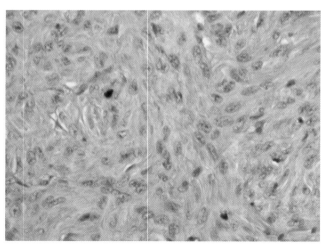

FIGURE 92.6 MIB-1 cell cycle labeling is very low.

Although pituicytoma is strongly immunoreactive for S-100 protein, no abundant reticulin fibers are seen in the tumor between individual tumor cells, as would be expected in schwannoma. No meningothelial, ependymal, or Schwann cell features are found on ultrastructural studies. An origin from specialized glial cells known as "pituicytes" is thought most likely.

References

1. Brat DJ, Scheithauer BW, Fuller GN, et al. Newly codified glial neoplasms of the 2007 WHO Classification of Tumours of the Central Nervous System: angiocentric glioma, pilomyxoid astrocytoma and pituicytoma. Brain Pathol 2007;17:319–24.
2. Brat DJ, Scheithauer BW, Staugaitis SM, et al. Pituicytoma: a distinctive low-grade glioma of the neurohypophysis. Am J Surg Pathol 2000;24:362–8.
3. Ulm AJ, Yachnis AT, Brat DJ, et al. Pituicytoma: report of two cases and clues regarding histogenesis. Neurosurgery 2004;54:753–7.

Case 93: Pituitary Adenoma with Apoplexy

CLINICAL INFORMATION

The patient is a 54-year-old male who presents with sudden onset of visual loss and is found to have a sellar region mass. Emergent surgical excision is undertaken, and histologic sections are reviewed.

OPINION

Sections show tissue fragments with a heterogeneous appearance. Zones of necrotic tissue of varying ages, some with complete loss of nuclear detail, are bordered by granulation tissue and aggregates of cytologically bland, monotonous epithelial cells. The latter manifest small amounts of cytoplasm and absence of mitotic activity.

We consider the lesion to be a pituitary neoplasm, and after special immunostaining, characterize it as follows: **Pituitary Mass, Excision—Pituitary Adenoma with Massive Necrosis and Focal Hemorrhage, Clinically Pituitary Apoplexy (Weak Gonadotroph Cell Adenoma).**

COMMENT

Pituitary apoplexy today is usually caused by hemorrhage and/or necrosis into an underlying pituitary adenoma. Apoplexy can be either a clinical emergency, as in this case, or an occult occurrence, with intratumoral hemorrhage and/or necrosis discovered only on preoperative neuroimaging studies or as significant hemosiderin pigment deposits on histopathologic examination by the pathologist.

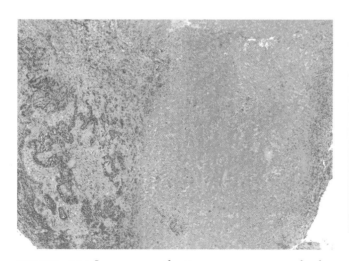

FIGURE 93.1 Lower-magnification appearance of the resected tissue shows a broad zone of eosinophilic necrotic tissue, adjacent to which there are nests of small blue cells.

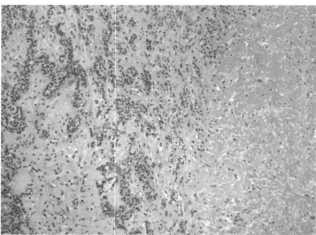

FIGURE 93.2 Low-power magnification allows identification of the "small blue cells" and verifies that they are epithelial cells, not lymphocytes. Early organization of the necrosis is underway, with influx of fibroblasts.

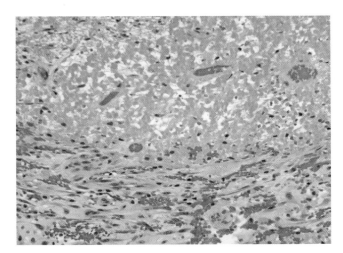

FIGURE 93.3 Intermediate-power magnification shows the preservation of a pituitary adenoma architectural pattern within the coagulative necrosis; note brisk surrounding granulation tissue response.

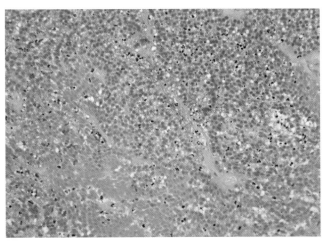

FIGURE 93.4 Intermediate-power magnification of a recently necrotic portion of the adenoma allows discernment of nuclear detail and verifies the absence of normal anterior pituitary gland architecture.

DISCUSSION

Pituitary apoplexy is almost always the result of bleeding into, or infarction of, a pituitary adenoma. The swelling and mass effect within the pituitary adenoma compresses surrounding structures and results in sudden severe headache, nausea and vomiting, visual defects, oculomotor palsies, and impairment in pituitary function. Although supportive therapy alone (including steroids) may result in clinical improvement, some patients required urgent surgical decompression of their mass. Most pituitary tumor apoplexy is spontaneous, but precipitating factors have included pituitary endocrine stimulation testing, surgery (especially coronary artery surgery), and coagulopathy. Rarely, apoplexy may be a result

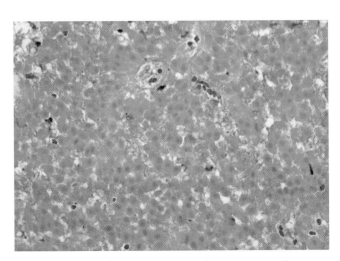

FIGURE 93.5 High-power view of an area with more advanced necrosis and greater loss of cell detail.

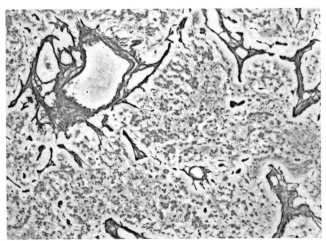

FIGURE 93.6 Reticulin stain of the necrotic adenoma shows the expected disruption of normal acinar pattern and looks identical to what a reticulin stain shows in a non-apoplectic adenoma.

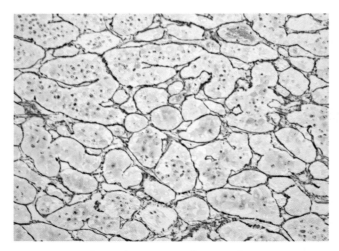

FIGURE 93.7 Reticulin stain of normal anterior pituitary gland from another patient, for comparison with Figure 93.6.

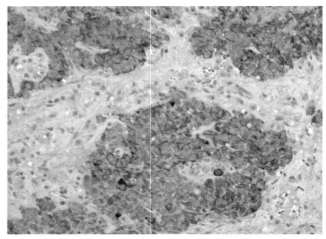

FIGURE 93.8 CAM5.2 immunostaining is seen in the preserved, viable aggregates of adenoma cells.

of bleeding into a Rathke cleft cyst or other sellar region mass.

Pituitary adenomas with several different types of hormonal secretory patterns may present with apoplexy, including growth hormone-secreting adenomas, corticotrophin-secreting adenomas, and clinically nonfunctioning adenomas, including those with patchy weak immunostaining for alpha subunit, follicle-stimulating hormone (FSH), or

luteinizing hormone (LH) (i.e., weak gonadotroph cell adenomas), such as this one.

Histologically, either necrosis or hemorrhage, or both, may be present in cases of apoplexy. The necrosis may be of slightly differing ages and may show varying degrees of preservation of nuclear detail and architectural pattern, but usually the basic

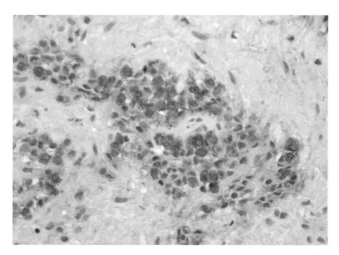

FIGURE 93.9 Synaptophysin immunostaining is seen in the preserved, viable aggregates of adenoma cells.

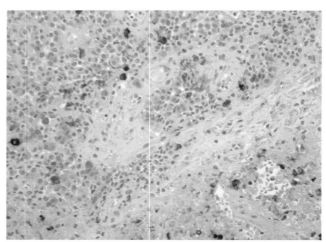

FIGURE 93.10 Immunostaining for alpha subunit in the viable adenoma (upper left), as well as in a few of the cells in necrotic areas (lower right); the latter should be interpreted with caution, unless the staining is also seen in the viable cells.

architectural outline of the adenoma can be detected. Often, the necrosis appears subacute in age and may show a modest neutrophilic cell response, similar to the cellular response seen in other infarctions of 48–96 hours in duration. At the edge of the necrotic areas, granulation tissue, hemosiderin deposits, and residual clusters of viable adenoma may be found.

Even within the necrotic areas, the alteration in reticulin pattern that is diagnostic for pituitary adenoma can still be detectable for a considerable length of time and allow confident diagnosis of an underlying adenoma. Loss of reticulin pattern is the hallmark of an adenoma and contrasts with the honeycomb pattern of reticulin outlining normal acini in non-adenomatous anterior pituitary gland. Small viable islands of adenoma are often found and should not be mistaken for lymphocytes or histiocytes. The viable adenoma retains co-expression of CAM5.2 and synaptophysin, verifying the diagnosis of pituitary adenoma. Immunostaining for these antibodies, or any of the anterior pituitary hormones is, of course, less interpretable in necrotic portions of the lesion, but in the most acute/recent areas of necrosis, some bona fide immunostaining may be retained in some of the adenoma cells.

References

1. Binning MJ, Liu JK, Gannon J, et al. Hemorrhagic and non-hemorrhagic Rathke cleft cysts mimicking pituitary apoplexy. J Neurosurg 2008;108:3–8.
2. Kleinschmidt-DeMasters BK, Lillehei KO. Pathological correlates of pituitary adenomas presenting with apoplexy. Hum Pathol 1998;29:1255–65.
3. Nawar RN, AbdelMannan D, Selman WR, et al. Pituitary tumor apoplexy: a review. J Intens Care Med 2008;23:75–90.
4. Nielsen EH, Lindholm J, Bjerre P, et al. Frequent occurrence of pituitary apoplexy in patients with non-functioning pituitary adenoma. Clin Endo 2006;64:319–22.
5. Semple PL, Jane JA, Lopes MBS, et al. Pituitary apoplexy: correlation between magnetic resonance imaging and histopathological results. J Neurosurg 2008;108:909–15.

Case 94: Pituitary Adenoma in an Ectopic Site

CLINICAL INFORMATION

The patient is a 56-year-old male with a lesion of the left cavernous sinus/posterior sphenoid area, found on work-up for headache. The lesion has been followed by multiple MRI scans, has shown no change in size over time, and does not fill the cavernous sinus. The patient does not have cranial nerve palsies. According to the patient's neurosurgeon, there is no well-defined intrasellar or pituitary region mass, and systemic metastatic work-up is negative. Prior to surgery, the patient has undergone an extensive endocrinologic work-up that shows a mildly elevated prolactin of 28 ng/dl. A decision is made to biopsy the lesion.

OPINION

Biopsies show fibrous tissue, in which are embedded nests of monomorphic epithelial cells. These nests show neither necrosis or mitotic activity, and cells manifest bland nuclei and scant cytoplasm.

We consider the biopsy as representing a pituitary adenoma, albeit in the wall of the cavernous sinus and not the pituitary gland. We characterize it as follows: **Left Cavernous Sinus, Biopsy—Pituitary Adenoma, Ectopic.**

COMMENT

By immunohistochemistry, the adenoma displayed diffuse immunoreactivity for prolactin, explaining the mild elevation noted preoperatively.

DISCUSSION

The usual site of pituitary adenomas is the sellar region, although adenomas can occasionally arise

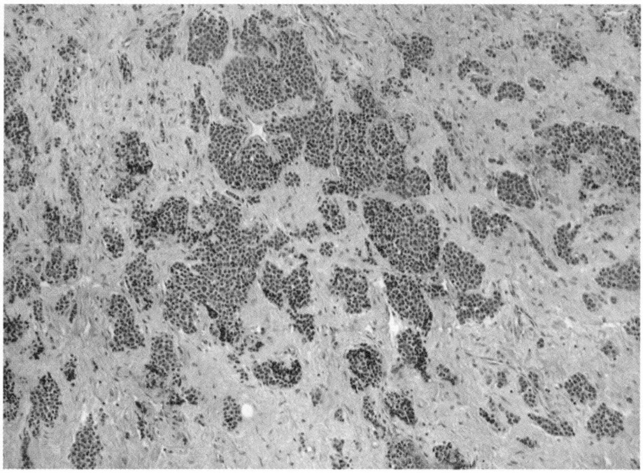

FIGURE 94.1 Nests of monomorphic cells are seen embedded within the connective tissue of the dura.

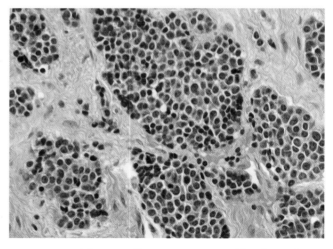

FIGURE 94.2 Intermediate-power magnification shows absence of necrosis, mitotic activity, as well as a fibrillar matrix.

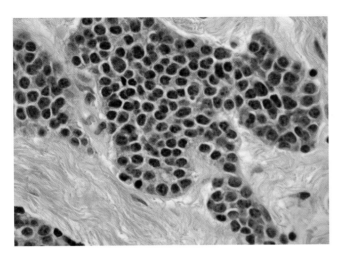

FIGURE 94.3 High-power magnification highlights the endocrine features of the cells, with clumpy coarse nuclear chromatin pattern and moderate amounts of cytoplasm.

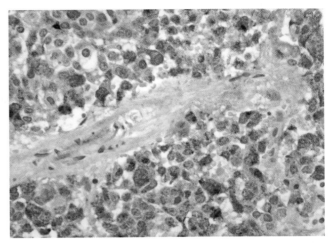

FIGURE 94.4 Diffuse immunoreactivity for prolactin is seen.

anywhere along the migration pathway followed by the craniopharyngeal duct/Rathke pouch during the embryologic period. Reported ectopic sites for pituitary adenoma include the sphenoid sinus, cavernous sinus, third ventricle, and even nasopharynx.

Sections show small clusters of monomorphic cells within the fibrotic dura. The small cells manifest prominent nucleoli, clumpy nuclear chromatin, and moderate amounts of chromophobic cytoplasm by periodic acid Schiff/Orange G stain. No ganglion cell differentiation is identified, and no fibrillar matrix is interspersed within the cell clusters, as might be seen in an olfactory neuroblastoma. Immunostains show the tumor to be positive for synaptophysin and pan-cytokeratin—as can be seen with pituitary adenomas in any site—and negative for GFAP and CD45 (leukocyte common antigen). Additional immunostains showed no encirclement of cell nests by S-100 positive cells, as might be seen with a paraganglioma.

An immunoperoxidase panel for anterior pituitary hormones showed strong, diffuse immunoreactivity for prolactin, with negative immunoreactivity for other pituitary hormones, including growth hormone. MIB-1 cell cycle labeling index was negligible.

References

1. Collie RB. Collie MJ. Extracranial thyroid-stimulating hormone-secreting ectopic pituitary adenoma of the nasopharynx. Otolaryngology—Head & Neck Surgery 2005;133: 453–4.
2. Gondim JA, Schops M, Ferreira E, et al. Acromegaly due to an ectopic pituitary adenoma in the sphenoid sinus. Acta Radiologica 2004;45:689–91.
3. Hou L, Harshbarger T, Herrick MK, et al. Suprasellar adrenocorticotropic hormone-secreting ectopic pituitary adenoma: case report and literature review. Neurosurgery 2002;50:618–25.
4. Kleinschmidt-DeMasters BK, Winston KR, Rubinstein D, et al. Ectopic pituitary adenoma of the third ventricle. Case report. J Neurosurg 1990;72:139–42.
5. Mitsuya K, Nakasu Y, Nioka H, et al. Ectopic growth hormone-releasing adenoma in the cavernous sinus—case report. Neurologia Medico-Chirurgica 2004;44:380–5.

Case 95: Metastatic Small Cell Carcinoma of Lung

CLINICAL INFORMATION

The patient is a 54-year-old male with known diagnosis of small cell lung cancer and previously diagnosed brain metastases. He has been treated in the past with whole-brain irradiation, in addition to stereotactic radiosurgery. However, over the previous months, there has been slow but progressive increase in the size of the right frontal and right temporal brain lesions. Resection of both lesions is undertaken, and histologic sections are reviewed.

OPINION

Extensively necrotic tissue is seen, containing small collections of small malignant cells with hyperchromatic nuclei and scant cytoplasm. The tumor is relatively sharply demarcated from the surrounding gliotic brain tissue. Necrosis in the lesion is associated with fibrinoid vascular necrosis and other features of radiation-induced damage.

We consider the pathology to be that of a metastatic carcinoma and characterize it as follows: **Right Frontal Lobe and Right Temporal Lobe, Excision—Metastatic Small Cell Carcinoma of Lung, with Extensive Radionecrosis.**

COMMENT

This tumor is particularly necrotic as a result of the patient having received both whole-brain radiation and stereotactic radiosurgery prior to removal of his brain metastases. The continued growth of the lesions, despite therapy in this patient, is attributable to residual nests of viable, growing tumor cells.

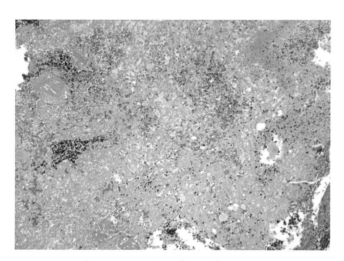

FIGURE 95.1 Low-power view shows the extensive necrosis in this lesion as a result of prior treatment with stereotactic radiosurgery; note small islands of viable tumor cells.

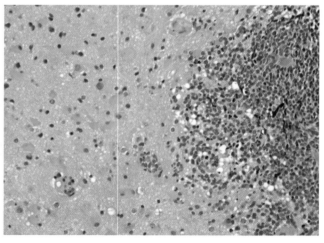

FIGURE 95.2 Low-power view shows the sharp interface between the viable metastatic tumor and the adjacent gliotic brain, rather than individual tumor cell infiltration, as would be seen with most primary high-grade neoplasms of brain.

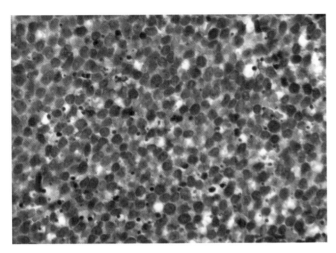

FIGURE 95.3 High-power magnification shows tumor cell monotony, high nuclear-to-cytoplasmic ratio, and mitoses in this metastatic small cell carcinoma of lung.

DISCUSSION

Lung is the most common primary source for metastases to the brain in adults. Adenocarcinomas and small cell carcinomas of lung are particularly prone to central nervous system spread. Most metastatic lesions to the central nervous system parenchyma tend to be well circumscribed, in contrast to the infiltrative pattern of most high-grade primary brain tumors, such as ana-

plastic astrocytoma and glioblastoma. Metastases tend to display central necrosis as they outstrip their blood supply, often with preservation of cuffs of tumor cells around the surviving blood vessels. Pseudopalisading necrosis is seldom seen in metastatic lesions of any kind but is typically found in many glioblastomas.

Small biopsies of metastatic small cell carcinoma of the lung to the brain or spinal cord may prompt consideration of a primary embryonal tumor of the central nervous system, such as medulloblastoma or primitive neuroectodermal tumor (PNET). Fortunately, embryonal tumors are uncommon in adults, in comparison to metastases. Primitive neuroectodermal tumors usually lack sharp circumscription and may additionally show recognizable glial elements, rosettes, or neuronal differentiation in the tumor.

Immunohistochemical profiles of medulloblastoma/PNET only minimally overlap with metastatic small cell carcinoma of lung. Both primary neuroectodermal tumors and metastatic small cell carcinoma of lung can be immunoreactive for CD56 (NCAM, neural cell adhesion molecule), but usually only primitive neuroectodermal tumors, such as medulloblastoma or supratentorial PNET, are

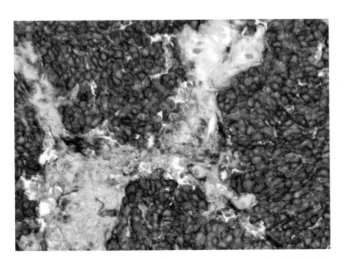

FIGURE 95.4 Immunohistochemical reaction for CD56 is strong and diffuse.

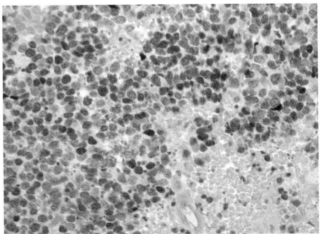

FIGURE 95.5 Immunohistochemical reaction for TTF-1 is seen in tumor nuclei.

immunoreactive for synaptophysin. Metastatic small cell carcinomas may be immunoreactive for CAM5.2 but often are not for CK7 or CK20. The combination of immunoreactivity for thyroid transcription factor-1 (TTF-1) and CD56 (with or without immunoreactivity for CAM5.2) suggests metastatic small cell carcinoma of the lung.

CAM5.2 is a good discriminator between primary and metastatic high-grade tumors in brain. CAM5.2 immunoreactivity is rare in GBM and usually only focal when present. Immunoreactivity for AE1/AE3, in contrast, is seen in up to 95.7% of GBMs because of cross reactivity of this antibody with GFAP. Thus, AE1/AE3 does not provide a good screening tool for distinguishing primary from metastatic tumors of the central nervous system.

References

1. Becher MW, Abel T, Thompson RC, et al. Immunohistochemical analysis of metastatic neoplasms of the central nervous system. J Neuropathol Exp Neurol 2006;65:935–44.
2. Oh D, Prayson RA. Evaluation of epithelial and keratin markers in glioblastoma multiforme: an immunohistochemical study. Arch Path Lab Med 1999;123:917–20.
3. Prayson, RA. Non-glial tumors. In: Prayson RA, Editor. Neuropathology. Philadelphia, PA: Elsevier Churchill Livingstone;2005. p. 532–6.
4. Wesseling P, von Deimling A, Aldape KD. Metastatic tumours of the CNS. In: Louis DN, Ohgaki H, Wiestler OD, Cavenee WK, Editors. WHO Classification of Tumours of the Central Nervous System. Lyon, FR: IARC Press;2007. p. 248–51.

Case 96: Leukemic Involvement of the Central Nervous System

CLINICAL INFORMATION

The patient is a 29-year-old male who presents to the emergency department with right ankle pain and is found to have an elevated white blood cell count of 159,000/μl and thrombocytopenia, with a platelet count of 20,000/μl . Hours after admission to the hospital, the patient is found unresponsive, and an emergent CT scan reveals a massive intracerebral hemorrhage. Clot is evacuated, and histologic sections from the clot are reviewed.

OPINION

Sections show massive acute clot within brain parenchyma, containing sheets of discohesive neoplastic hematopoietic cells, with kidney bean-shaped to bi-lobed irregular nuclei, high nuclear-to-cytoplasmic ratio, and only mildly granular cytoplasm. Nucleoli are moderate in size. Myeloperoxidase reaction is strongly and diffusely positive.

We consider the lesion to be a hematopoietic neoplasm, and after special immunostaining and fluorescence in situ hybridization (FISH) studies, characterize it as follows: **Cerebral Hemispheric Clot, Evacuation—Acute Leukemia with Hemorrhage (Acute Promyelocytic Leukemia, Hypogranular Form).**

COMMENT

The clot likely occurred as a result of a combination of the very low platelet count coupled with the very high circulating white cell count in this patient. This period in acute leukemia, when the platelet count falls below 25,000/μl and the white count exceeds

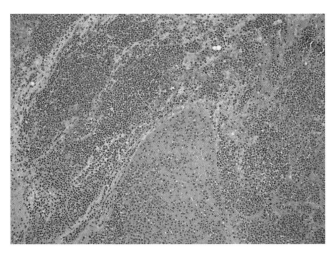

FIGURE 96.1 Lower-magnification appearance shows a clot within the brain parenchyma, accompanied by the sheets of neoplastic hematopoietic cells.

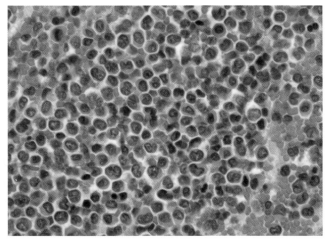

FIGURE 96.2 High-power magnification illustrates the kidney bean-shaped nuclei and hypogranular cytoplasm of the neoplastic hematopoietic cells.

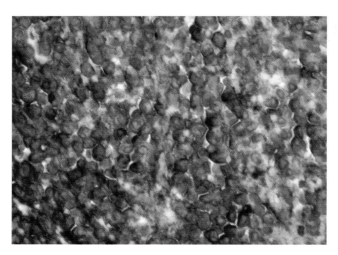

FIGURE 96.3 High-power magnification depicts the strong, diffuse, cytoplasmic immunoreactivity for myeloperoxidase in the tumor cells.

100,000/µl, has been termed the "critical period" for risk of central nervous system (CNS) hemorrhage.

DISCUSSION

Criteria for diagnosis and classification of leukemias involving the CNS are identical to those utilized in other tissues in the body. In this case, the histologic features were those of a myelocytic leukemia, with bean-shaped nuclei and abundant cytoplasm, rather than that of a B-cell lymphoma, with rounded nuclei and more prominent nucleoli. The immunohistochemical reaction for CD45RB (leukocyte common antigen) was patchy, and no staining for CD20 (B-cell marker) was detected. In contrast, the cytoplasmic reaction for myeloperoxidase was diffuse, strong, and almost obliterated the nuclear detail of the cells. In addition, FISH was performed to look for the PML/RARA rearrangement associated with the (15;17)(q22;q21.1) translocation found in acute promyelocytic leukemia, and it was found in this case. The cytoplasm is relatively hypogranular in this example but may show coarse granulation in some examples of acute promyelocytic leukemia.

Leukemias of several different types can involve the CNS. Direct tumor involvement manifests as intraparenchymal or extra-axial mass lesion(s) or as infiltrations of the leptomeninges or dura. CNS hemorrhage is less common. However, in cases where there is extensive systemic and bone marrow involvement by the leukemia, coagulopathy and thrombocytopenia can result, and CNS hemorrhage may be the cause of demise, as it was in this patient soon after his clot evacuation.

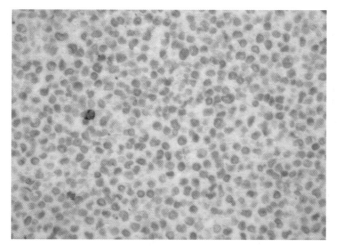

FIGURE 96.4 High-power magnification shows the absence of immunostaining for the B-cell marker CD20 in the tumor cells.

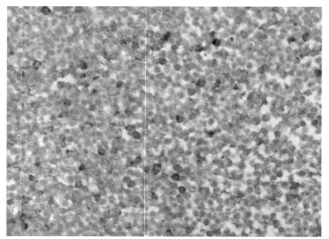

FIGURE 96.5 As is the case with most acute promyelocytic leukemias, only patchy weak immunoreactivity for CD45RB (leukocyte common antigen) is present.

The most likely leukemia types to develop CNS hemorrhage are, in descending order of frequency, acute myeloblastic leukemia, blastic phase of chronic myelogenous leukemia, and lymphoblastic leukemia (ALL). Acute promyelocytic leukemia constitutes a minority (5–8%) of all acute myelogenous leukemias. The current case is unusual, in that the patient had severe thrombocytopenia and massively elevated white blood cell count on his initial clinical presentation and developed CNS bleeding within hours after hospital admission. Similar cases of intracerebral hemorrhage as the first clinical manifestation of acute promyelocytic leukemia have been reported; however, CNS hemorrhage may also develop during relapse or as a late complication of radiation therapy, in children with ALL who have received whole-brain radiotherapy. The hemorrhage in the latter instance develops years after cranial irradiation treatment and is a result of the formation of intracerebral cavernous malformations that subsequently rupture.

References

1. Chamberlain MC. Leukemia and the nervous system. Curr Oncol Reports 2005;7:66–73.
2. Glass J. Neurologic complications of lymphoma and leukemia. Sem Oncol 2006;33:342–7.
3. Larson JJ, Ball WS, Bove KE, et al. Formation of intracerebral cavernous malformations after radiation treatment for central nervous system neoplasia in children. J. Neurosurg 1998;88:51–6.
4. Marcheta MP, Kok Shun J, Liu Yin JA. Central nervous system relapse of acute promyelocytic leukaemia in a patient with cerebral haemorrhage at diagnosis. Brit J Haematol 2001;114:954–5.
5. Nowacki P, Zdziarska B, Fryze C, et al. Co-existence of thrombocytopenia and hyperleukocytosis ("critical period") as a risk factor of haemorrhage into the central nervous system in patients with acute leukaemias. Haematologia 2002;31:347–55.

CLINICAL INFORMATION

The patient is a 58-year-old male who first develops diplopia about 1 year ago but puts off seeking medical attention until the onset of blurred vision 2 months ago. Physical examination shows his visual acuity to be 20/40 on the left and 20/20 on the right. Examination of cranial nerves III, IV, and VI reveal a lack of upward gaze on the left side, as well as anisocoria, with the left pupil being larger than the right. Neuroimaging studies demonstrate a large, enhancing mass in the sellar and suprasellar regions, posterior to the clivus and to the left of midline. The decision is made to attempt surgical debulking of the lesion, and histologic sections are available for review.

OPINION

Biopsies show a moderately hypercellular, slightly lobulated mass, with epithelioid cells arranged in cords and rows. Cells are contiguous to each other and show touching borders, rather than being arranged in individual lacunae. Many cells manifest a vacuolated cytoplasm (physaliphorous cells), and cells are embedded in abundant, extracellular, gray-blue mucin. Mitoses or necrosis are not seen, but slight nuclear atypia is apparent.

After immunohistochemical studies, we consider the resected lesion as representing a bone-based mass and characterize it as follows: **Left Clivus, Resection-Chordoma**.

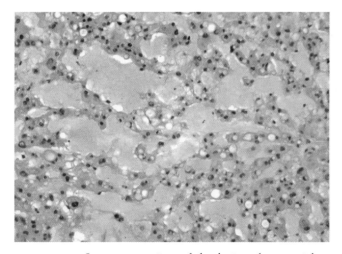

FIGURE 97.1 Low-power view of the lesion shows epithelioid cells arranged in rows and cords and embedded in a mucinous matrix.

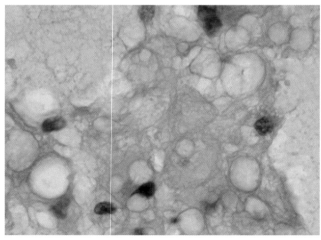

FIGURE 97.2 High-power magnification illustrates the extensive vacuolization within tumor cytoplasm and absence of mitotic activity.

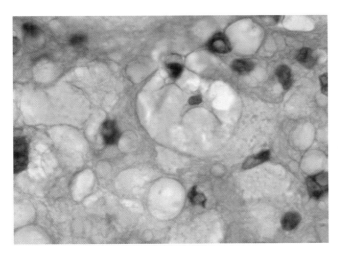

FIGURE 97.3 High-power magnification highlights occasional, very large, physaliphorous cells and modest nuclear atypia.

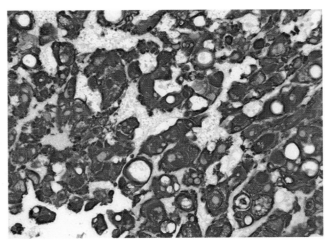

FIGURE 97.4 Chordomas are generally strongly and diffusely immunoreactive for keratin (AE1/AE3).

COMMENT

Chordomas are relatively uncommon tumors, but about a third of them occur in the clivus or spheno-occipital region.

DISCUSSION

Chordoma is a tumor of notochordal derivation that can occur anywhere along the neural axis, including skull base, sacrococcygeal region, and vertebral bodies. Virtually all involve intraosseous sites, and most cause significant bone destruction. Symptoms relate to the location of the lesion, and in the skull base, problems with visual acuity, cranial nerve palsies of cranial nerves III, IV, and VI (resulting in diplopia), and headache are typical symptoms.

In the skull base, chordomas must be differentiated from chondrosarcomas, almost all of which are well differentiated. In addition, a variant denoted as chondroid chordoma was first described in 1973

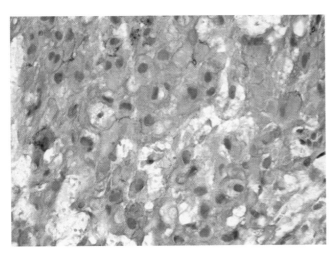

FIGURE 97.5 Chordoma may show far more focal immunoreactivity for EMA.

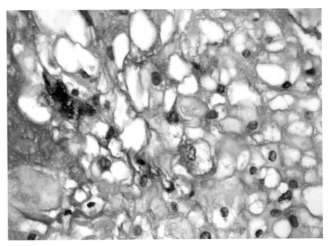

FIGURE 97.6 Chordoma may also be only focally positive for S-100 protein.

and is characterized by varying amounts of cartilaginous elements, admixed with more typical chordoma. The existence of this lesion has been debated and contested ever since. Nevertheless, the salient point is that making the distinction between tumors with and without a chordoma element is important. Despite the deceptive nomenclature of the lesions, chordoma of the skull base manifests a significantly worse prognosis than well-differentiated skull base chondrosarcoma.

Because these tumors can seldom be gross totally resected, sometimes rather limited-sized or poorly preserved surgical specimens are received by the pathologist. Immunohistochemical staining then becomes important in making the distinction. Keratin (AE1/AE3) stains are the best discriminator between chordoma and chondrosarcoma, because keratin is positive in nearly 100% of the former and 0% of the latter. Both usually show S-100 protein immunoreactivity, and chordoma, additionally, is positive for EMA. However, not all cases show S-100 immunoreactivity, and some studies have shown EMA immunoreactivity in chondrosarcomas of skull base. Thus, other antibodies have been sought to distinguish these lesions. Brachyury in some studies has been found in a high (>80%) percentage of chordomas, but not in chondrosarcoma. In contrast, podoplanin is found in a similar high percentage of chondrosarcomas of skull base, but not chordomas.

Only a minority of chordomas metastasize to distant sites. Unfortunately, histologic features poorly predict which tumors will manifest this behavior.

References

1. Heffelfinger MJ, Dahlin DC, MacCarty CS, et al. Chordomas and cartilaginous tumors at the skull base. Cancer 1973;32:410–20.
2. Oakley GJ, Fuhrer K, Seethala RR. Brachyury, SOX-9, and podoplanin, new markers in the skull base chordoma vs. chondrosarcoma differential: a tissue microarray-based comparative analysis. Mod Pathol 2008;21:1461–9.
3. Prayson RA. Non-Glial Tumors. In: Prayson RA, Editor. Neuropathology. Philadelphia, PA: Elsevier Churchill Livingstone;2005. p. 503–4.

Case 98: Metastatic Papillary Carcinoma of the Thyroid

CLINICAL INFORMATION

The patient is a 56-year-old female who presents with a history of papillary thyroid cancer, diagnosed 2 years previously. At the time of initial surgery, the patient has metastases noted in several lymph nodes. Most recently, the patient presents with episodes of confusion. On imaging, a right temporal lobe mass, measuring 1.6 cm, is identified. The lesion is excised, and histologic sections are reviewed.

OPINION

Histologic sections show a lesion that is sharply demarcated from the adjacent gliotic parenchyma. The lesion itself is marked by a tumor that demonstrates a papillary architectural pattern. Fibrovascular cores are lined by tumor cells. The tumor cells show nuclear clearing and occasional nuclear grooves. Rare mitotic figures are seen. Adjacent to the tumor is a large area of geographic necrosis. Focal microcalcifications are seen in viable tumor. On immunohistochemical analysis, the tumor demonstrates positive staining, with antibody to thyroglobulin and to thyroid transcription factor-1 (TTF-1).

We consider the lesion to be a metastatic neoplasm and characterize it as follows: **Right Temporal Lobe, Excision—Metastatic Papillary Carcinoma of the Thyroid.**

COMMENT

The tumor is consistent with a metastasis from the patient's previously diagnosed papillary carcinoma of the thyroid. Thyroglobulin and TTF-1 immunoreactivity support an origin of the metastasis from the thyroid tumor.

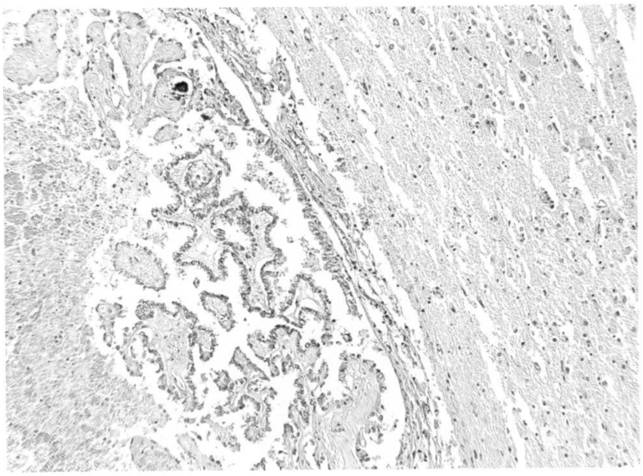

FIGURE 98.1 The interface between the tumor and the adjacent gliotic brain parenchyma is sharply delineated, typical of a metastasis.

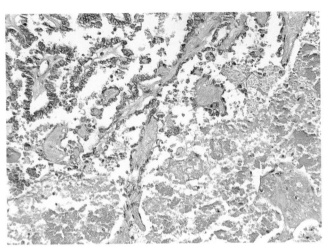

FIGURE 98.2 Intermediate magnification showing geographic necrosis adjacent to a papillary neoplasm.

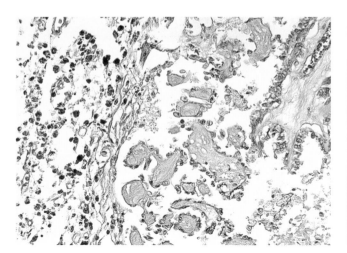

FIGURE 98.3 Focal hemosiderin deposition indicates previous hemorrhage associated with the tumor.

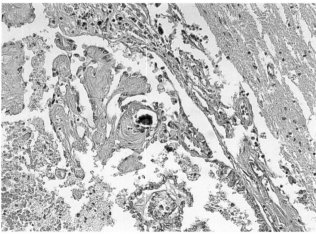

FIGURE 98.4 Focal calcifications are seen in papillary areas of the tumor.

DISCUSSION

Metastatic disease from the thyroid gland is relatively uncommon. Most frequently, tumors that metastasize to the CNS include primaries from the lung, breast, kidney, and skin (melanoma). Metastases are frequently (although not always) multifocal. The tumor in this case presents as a single mass. Morphologically, metastases, in contrast to gliomas, are well circumscribed, in that there is often a sharp interface between the tumor and the adjacent gliotic parenchyma.

In many cases, determining the site of origin by examining the metastasis is not possible. In the current case, the history of previous papillary carcinoma of the thyroid and the papillary architecture and cytology of the metastatic tumor are useful in suggesting the site of origin. This impression was confirmed by immunohistochemical staining. Thyroglobulin is fairly specific for a thyroid carcinoma. TTF-1, although an excellent

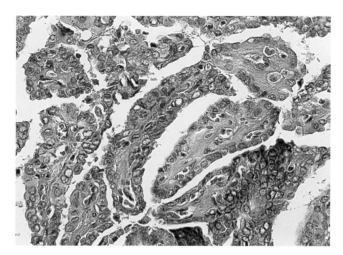

FIGURE 98.5 High-magnification appearance of the tumor shows nuclear clearing and occasional cleaved or grooved nuclei, cytologically consistent with papillary carcinoma of thyroid origin.

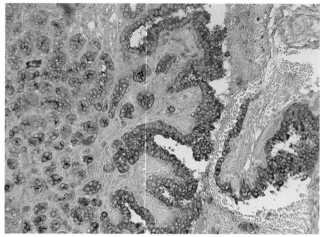

FIGURE 98.6 Thyroglobulin immunoreactivity is present in the tumor.

marker for thyroid cancer, is also well-known to stain a significant subset of metastatic tumors of pulmonary origin and therefore is not specific.

References

1. Aguiar PH, Agner C, Tavares FR, et al. Unusual brain metastases from papillary thyroid carcinoma: case report. Neurosurgery 2001;49:1008–13.

2. DeYoung BR, Wick MR. Immunohistologic evaluation of metastatic carcinomas of unknown origin: an algorithmic approach. Semin Diagn Pathol 2000;17:184–93.

3. Oliveira AM, Tazelaar HD, Myers JL, et al. Thyroid transcription factor-1 distinguishes metastatic pulmonary from well-differentiated neuroendocrine tumors of other sites. Am J Surg Pathol 2001;25:815–19.

Case 99: Leptomeningeal Carcinomatosis

CLINICAL INFORMATION

The patient is a 52-year-old male with a diagnosis of stage IV non-small cell lung cancer metastatic to bone. Approximately 1 month prior to surgery, the patient began to have symptoms of difficulty with memory and with dragging both feet when walking. This led to an MRI that showed meningeal enhancement, but no mass lesions in the brain. As a result of persistent symptoms, a decision is made to biopsy the patient, and histologic sections are reviewed.

OPINION

Biopsies of cerebral cortex show leptomeninges and Virchow-Robin spaces, filled with metastatic neoplastic cells. These cells are arranged in cohesive groups, and where small, cortical, rounded metastases are formed in the superficial cortex, gland formation is evident in the metastatic adenocarcinoma. High power shows cells with large vesicular nuclei, prominent nucleoli, and vacuolated, mucin-filled cytoplasm. An additional biopsy of overlying dura was negative for tumor cells.

We consider the biopsy to be metastatic carcinoma, with involvement of the leptomeninges, and characterize it as follows: **Right Frontal Cortex, Biopsy—Leptomeningeal Carcinomatosis, Metastatic Non-Small Cell Carcinoma of Lung, WHO Grade IV.**

COMMENT

Leptomeningeal carcinomatosis, synonymous with carcinomatous meningitis, often occurs without coexistent parenchymal brain metastases or dural involvement.

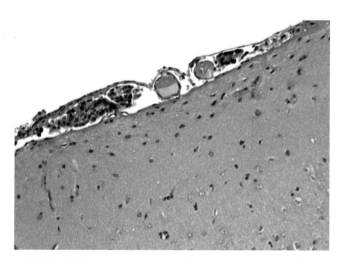

FIGURE 99.1 Section of cerebral cortex, shown at intermediate magnification, demonstrates clusters of metastatic neoplastic cells confined to the subarachnoid space.

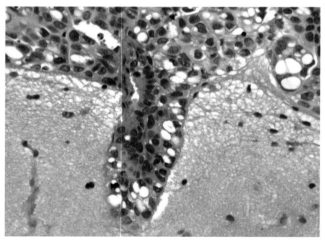

FIGURE 99.2 Adjacent sections show a thicker layer of tumor cells in the meninges that dips down into cortex along Virchow-Robin spaces; note reactive gliosis in underlying subpial tissue.

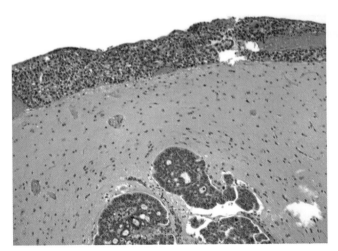

FIGURE 99.3 In some areas, the metastatic tumor forms small nodules of growth, where it has broken out from Virchow-Robin spaces; here, the gland formation in this metastatic adenocarcinoma of lung is readily apparent.

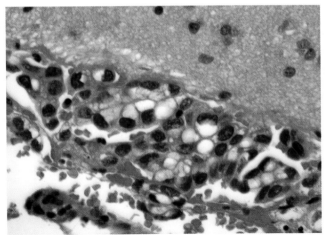

FIGURE 99.4 High-power magnification illustrates the large vesicular nuclei, prominent nucleoli, and abundant intracytoplasmic mucin in this metastatic adenocarcinoma.

DISCUSSION

Leptomeningeal spread of cancer to the brain usually is as a result of spread from a lung or breast primary. However, leptomeningeal carcinomatosis has been reported with virtually every systemic tumor type, including carcinomas of the ovary, prostate, urinary bladder, gallbladder, fallopian tube, stomach, kidney, and cervix, and cutaneous melanoma.

Neuroimaging features in classic examples show diffuse enhancement, with gadolinium administration in the subarachnoid space, including the cisterns around the midbrain, the sylvian fissures, or cerebellar and cerebral sulci. Hydrocephalus can be seen. However, neuroimaging features can be far more subtle, prompting clinicians to obtain cerebrospinal fluid for cytologic examination. Although positive cytologic findings establish the diagnosis, false-negative cerebrospinal fluid (CSF) cytologic results are common. According to Glantz et al., false-negative results can be minimized by "1) withdrawing at least 10.5 mL of CSF for cytologic analysis; 2) processing the CSF specimen immediately; 3) obtaining CSF from a site of known leptomeningeal disease; and 4) repeating this procedure once if the initial cytology is negative." Some workers have advocated the use of immunohistochemistry to increase recognition of malignant cells.

References

1. Abdo AA, Coderre S, Bridges RJ. Leptomeningeal carcinomatosis secondary to gastroesophageal adenocarcinoma: a case report and review of the literature. Can J Gastroenterol 2002;16:807–11.
2. Bendell JC, Domchek SM, Burstein HJ, et al. Central nervous system metastases in women who receive trastuzumab-based therapy for metastatic breast carcinoma. Cancer 2003;97:2972–7.
3. Cone LA, Koochek K, Henager HA, et al. Jennings LM. Leptomeningeal carcinomatosis in a patient with metastatic prostate cancer: case report and literature review. Surg Neurol 2006;65:372–5.
4. Glantz MJ, Cole BF, Glantz LK, et al. Cerebrospinal fluid cytology in patients with cancer: minimizing false-negative results. Cancer 1998;82:733–9.
5. Lee JL, Kang YK, Kim TW, et al. Leptomeningeal carcinomatosis in gastric cancer. J Neurooncol 2004;66:167–74.
6. Lisenko Y, Kumar AJ, Yao J, et al. Leptomeningeal carcinomatosis originating from gastric cancer: report of eight cases and review of the literature. Am J Clin Oncol 2003;26:165–70.
7. Thomas JE, Falls E, Velasco ME, et al. Diagnostic value of immunocytochemistry in leptomeningeal tumor dissemination. Arch Pathol Lab Med 2000;124:759–61.

Case 100: Dural Carcinomatosis

CLINICAL INFORMATION

The patient is a 60-year-old female with known stage IV breast cancer. She was recently seen by her oncologist, with complaints of feeling dizzy and weak with progressive nausea and vomiting. She also complains of diffuse bone pain. CT/positron emission tomography (PET) scan of her body demonstrates new metastatic disease in her bones, liver, and lung. MRI of her brain demonstrates increased intracranial pressure, midline shift of approximately 1 cm, and a left frontal subdural bleed. Because of progressive symptoms, she undergoes semi-emergent left frontal craniotomy, for drainage of the acute-on-chronic subdural clot; biopsy of thickened dura is also undertaken. Histologic sections of dura are reviewed.

OPINION

Biopsies show thickened, fibrotic dura, containing clusters of metastatic tumor cells with the cribriform features of breast carcinoma. The tumor is strongly and diffusely immunoreactive for CK7, negative for CK20, and shows estrogen receptor positive (3+) in 96% tumor cell nuclei, negative nuclear immunostaining for progesterone receptor, and Her2/neu protein overexpression (score of 3+) in 50% of invasive carcinoma cells.

We consider the biopsy as representing metastatic tumor to dura and characterize it as follows: **Left Frontal Dura, Biopsy—Dural Carcinomatosis, Clinically Associated with Acute and Subacute Subdural Hematoma, Secondary to Metastatic Adenocarcinoma of Breast.**

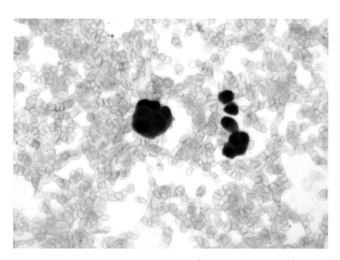

FIGURE 100.1 Intraoperative touch preparation, taken of the surgical specimen sent out or frozen section consultation, shows metastatic adenocarcinoma.

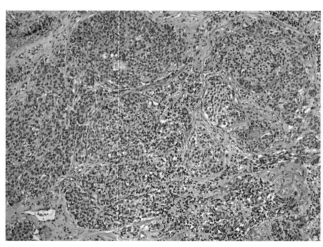

FIGURE 100.2 Permanent specimen of dura shows nests of metastatic tumor cells throughout the tissue.

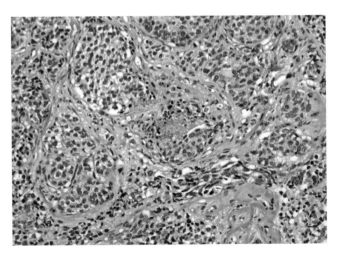

FIGURE 100.3 Focal necrosis is seen within the metastatic tumor cell nests.

COMMENT

Dural carcinomatosis often occurs as a late-stage complication in patients who also manifest bone and other systemic metastatic disease. Patients with systemic carcinomas who present with acute or subacute subdural hematomas should be suspected of having dural tumor involvement.

DISCUSSION

Dural metastases are usually more discrete masses, rather than diffuse, involving dura in a thickened, diffuse layer of tumor. The most common tumor types to involve the dura are breast carcinoma (as this case), prostate cancer, lung cancer, and hematopoietic tumors. Even at biopsy or autopsy tissue examination, less than one-half of cases show coexistent brain parenchymal metastatic disease. Both antecedent pulmonary lymphangitic spread and bony disease seem to be associated with development of dural metastatic disease. Hence, usually the patient is known to have systemic malignancy before presenting with dural involvement, making the diagnosis easier for the pathologist.

Nevertheless, documentation of identity of the metastatic tumor with the alleged primary neoplasm is important. An algorithmic approach for the work-up of metastatic disease of known type to the CNS has been outline by Becher et al. This involves a "first round" of antibodies for epithelial tumors or known adenocarcinomas, using CAM5.2, CK7, CK20, and thyroid transcription factor-1

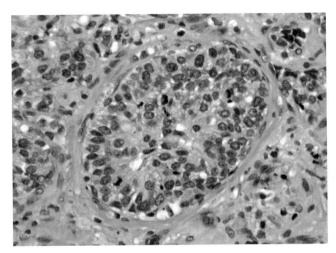

FIGURE 100.4 High-power magnification demonstrates cells with high nuclear-to-cytoplasmic ratio and many mitoses.

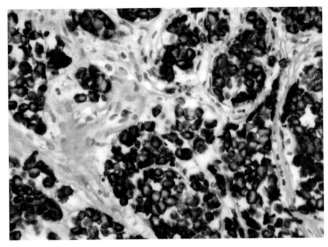

FIGURE 100.5 Tumor is strongly and diffusely immunoreactive for cytokeratin 7, but it was negative for CK20.

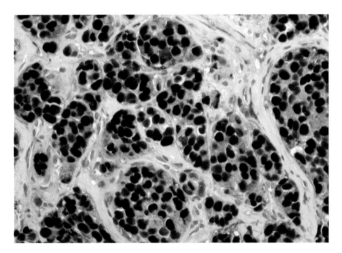

FIGURE 100.6 Strong, 3+, nuclear immunoreactivity is seen for estrogen receptor.

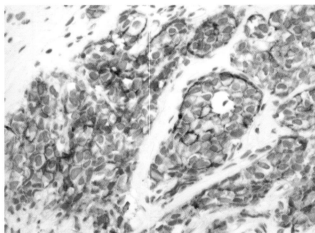

FIGURE 100.7 Strong membranous immunostaining is found for Her2neu indicative of overexpression of protein.

(TTF-1). Tumors that are positive for CAM5.2 and CK7 and negative for CK20 are then additionally immunostained for GCFDP-15, estrogen receptor, and CA125, to differentiate breast carcinoma from endometrial carcinoma. In contrast, for very poorly differentiated CNS metastases, the suggested initial battery of immunostains is broader and includes GFAP, CAM5.2, synaptophysin, CK7, CK20, Melan-A, CD3, and CD20.

References

1. Becher MW, Abel T, Thompson RC, et al. Immunohisto-chemical analysis of metastatic neoplasms of the central nervous system. J Neuropathol Exp Neurol 2006;65:935–44.
2. Jamjoom AB. Cast IP. Subdural haematoma [sic] caused by metastatic duralcarcinomatosis. Br J Neurosurg 1987;1:385–8.
3. Kleinschmidt-DeMasters BK. Dural metastases. A retro-spective surgical and autopsy series. Arch Pathol Lab Med 2001;125:880–7.
4. Minette SE. Kimmel DW. Subdural hematoma in patients with systemic cancer. Mayo Clinic Proc 1989;64:637–42.

Case 101: Mesenchymal Chondrosarcoma

CLINICAL INFORMATION

The patient is a 39-year-old female who presents with severe thoracic region pain. Preoperative neuroimaging shows a tumor anterior to the spinal cord, at the T4-5 level, with significant cord compression. The decision is made to resect portions of the mass. Intraoperatively, no intradural tumor was identified by the neurosurgeon.

OPINION

Sections show a hypercellular neoplasm, punctuated by staghorn blood vessels and composed of small, elongated to comma-shaped nuclei with scant cytoplasm. The tumor is attached to dense connective tissue and associated with reactive cartilage and bone. However, in addition, there are islands of more cytologically atypical and irregular cartilage and bone, blending intimately with undifferentiated myxoid tissue and undifferentiated tumor composed of small blue cells.

We consider the tumor to be a sarcoma and characterize it as follows: **Spinal Thoracic T4–5 Levels, Excision—Mesenchymal Chondrosarcoma.**

COMMENT

Mesenchymal chrondrosarcoma is a rare neoplasm, constituting 10% or less of all chrondrosarcomas.

DISCUSSION

Mesenchymal chrondrosarcoma has a peak incidence in young adults in the second and third decades. Maxilla, mandible, orbit, ribs, ilium, and vertebrae (as in this case) are the most frequent bony sites of involvement. Soft tissue may also be the primary site of involvement, or tumor may break through bone

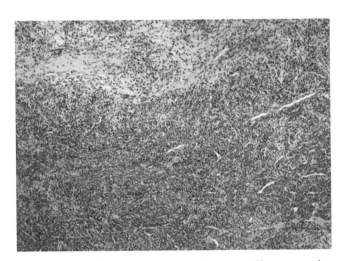

FIGURE 101.1 Low-power magnification illustrates the sheets of undifferentiated small blue cells.

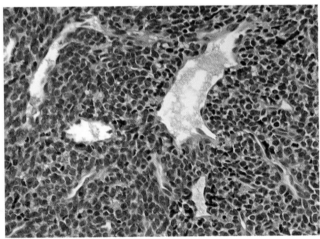

FIGURE 101.2 High-power magnification shows the staghorn blood vessels typically seen in this tumor type.

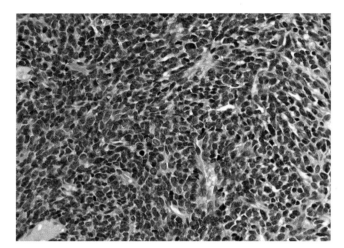

FIGURE 101.3 Cells manifest oval nuclei, with hyperchromasia and inconspicuous nucleoli; cytoplasm is virtually nondetectable. Cells form cushions that jut into blood vessels, but the actual tumor cells do not line vessel walls.

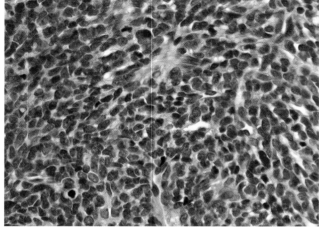

FIGURE 101.4 Mitotic activity is brisk, although necrosis is often not present.

and extend into adjacent soft tissues. Meninges represent one of the most common extraskeletal sites of involvement. Within the CNS, the intracranial compartment is more commonly affected than intraspinal areas.

Histologically, the tumor is composed of sheets of highly undifferentiated, small, round cells, inter-

rupted by islands of well-differentiated hyaline cartilage. The transition between the two is often subtle. The small blue cell portion of the tumor is usually composed of round-to-oval cells with scant cytoplasm, but spindled areas can be present. The small blue portion of the tumor most closely resembles hemangiopericytoma (HPC) or Ewing sarcoma. Staghorn blood vessels often simulate those seen in HPC. However, the presence of cartilage rules out Ewing sarcoma and usually HPC of the CNS as well.

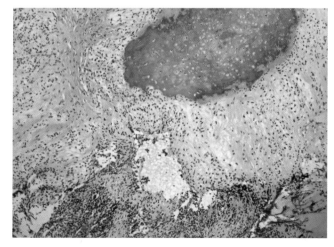

FIGURE 101.5 Transition between the small blue cells, slightly myxoid areas, abnormal osteoid, and cartilage can be identified.

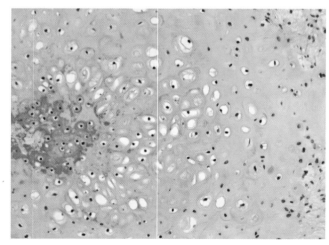

FIGURE 101.6 High-power view shows hyaline cartilage islands.

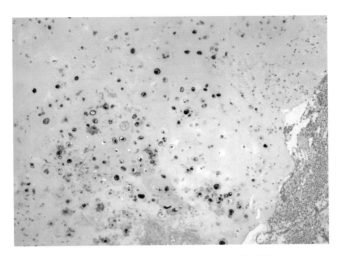

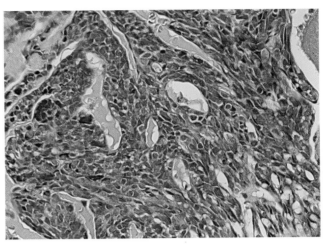

FIGURE 101.7 The cartilage component is S-100 immuno-reactive.

FIGURE 101.8 The malignant, undifferentiated small blue cell component is immunoreactive for CD99.

Immunoreactivity for vimentin and CD99 in the small cell component can be seen in mesenchymal chondrosarcoma, HPC, and Ewing. Chondroid areas are immunoreactive for S-100 protein. Osteoid and bone can also be found.

References

1. Devoe K, Weidner N. Immunohistochemistry of small round-cell tumors. Sem Diagn Pathol 2000;17:216–24.

2. Nakashima Y, Park YK, Sugano O. Mesenchymal chondrosarcoma. In: Fletcher CDM, Unni KK, Mertens F, Editors. WHO Classification of Tumours: Tumours of Soft Tissue and Bone. Lyon, FR: IARC Press;2002. p. 255–6.

3. Rajaram V, Brat DJ, Perry A. Anaplastic meningioma versus meningeal hemangiopericytoma: immunohistochemical and genetic markers. Hum Pathol 2004;35:1413–8.

4. Rushing EJ, Armonda RA, Ansari Q, et al. Mesenchymal chondrosarcoma: a clinicopathologic and flow cytometric study of 13 cases presenting in the central nervous system. Cancer 1996;77:1884–91.

INDEX